A Guide to Medical Surgical Nursing

Srinanda Ghosh MN (Master of Nursing)
Principal
Woodlands College of Nursing
Kolkata, West Bengal, India

Manashi Sengupta MSc (Nursing)
Professor
Sankar Madhab College of Nursing
Guwahati, Assam, India

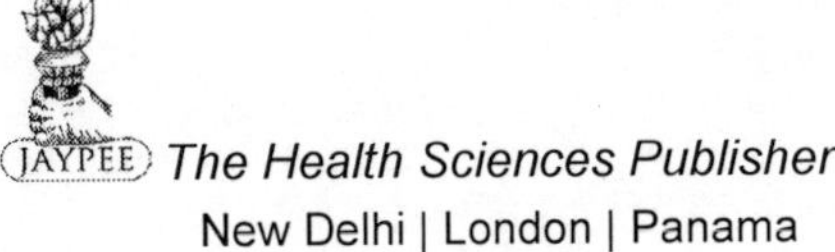
The Health Sciences Publisher
New Delhi | London | Panama

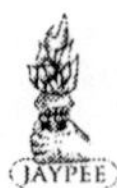

Jaypee Brothers Medical Publishers (P) Ltd

Headquarters
Jaypee Brothers Medical Publishers (P) Ltd
4838/24, Ansari Road, Daryaganj
New Delhi 110 002, India
Phone: +91-11-43574357
Fax: +91-11-43574314
Email: jaypee@jaypeebrothers.com

Overseas Offices
J.P. Medical Ltd
83 Victoria Street, London
SW1H 0HW (UK)
Phone: +44 20 3170 8910
Fax: +44 (0)20 3008 6180
Email: info@jpmedpub.com

Jaypee-Highlights Medical Publishers Inc
City of Knowledge, Bld. 235, 2nd Floor, Clayton
Panama City, Panama
Phone: +1 507-301-0496
Fax: +1 507-301-0499
Email: cservice@jphmedical.com

Jaypee Brothers Medical Publishers (P) Ltd
17/1-B Babar Road, Block-B, Shaymali
Mohammadpur, Dhaka-1207
Bangladesh
Mobile: +08801912003485
Email: jaypeedhaka@gmail.com

Jaypee Brothers Medical Publishers (P) Ltd
Bhotahity, Kathmandu
Nepal
Phone: +977-9741283608
Email: kathmandu@jaypeebrothers.com

Website: www.jaypeebrothers.com
Website: www.jaypeedigital.com

Inquiries for bulk sales may be solicited at: jaypee@jaypeebrothers.com

A Guide to Medical Surgical Nursing

First Edition: 2017, Reprint: 2024

ISBN: 978-93-86150-56-1

Printed in India

Dedicated to

Our students

Preface

At last by the grace of Almighty God we have been able to bring out the first edition of *A Guide to Medical Surgical Nursing.*

Medical Surgical Nursing is a major subject to be studied in any basic nursing curriculum prescribed by Indian Nursing Council. Knowledge of this subject paves way in learning other branches of nursing. Number of books with multiple volumes have been written on this subject. In our experience, we have found that students get lost in those volumes of books.

This book has been presented in a simple, comprehensive, pointwise and student-friendly manner. The style of presentation would not only make it easy for students to understand the subject in a better manner but would also help them to quickly review and revise the subject before examination.

This book also has been written by keeping in mind the need of the students to know in detail about the nursing management of patient with systemwise various disease conditions. If the students gain this nursing knowledge, it can be utilized in taking care of individual patient in health care settings.

Further to make learning simple and interesting, tables, flow charts, diagrams have been included. If it finds favor with the students and teachers in all aspect, we will consider our efforts to have been worthwhile.

Srinanda Ghosh
Manashi Sengupta

Acknowledgments

Our grateful acknowledgment and deep appreciation to all those who have provided sustained help and support all through in bringing out the title *A Guide to Medical Surgical Nursing*.

All our friends, colleagues, well-wishers as well as our family members, deserve warm and sincere thanks for their kind cooperation and encouragement in this humble endeavor.

We would be failing in our duty if we do not place on record our sincere gratitude to Shri Jitendar P Vij, (Group Chairman), Jaypee Brothers Medical Publishers (P) Ltd, New Delhi, India for publishing this book and also the staff members of Kolkata production unit of Jaypee Brothers Medical Publishers (P) Ltd, for their constant encouragement, support and cooperation to complete this book.

Contents

1

Nursing Management of Patients with Disorders of Neurological System

NURSING ASSESSMENT OF PATIENTS WITH NEUROLOGICAL DISORDERS

Assessment

Subjective data

Obtain a complete history of trauma or falls that may involve the head or spinal cord.

- **History of present illness**: Pain, seizures, dizziness, vertigo, visual disturbances, weakness and abnormal sensation.
- **Medications**: History of past and present use of medication, specially use of sedative, opioids, tranquilizers and mood-elevating drugs.
- **Surgery or other treatment**: Surgery involving any part of the nervous system, such as the head, spine or sensory organs. Any exposure to toxic agents during perinatal period—Viruses, alcohol, tobacco, drugs and radiation.

Objective data

- **Physical examination**: Determine the presence, location and nature of disease. The 15 point GCS is the classic tool for patients who have deficit in eye opening, verbal ability or motor function.
- **Mental status**: Alert and oriented, orderly thought process, appropriate mood and affect.
- **Cranial nerves**: Smell intact to soap and coffee. Visual fields acuity 20/20 in both eyes; intact extraocular movement; no nystagmus; pupils equal, round reactive to light and accommodation; intact facial sensation to touch and pinprick facial movement full, intact gag and swallow reflex, symmetric evaluation with head turning and shrugging of shoulders against resistance; midline protrusion of tongue.
- **Motor system**: Normal gait and station, normal walk, negative Romberg's test, normal and symmetric muscle bulk, tone strength smooth performance of finger, nose, heel and skin movements
- **Reflexes**: Biceps, triceps, brachioradiali, patellar and Achilles tendon reflexes 2+ bilateral, down going toes with plantar stimulation.

Diagnostic Tests

CSF analysis

- **Lumbar puncture**: CSF is aspirated by needle insertion in L_3 to L_4 or L_4 to L_5 interspace to assess many CNS diseases.

Radiology

- **Skull and spine X-ray**: Simple X-ray of skull and spinal column is done to detect fractures, bone erosion, calcification and abnormal vascularity.
- **Cerebral angiography**: Serial X-ray visualization of intracranial and extracranial blood vessels is performed to detect vascular lesions and tumor of brain.
- **CT scan**: CT scans of several levels or thin cross sections of body parts are done to detect problems such as hemorrhage, tumor, cysts, edema, infarction, brain atrophy and other abnormalities.
- **MRI**: Imaging of brain, spinal cord and spinal canal, by means of magnetic energy. It is used in detection of stroke, multiple sclerosis, tumor, trauma, herniation and seizures.

ELECTROGRAPHIC STUDIES

Electroencephalography (EEG)

Electrical activity of brain is recorded by scalp electrodes to evaluate seizures disorders, cerebral disease.

Electromyography (EMG) and Nerve Conduction Study

Electrical activity associated with nerve skeletal muscle is recorded by insertion of needle electrodes to detect muscle and peripheral nerve disease.

HEAD INJURY

Definition

Any injury to the scalp, skull or brain.

Incidence

Trauma is the most common cause of death in the United States. Approximately 1.4 million people receive treatment from head injuries every year. 2,35000 are hospitalized, 86,000 have permanent disabilities and 50,000 people die.

Causes

- Motor vehicle crashes
- Violence
- Falls.

Risk Factors

- Age 15 to 24 years
- Male
- Children younger than 5 years
- Very old, older than 75 years.

Types

Scalp injury

Minor head injury. Scalp bleeds profusely when injured. It may result in abrasion (brush wound), contusion (laceration, or hematoma) beneath the layers of tissue of the scalp (subgaleal hematoma).

Skull fractures

A break in the continuity of the skull caused by forceful trauma. Classified as simple, communited, depressed or basilar. A simple (linear) fracture is a break in the continuity of the bone. A communited skull fracture refers to splintered or multiple fracture line. When bone fragments are embedded into brain tissue the fracture is depressed. A fracture of the base of the skull is called a basilar skull fracture.

Brain injuries

The terms open, closed, contusion and concussion are often applied to brain injuries. Open injuries are those that penetrate the skull. Close injuries are blunt trauma.

Concussion—It is a head trauma that may result in loss of consciousness for 5 minutes or less. If the brain tissue in the frontal lobe is affected, the patient may exhibit bizarre irrational behavior, whereas involvement of the temporal lobe can produce temporary amnesia or disorientation. Patient may be hospitalized overnight for observation. Treatment involves observing the patient for headache, dizziness, lethargy irritability and anxiety. These symptoms after injury referred to as postconcussion syndrome.

Contusion—It is associated with more extensive damage than that from concussions. There are multiple areas of small hemorrhage and bruised in the brain tissue. Patient may lie motionless, with a faint pulse, shallow respirations, cool and pale skin. The blood pressure and the temperature are subnormal and the clinical picture is similar to shock. Patient with severe brain damage have abnormal motor function, abnormal eye movement, elevated intracranial pressure (ICP), disability and death. Residual headache and vertigo are common and impaired mental function or seizures may occur as a irreversible cerebral damage.

Intracranial hemorrhage

Hematomas (collection of blood) that develops within the cranial vault are the most serious brain injuries. A hematoma may be epidural (above the dura), subdural (below the dura) or intracerebral (within the brain).

Epidural/Extradural hematoma

- After a head injury, blood may collect in the epidural (extradural) space between the skull and the dura. This can result from a skull fracture that causes a rupture or laceration of the middle meningeal artery.
- Symptoms include a momentary loss of consciousness occurs at a time of injury followed by an interval of apparent recovery (lucid interval). During this interval compensation for the absorption of CSF and decreased intravascular volume to maintain a normal ICP.
- When this mechanism fails a small increase in the volume of the blood clot produces a marked elevation in ICP. Signs of compression appears (such as deterioration of consciousness, signs of focal neurologic deficit, dilation and fixation of a pupil or paralysis of an extremity).

Subdural hematoma: Subdural hematoma is a collection of blood between the dura and the brain. Common cause is trauma but can occur as a result of coagulopathies or rupture of an aneurysm. It results as acute, subacute, chronic and intracerebral hemorrhage and hematoma.

- **Acute and subacute subdural hematoma (SDH)**: Acute SDH are associated with major head injury involving contusion or laceration. Clinical symptoms develop over 24 to 48 hours. It includes changes in the level of consciousness (LOC) pupillary signs and hemiparesis. Coma, increase blood pressure, decrease heart rate and slowing respirations are all signs of rapidly expanding mass requiring immediate intervention.
- **Subacute SDH**: Subacute SDH are results of less severe contusions and head trauma. Manifestations begin between 48 hours and 2 weeks after the injury. Signs and symptoms are similar with acute SDH.
- **Chronic SDH**: It can develop from minor head injuries and are seen most frequently in the elderly and alcoholic clients. Clients experience atrophy of the brain, which results in stretching

of the bridging veins and an increase in the size of the subdural space. These stretched veins easily ruptured in a fall; even if the fall does not result in other injuries. The time between injury and onset of symptom can be lengthy (e.g. 3 weeks to months).The blood within the brain changes in character within 2 to 4 days, becoming thicker and darker. Symptoms include severe headache off and on, alternating focal neurologic signs; personality changes, mental deterioration and focal seizures.

- **Intracerebral hemorrhage and hematoma:** It is bleeding into the substance of the brain. It is commonly seen in head injuries when force is exerted to the head over a small area (missile injuries, bullet wounds, stab injuries). These hemorrhage within the brain results from—
  - Systemic hypertension causing degeneration and rupture of a vessel.
  - Rupture of a saccular aneurysm.
  - Vascular anomalies.
  - Intracranial tumors.
  - Bleeding disorders such as leukemia, hemophilia, aplastic anemia, etc.
  - Complications of anticoagulant therapy.

Pathophysiology

- Damage of the brain from traumatic injury takes two form—primary injury and secondary injury.
- Primary injury is the initial damage to brain, that result from the traumatic event.
- Primary injury includes contusions, lacerations and ruptures blood vessels due to impact, acceleration/deceleration or foreign object penetration.
- Secondary injury evolves over the ensuring hours and days after the initial injury and is due primarily to unchecked cerebral edema, ischemia and the chemical changes associated with direct trauma to the brain.
- Inflammation leads to cerebral edema and increase ICP.
- Diffuse hemorrhage occurs if there is learning of several small vessels within the brain.
- Whenever pressure is increase within the brain, the brain become hypoxic leading to brain tissuc ischemia.
- Cells within the brain becomes anoxic and cannot metabolize properly, producing ischemia, infarction, irreversible brain damage and eventually brain death.

Diagnostic Studies

- A thorough and rapid physical examination and evaluation of neurologic status detects obvious brain injuries.
- CT Scan—It is the best diagnostic test to evaluate craniocerebral trauma because it allows rapid diagnosis and intervention in the acute setting.
- MRI, PET scan may be used in the diagnosis and differentiation of head injuries.
- A cervical spine X-ray series or CT scan of the spine may also be indicated since cervical spine trauma often occurs concomitantly with head injury.
- Cerebral angiography is used to identify supratentorial, extracerebral and intracerebral hematomas and cerebral contusions.

Management

Goals

- Prompt recognition and treatment of hypoxia.
- Control of increasing ICP.
- Stabilization of other conditions.

Treatment of increased ICP

- Initial management is based on the principle of preventing secondary injury and maintaining adequate cerebral oxygenation with hyperventilation by mechanical ventilator or by bagmask ventilation.
- Fluids are administered intravenously to stabilize blood pressure.
- Surgery is required for evacuation of blood clots, debridement and elevation of depressed fractures of the skull, and suture of severe scalp lacerations.
- The patient is cared in the intensive care unit.
- ICP is monitored closely; if increased, it is managed by maintaining adequate oxygenation elevating the head of the bed, and maintaining normal blood volume.

Treatment of skull fractures

- The treatment of skull fractures is usually conservative.
- For depressed fractures and fractures with loose fragments, a craniotomy is necessary to elevate the depressed bone and remove the free fragments.
- If large amounts of bone are destroyed, the bone may be removed (craniotomy) and a cranioplasty will be needed later.
- Treatment of large acute subdural and epidural hematoma or those with associated significant neurologic impairment:
  - The blood must be removed through surgical evacuation. A craniotomy opening is generally performed to visualize and allow control of the bleeding vessels.
  - Burr hole openings may be used in an extreme emergency for a more rapid decompression, followed by a craniotomy.
  - A drain is generally placed post-operatively for several days to prevent reaccumulation of blood.

Supportive measures

- Treatment also includes ventilator support, seizure prevention, fluid and electrolyte maintenance, nutritional support and management of pain and anxiety.
- Comatose patients are intubated and mechanically ventilated to ensure adequate oxygenation and protect the airway.

NURSING MANAGEMENT

Nursing Assessment

Subjective data

Immediate health history including history of trauma/accident and its causes. History of unconsciousness or amnesia after a head injury. Any significant past medical and surgical history. Any history of alcohol intake or ingestion of other drugs before injury.

Objective data

Monitor the patient for tachycardia or bradycardia, hypothermia or hyperthermia, Glasgow coma score below 8, signs of hypoxia such tachypnea, low oxygen saturation, low blood pressure, deterioration in level of consciousness, abnormal pupillary reaction to light, diminished or absent of corneal and gag reflex as well as motor function.

Nursing Diagnoses

- Ineffective airway clearance and impaired gas exchange related brain injury.
- Ineffective cerebral tissue perfusion related to increased ICP.
- Deficient fluid volume related to decreased LOC and hormonal dysfunction.

- Acute pain (headache) related to trauma and cerebral edema.
- Hyperthermia related to increased metabolism, infection and loss of cerebral integrative function secondary to possible hypothalamic injury.
- Disturbed thought process related to brain injury.
- Deficient knowledge about brain injury, recovery and the rehabilitation process.

Planning Outcomes/Goals

Maintenance of a Patent Airway

- Maintain adequate CPP.
- Maintain fluid and electrolyte balance.
- Minimize pain and discomfort.
- Maintain normal body temperature.
- Improve thought process and knowledge level.

Nursing Interventions

Maintenance of a patent airway

- Monitor respiratory rate and pattern.
- Anticipate need for intubation if gag reflex is impaired or absent.
- Assume neck injury with head injury.
- Maintain patent airway using suctioning, or introducing airway device.
- Position patient with head end elevated to 30°.
- Assist with endotracheal intubation or tracheostomy as required.
- Check and document ventilator parameters.
- Monitor oxygenation with pulse oximetry to know about oxygen status.
- Provide oxygen support as needed.

Maintain adequate cerebral prefusion pressure

- Monitor vital signs, level of consciousness, oxygen saturation, cardiac rhythm, GCS score, pupil size and reactivity.
- Administer oxygen via nonrebreather mask.
- Establish IV access with large bore cannula to infuse normal saline or Ringer's lactate solution.
- Control external bleeding with sterile pressure dressing.
- Assess for rhinorrhea, otorrhea, and scalp wounds.
- Remove patient's clothing.
- Maintain patient warmth using blankets, warm IV fluids, overhead warming lights, warm humidified oxygen.
- Maintain blood pressure with inotropic medications as ordered to ensure oxygenation to brain tissue.

Maintains fluid and electrolytes within normal limits

- Monitor acid-base balance, fluid intake and output, and electrolyte results.
- Assess fluid volume status to avoid hypovolemia and hypervolemia.
- Provide fluid and electrolytes via IV access until the patient is able to take liquids by mouth.

Minimize pain and discomfort

- Assess the level of pain through pain rating scale.
- Promote bed rest.
- Change the position as desired by the patient or according to patient condition.
- Administer analgesics as ordered.

Maintenance of normal body temperature

- Check and record temperature at regular intervals.
- Give tepid sponge.
- Administer antipyretic as ordered.

Improve thought process and knowledge level

- Assess the thought process and knowledge and understanding level of patients.

- Encourage the patient to ventilate his feelings.
- Explain rationales before doing any procedure.
- Reinforce the patient for participating in activities of daily living.
- Report significant other about day-to-day prognosis of the patient.

GUILLAIN-BARRÉ SYNDROME (GBS)

Definition

Guillain-Barré syndrome (GBS)

It is an inflammatory disorder of the peripheral nerves.

- The peripheral nerves convey sensory information (e.g. pain, temperature) from the body to the brain and motor (i.e. movement) signals from the brain to the body.
- GBS is characterized by weakness and numbness or tingling in the legs and arms, and possible loss of movement and feeling in the legs, arms, upper body, and face.
- Chronic inflammatory demyelinating polyradicalneuropathy (CIDP), is a related form of Guillain-Barré syndrome.

Incidence

- Guillain-Barré syndrome is a rare disorder.
- Its frequency is about 1 to 2 cases in every 100,000 people per year in the United States.
- Men and women, young and old, are equally prone to contracting GBS.

Causes

Guillain-Barré syndrome is not hereditary or contagious. Causes of GBS are not known; however, in about half of all cases the onset of the syndrome follows a viral or bacterial infection, such as the followings:

- Flu and common cold.
- Gastrointestinal viral infection.
- Infectious mononucleosis.
- Viral hepatitis.
- Campylobacteriosis (usually from eating undercooked poultry).
- Porphyria (rare disease of red blood cells).
- A small number of cases have been known to occur after a medical procedure, such as minor surgery. Guillain-Barré syndrome may be an **autoimmune disorder** in which the body produces antibodies that damage the myelin sheath that surrounds peripheral nerves.
- The **myelin sheath** is a fatty substance that surrounds axons. It increases the speed at which signals travel along the nerves.

Clinical Manifestations

- Numbness or tingling (paresthesia) in the toes and fingers, with progressive weakness in the arms and legs.
- Some patients experience paresthesia only in their toes and legs; others only experience symptoms on one side of the body.
- The symptoms may stay in this phase, causing only mild difficulty in walking, requiring crutches or a walking stick.
- The illness progresses, leading to complete paralysis of the arms and legs.
- About one quarter of the time, the paralysis continues up the chest and freezes the breathing muscles, leaving the patient dependent on a ventilator.
- If the swallowing muscles are also affected, a feeding tube may be needed. In CIDP, the course of illness is longer and respiratory failure is much more unlikely.

Diagnostic Tests

- As the cause and symptom is unknown, GBS can be difficult to diagnose.

- If the symptoms occur uniformly across the body and progress rapidly, the diagnosis is easier.
- Observation of the patient's symptoms and an evaluation of the medical history provide the basis for diagnosis of Guillain-Barré syndrome.

Three tests can confirm a diagnosis of Guillain-Barré syndrome.

Lumbar puncture (spinal tap)

The patient is given local anesthsia. Once the anesthesia has taken effect, a needle is inserted between two lower (lumbar) vertebrae and a sample of cerebrospinal fluid is drawn. An elevated level of protein in the fluid is characteristic of GBS.

Electromyogram (EMG)

This is an effective diagnostic tool because it records muscle activity and can show the loss of reflexes due to the disease's characteristic slowing of nerve responses.

Nerve conduction velocity (NCV)

This test is performed with EMG, and together, they are often referred to as **EMG/NCV studies**. NCV records the speed at which signals travel along the nerves.

Management

Goals

To reduce symptoms, offer immunotherapy to shorten the duration of the disease, and maintain the body's muscles.

GBS is considered a medical emergency and most patients are admitted to **intensive care unit** soon after diagnosis.

Treat respiratory failure

- Increasing muscular paralysis can temporarily affect the chest muscles, causing shortness of breath.
- The patient may be required to be put on a ventilator. The ventilator helps to stabilize and assist the patient's respirations.
- Most patients may only need to be on a ventilator for 1 to 2 weeks, while others will need it for longer periods of time.
- The patients that need mechanical ventilation for increased periods of time may need a tracheostomy.
- Frequent suctioning may be required. This is done through the tracheostomy tube or the endotracheal tube.

Sedation and pain medications

- Many people require light sedation to help prevent them from fighting against the ventilator or pulling at the ventilator tubing. Pain medication is also crucial at this point. Patients still have pain and need to be properly medicated. This may also help reduce anxiety.

Communication is vital for patients who are on mechanical ventilator

- Effective communication must be established between the patient, family, medical and nursing staff.
- The patient should be involved in the decision-making process regarding their treatment and care.
- Communication can be sought out by using alphabet boards, pictures, dry erase boards, or pencil and paper.
- Some patients are only able to shake their head or blink their eyes for yes and no answers.

Cardiac Monitoring—The patient should be monitored for arrhythmias, and chanes in blood pressure. These changes can reflect peripheral autonomic nervous system involvement.

- GBS and CIDP are treated with plasmapheresis or immunoglobulin. Corticosteroids may be used to treat CIDP but are not used to treat GBS, as it worsens rather than improves the condition.

Plasmapheresis

Patients diagnosed early in the course of the disease and those who are acutely ill often respond well to blood plasma exchange (plasmapheresis).

- In this procedure, blood is withdrawn and passed through a series of filters that separate the different types of blood cells.
- The blood cells are then suspended in donor or synthetic plasma and returned to the patient's body.
- Plasmapheresis is thought to remove the substances that damage myelin. It can shorten the course of GBS, alleviate symptoms, and prevent paralysis.

Immunoglobulin

Large doses of immunoglobulin given intravenously can help shorten the duration of symptoms.

Medications

- Muscle and joint pain can be treated with aspirin. If necessary, stronger pain medication (e.g. acetaminophen with codeine) may be prescribed. Muscle spasms can be controlled with relaxants such as diazepam (Valium).
- In the later stages of rehabilitation, lingering sensation problems can be treated with tricyclic antidepressants or anticonvulsants such as gabapentin (Neurontin).
- Corticosteroids, is used to treat the symptoms of autoimmune disorders, actually it worsens Guillain-Barré syndrome and should not be used. They are sometimes used to treat CIDP.

Physical Therapy

- Before recovery begins, caregivers move the patient's arms and legs to prevent stiffness.
- After symptoms subside, the rehabilitation team will prescribe an active exercise routine to help regain muscle strength and independence.
- Training with adaptive devices, such as a wheelchair or braces, give the patient mobility.

Hydrotherapy

Whirlpool therapy (hydrotherapy) may help to relieve pain and be useful in retraining the movement of affected limbs.

Counseling

Counseling often is suggested to reassure the patients diagnosed with GBS or CIDP and to help them feel positive about their treatment and recovery.

Prognosis

- Patients may remain in the hospital for several months and recovery may take a year or more.
- Most patients recover completely, but some have residual weakness, numbness, and occasional pain.
- A small number are unable to resume their normal occupation.
- Fewer than 5% of GBS patients die. Those fatalities usually result from cardiovascular or respiratory complications.
- Death resulting from CIDP is rare.

NURSING MANAGEMENT

Nursing Assessment

Subjective data

Weakness of lower limbs, fingers and toes, ascending paralysis.

Objective data

During the routine assessment the nurse must monitor the ascending paralysis; assess respiratory functions; monitor arterial blood gas, assess the gag, corneal, and swallowing reflexes. Monitoring blood pressure and cardiac rate and rhythm is also important because during acute phase there is evidence of cardiac dysrhythmias.

Nursing Diagnoses

- Impaired spontaneous ventilation related to progression of disease process resulting in respiratory muscle paralysis.
- Risk for aspiration related to dysphagia.
- Acute pain related to parathesias, muscle aches and cramps and hyperthesias.
- Impaired verbal communication related to intubation or paralysis of the muscles of speech.
- Self care deficit related to inability to use muscles to accomplish activities of daily living.

PLANNING OUTCOMES/GOALS

- Maintain adequate ventilation.
- Be free from aspiration.
- Be pain-free or have pain controlled.
- Maintain an acceptable method of communication.
- Maintain adequate nutritional intake.
- Return to usual physical functioning.

Nursing Interventions

General nursing care

Respiratory—Observe for changes in respiratory pattern, shortness of breath, dyspnea, and suction increased secretions.

Cardiac—Look for changes in cardiac rhythms, increased ectopic beats and blood pressure. Assess for chest pain or discomfort.

Gastric feeding—The head of the bed should be elevated 30 to 45 degress to help decrease the risk of aspiration.

Mouth—The nurse should look for drooping and or drooling from the mouth, and complaints of dysphagia.

Bowels—Bowel movements should be documented. Nausea and/or vomiting could be signs of constipation. Medications should be ordered routine or prn (when required) to help prevent constipation.

Bladder—The bladder can temporarily lose its ability to squeeze and empty itself, which can lead to urinary retention. If this happens a foley catheter should be inserted. Daily foley and perineal care should be done routinely to help prevent urinary tract infections.

Skin—The patient's skin should be inspected every shift for potential breakdown. Patients should be turned and repositioned every 2 hours to decrease the risk of pressure ulcers and promote circulation. Feet and hands should be assessed for foot or wrist drop.

DEEP VEIN THROMBOSIS (DVT)

Bedridden patients are at high risk for developing DVT. Prophylactic antithrombolytics should be ordered such as subcutaneous heparin 5,000 units BID or twice daily.

Physical Therapy

- Arrangements for physical therapy should be initiated as soon as possible for the patient to have optimal recovery.
- Caregivers may need to be taught how

to manually move the patient's arms and legs to help keep the muscles flexible and strong.
- Whirlpool therapy may help to relieve pain. Once discharged the patient should be sent home with an active exercise routine to help regain muscle strength.
- Patients should be evaluated for splints, walking aids and rehabilitation.

Psychological Support and Communication

- Patients and family members need to be involved in all aspects of care.
- The patient should be allowed to communicate his or her feelings of frustration, pain, anxiety, isolation, and low self-esteem.
- Counseling and medication to help deal with these feelings may be necessary for a while for both patient and family.

PARKINSON'S DISEASE

Definition

- Parkinson's disease is a chronic, progressive neurodegenerative movement disorder.
- Tremors, rigidity, slow movement (bradykinesia), poor balance, and difficulty walking (called Parkinsonian gait) are primary symptoms of Parkinson's disease
- Idiopathic Parkinson's disease is the most common form of Parkinsonism, a group of movement disorders that have similar features and symptoms.
- Parkinson's results from the degeneration of dopamine-producing nerve cells in the brain, specifically in the substantia nigra and the locus coeruleus.
- Dopamine is a neurotransmitter that stimulates motor neurons, those nerve cells that control the muscles. When dopamine production is depleted, the motor system nerves are unable to control movement and coordination.
- Parkinson's disease patients have lost 80% or more of their dopamine-producing cells by the time symptoms appear.

Incidence and Prevalence

- Parkinson's disease affects 1 to 1½million people in the United States.
- The disorder occurs in all races but is somewhat more prevalent among Caucasians.
- Men are affected slightly more often than women.
- Symptoms of Parkinson's disease may appear at any age, but the average age of onset is 60.
- It is rare in people younger than 30 and risk increases with age.
- It is estimated that 5% to 10% of patients experience symptoms before the age of 40.

Risk Factors

- A genetic predisposition for Parkinson's disease is possible, with the onset of disease and its gradual development dependent on a trigger, such as trauma, other illness, or exposure to an environmental toxin.
- The risk increases with age, as Parkinson's disease generally manifests in the middle or late years of life.

Causes

The cause of Parkinson's disease is unknown. Many researchers believe that several factors combined are involved:

- Free radicals
- Accelerated aging
- Environmental toxins
- Genetic predisposition.

Pathophysiology

- It may be the free radicals—unstable and potentially damaging molecules that lack on electron—are involved in the degeneration of dopamine-producing cells.
- Free radicals add an electron by reacting with nearby molecules in a process called **oxidation**, which can damage nerve cells.
- Chemicals called antioxidants normally protect cells from oxidative stress and damage.
- If antioxidative action fails to protect dopamine-producing nerve cells, they could be damaged and, subsequently, Parkinson's disease could develop.
- Dysfunctional antioxidative mechanisms are associated with older age as well, suggesting that the acceleration of **age-related changes** in dopamine production may be a factor.
- Exposure to an **environmental toxin**, such as a pesticide, that inhibits dopamine production and produces free radicals and oxidation damage may be involved.

CLINICAL MANIFESTATIONS

Primary Symptoms

Bradykinesia

It is slowness in voluntary movement. It produces difficulty initiating movement as well as difficulty completing movement once it is in progress. The delayed transmission of signals from the brain to the skeletal muscles, due to diminished dopamine, produces bradykinesia.

Tremors

Tremors in the hands, fingers, forearm, or foot tend to occur when the limb is at rest but not when performing tasks. Tremor may occur in the mouth and chin as well.

Rigidity

Rigidity or stiff muscles, may produce muscle pain and an expressionless, mask-like face. Rigidity tends to increase during movement.

Poor balance

It is due to the impairment or loss of the reflexes that adjust posture in order to maintain balance. Falls are common in people with Parkinson's.

Parkinsonian gait

It is the distinctive unsteady walk associated with Parkinson's disease. There is a tendency to lean unnaturally backward or forward, and to develop a stooped, head-down, shoulders-drooped stance. Arm swing is diminished or absent and people with Parkinson's tend to take small shuffling steps (called festination). Someone with Parkinson's may have trouble starting to walk, appear to be falling forward as they walk, freeze in mid-stride, and have difficulty making a turn.

Secondary Symptoms

- Constipation.
- Difficulty swallowing (dysphagia)—saliva and food that collects in the mouth or back of the throat may cause choking, coughing, or drooling.
- Excessive salivation (hypersalivation).
- Excessive sweating (hyperhidrosis).
- Loss of bladder and/or bowel control (incontinence).
- Loss of intellectual capacity (dementia)—late in the disease.
- Psychosocial—anxiety, depression, isolation.

- Scaling, dry skin on the face and scalp (seborrhea).
- Slow response to questions (bradyphrenia).
- Small, cramped handwriting (micrographia).
- Soft, whispery voice (hypophonia).

Diagnostic Tests

- Diagnosis is based on symptoms and ruling out other disorders that produce similar symptoms.
- A patient must have two or more of the primary symptoms, one of which is a resting tremor or bradykinesia. In many cases, this diagnosis is made after observing that symptoms have developed and become established over a period.
- After a thorough neurological exam and medical history, the neurologist may order computerized tomography (CT scan) or magnetic resonance imaging (MRI scan) to meet the other criterion for a diagnosis of Parkinson's disease: ruling out disorders (e.g. brain tumor, stroke) that produce Parkinsonian symptoms.
- Some examples follows:
  - Medications—Antipsychotics (e.g. Hal-dol) and antiemetics (e.g. Compazine)
  - Multiple strokes
  - Hydrocephalus
  - Progressive supranuclear palsy—Degeneration of midbrain structures
  - Shy-Drager syndrome—Atrophy of central and sympathetic nervous systems
  - Wilson's disease—Copper excretion causes degeneration of the liver and basal ganglia
  - Blood and/or cerebrospinal fluid (CSF) analysis may be ordered to look for specific abnormalities associated with other disorders.

Medical Treatment

- There is no cure for Parkinson's disease. Treatment centers on the administration of medication to relieve symptoms.
- In some severe cases, a surgical procedure may offer the greatest benefit.

Medication

As the disease progresses, drug dosages may have to be modified and medication regimens changed. Sometimes a combination of drugs is given.

Levodopa and carbidopa combined (Sinemet)

It is the mainstay of Parkinson's therapy.

Levodopa is rapidly converted into dopamine by the enzyme dopa decarboxylase (DDC), which is present in the central and peripheral nervous systems. Much of levodopa is metabolized before it reaches the brain.

Carbidopa inhibits DDC. Combining levodopa with carbidopa increases the amount of levodopa that reaches the brain. Levodopa is most effective in treating bradykinesia and rigidity, less effective in reducing tremor, and often ineffective in relieving problems with balance.

Dopamine agonists

Dopamine agonists mimic dopamine's function in the brain. They are used primarily as adjuncts to levodopa/carbidopa therapy. They can be used as monotherapy but are generally less effective in controlling symptoms.

- Bromocriptine (Parlodel)
- Pergolide (Permax)
- Pramipexole (Mirapex)
- Ropinirole (Requip).

Amantadine (Symmetrel)

It is an antiviral drug with dopamine agonist properties. It increases the release of dopamine. It is often used to treat early-stage Parkinson's disease, either alone, with an anticholinergic drug, or with levodopa. Generally, it loses its effectiveness within 3 to 4 months.

MAO-B inhibitors

Dopamine is oxidized by monoamine oxidase B (MAO-B). Selegiline (Carbex) inhibits MAO-B, increasing the amount of available dopamine in the brain. MAO-B inhibitors boost the effects of levodopa.

Anticholinergics

Anticholinergics reduce the relative overactivity of the neurotransmitter acetylcholine to balance the diminished dopamine activity. This class of drugs is most effective in the control of tremor, and they are used as adjuncts to levodopa.

- Benztropine mesylate (Cogentin)
- Biperiden (Akineton)
- Diphenhydramine (Benadryl)
- Trihexyphenidyl (Artane).

COMT(catechol-O-methyltransferase) inhibitors

These new class of Parkinson's medications augment levodopa therapy by inhibiting the COMT enzyme, which metabolizes levodopa before it reaches the brain. Inhibiting COMT increases the amount of levodopa that enters the brain. These drugs are only effective when used with levodopa.

- Entacapone (Comtan)
- Tolcapone (Tasmar).

Carbidopa, levodopa, and entacapone are combined in Stalevo, which is indicated for patients who experience a reduced effectiveness of their PD medication.

Surgery

- Surgery is another method of controlling symptoms and improving quality of life when medication ceases to be effective or when medication side effects, such as jerking and dyskinesias, become intolerable.
- Only about 10% of Parkinson's patients are estimated to be suitable candidates.
- There are three surgical procedures for treating Parkinson's disease: ablative surgery, stimulation surgery or deep brain stimulation (DBS), and transplantation or restorative surgery.

Ablative surgery

- This procedure locates, targets, and then destroys (ablates) a clearly defined area of the brain affected by Parkinson's disease.
- The object is to destroy tissue that produces abnormal chemical or electrical impulses that produce tremors and dyskinesias.
- A heated probe or electrode is inserted into the targeted area.
- It is often difficult to estimate how much tissue to destroy and the amount of heat to use.
- It is always safer to burn a small area and risk the tremor returning or not being eliminated, rather than burning a larger region and risking serious complications such as paralysis or stroke.
- The patient remains awake during this procedure to determine if the tremor or dyskinesia has been eliminated.
- A local anesthetic is used to dull the outer part of the brain and skull.
- The brain is insensitive to pain, so it can be manipulated and probed without the patient feeling it.
- This type of surgery involves either pallidotomy or thalamotomy.

Pallidotomy—Ablation in the part of the brain called the globus pallidus—involves putting a hole (i.e. otomy) in the globus pallidus, the globe-shaped structure located deep inside the brain.

This procedure is performed to eliminate uncontrolled dyskinesias.

Thalamotomy—Ablation of brain tissue in the thalamus—involves creating an otomy in the thalamus. This structure is located below the globus pallidus. The procedure is performed to eliminate tremors.

Cryothalamotomy—A related procedure, uses a supercooled probe that is inserted into the thalamus to freeze and destroy areas that produce tremors.

Deep brain stimulation (DBS)

DBS targets the subthalamic nucleus, which is located below the thalamus and is difficult to reach, the globus pallidus, or the thalamus.

In DBS, the targeted region is inactivated, not destroyed, by an implanted electrode.

The electrode is connected via a wire running beneath the skin to a stimulator and battery pack in the patient's chest.

It is reversible—just turn off the current—and allows for precise calibrated symptom control.

The risk for hemorrhage or stroke is reduced, but the electrode can become infected, the simulator may have to be periodically programed, and the battery must be replaced every 5 years.

Battery replacement involves minor surgery.

Transplantation or restorative surgery

In transplantation, or restorative, surgery dopamine-producing cells are implanted into the striatum. The cells used for transplantation may come from one of several sources: the patient's body, human embryos, or pig embryos.

- Using **cells from the patient's body** has been unsuccessful because of an insufficient supply of dopamine cells and the inability of the implanted cells to survive.
- To use **fetal cells**, between three and eight embryos are needed per procedure, and even under the most favorable conditions, 90% of transplanted cells do not survive.
- This procedure is only moderately effective in some patients and usually in those younger than age 60.
- **Pig embryo cells** do survive transplantation and have an effect on symptoms.
- **Stem cells**, primitive cells that can grow into nerve cells, are able to survive and reproduce. Once they grow as nerve cells, they can be transformed into dopamine-producing cells.
- Stem cells are obtained from discarded blood in a newborn's umbilical cord, the bone marrow of an adult, or an aborted embryo.

NURSING MANAGEMENT

Nursing Assessment

Subjective data

Past health history—CNS trauma, cerebrovascular disorders, exposure to metals and carbon monoxide and encephalitis.

Medications—Use of major tranquilizers,

Functional health problems—Excessive salivation, dysphagia, weight loss, constipation, incontinence, excessive sweating, difficulty in initiating movements, frequent falls, insomnia, diffuse pain in head, and shoulders, depression, mood swings and hallucinations.

Objective data

Blank faces, slow and monotonous speech, dandruff, ankle edema, postural hypotension, drooling, tremor at night, aggravation of tremor with anxiety, absence in sleep, poor coordination, impaired postural reflexes, dysarthria, contractures, subtle dementia, bradykinesia and stooped posture.

Nursing Diagnoses

- Impaired physical mobility related to rigidity, bradykinesia, and akinesia as evidenced by difficulty in initiation of purposeful movements.
- Impaired verbal communication related to dysarthria, tremor, and bradykinesia as evidenced by decreased amount of communication, slow and slurred speech.
- Deficient diversional activity related to inability to perform usual leisure activities as evidenced boredom, lack of participation, restlessness and depression.
- Imbalanced nutrition less than body requirements related to dysphagia as evidenced by difficulty swallowing and chewing drooling, decreased gag reflex and weight loss.

PLANNING OUTCOMES/GOALS

- Uses physical exercise to prevent joint contracture and uses assistive devices appropriately for ambulation and mobility.
- Develop methods of communication that meet needs for interaction with others.
- Engages in diversional activities.
- Maintains nutritional intake adequate for metabolic needs.

Nursing Interventions

Uses physical exercise to prevent joint contracture and uses assistive devices appropriately for ambulation and mobility

- Assess the level of activities patient can perform.
- Assist patient with initial ambulation to determine degree of impairment and prevent injury.
- Consult physiotherapist about ambulation plan to facilitate safe ambulation.
- Provide appropriate assistive devices such as cane, walker or wheel chair for ambulation.

Develops methods of communication that meet needs for interaction with others

- Listen attentively to the patient.
- Use communication board for necessary communication.
- Encourage patient to repeat words to provide exercise.
- Refer to a speech therapist for specialized advice.

Engages in diversional activities

- Determine patient's interest for any activity.
- Assist patient to fulfill meaningful activities to meet individual needs.
- Monitor emotional, physical, social and spiritual responses to activity to evaluate effectiveness of interventions.
- Give counseling and psychological support.

Maintains nutritional intake adequate for metabolic needs

- Assess the nutritional need and body weight of the patient.
- Prescribe a balanced diet.
- Ensure that diet includes foods high in fiber content to prevent constipation.
- Assist patient to a sitting position before eating to promote swallowing and reduce risk of aspiration.
- Record intake and output.

BRAIN TUMORS

Definition

Primary brain tumors

A brain tumor is a localized intracranial lesion that occupies space within the skull.

A tumor usually grows as spherical mass, but it also can grow diffusely and infiltrate tissue.

Incidence—Secondary to metastatic, brain tumors develop from structures outside the brain and occur in 10% to 20% of patients with cancer.

Predisposing factors
- Increased intracranial pressure (ICP) and cerebral edema.
- Seizure activity and focal neurologic signs.
- Hydrocephalus.
- Altered pituitary function.
- Primary brain tumors originate from cells and structures within the brain.
- Brain tumors rarely metastasize outside the CNS, but metastatic lesions to the brain occur commonly from the lung, breast, pancreas, kidney and skin.

Cause—Unknown, the only known risk factor is exposure to ionizing radiation.

Secondary brain tumors

It is resulting from a metastasis from a malignant neoplasm elsewhere in the body.
- Brain tumors are generally classified according to the tissue from which they arise.

Types

The most common primary brain tumors originate in astrocytes. These tumors are called gliomas (e.g. astrocytoma, glioblastoma and multiforme) and account for 65% of primary brain tumors (Table 1.1).

Pathophysiology

- More than half of the brain tumors are malignant; they infiltrate the brain parenchyma and are not amenable to complete surgical removal.
- Other tumors may be histologically benign but are located such that complete removal is not possible.
- Unless treated all brain tumors eventually cause death from increasing tumor volume leading to increased ICP.
- Brain tumors rarely metastasize outside the central nervous system because they are contained by structural (meninges) and physiologic (blood brain) barriers.

Clinical Manifestations

The rate of growth and the appearance of manifestations depend on the location, size and mitotic rate of the cells of the tissue of origin. Wide range of possible clinical manifestations is associated with brain tumors.
- Headache: Tumor related headache tend to be worse at night and may awaken the patient. Usually dull in nature and constant but occasionally throbbing.
- Seizures: Seizures are common in gliomas and brain metastasis.
- Nausea and vomiting due to increased ICP.
- Cognitive dysfunction, including memory problems and mood or personality changes present in brain metastasis.
- Muscle weakness, sensory losses, aphasia, and visuospatial dysfunction.
- As the brain tumors expand, it may also produce manifestations of increased ICP, cerebral edema, or obstruction of the CSF pathways.

Table 1.1: Type of brain tumors with the tissue of origin

Type	Tissue of origin
Gliomas	
Astrocytoma	Supportive tissue,glial cells,and astrocytes
Glioblastoma multiforme	Primitive stem cell (glioblast)
Oligodendroglioma	Oligodendrocytes
Ependymoma	Ependymal epithelium
Medulloblastoma	Primitive neuroectodermal cell
Meningogioma	Meninges
Acoustic neuroma	Cells that form myelin sheath around nerves; Commonly affects cranial nerve VII
Pituitary adenoma	Pituitary gland
Hemangioblastoma	Pituitary gland
Pituitary central nervous system	Lymphocytes
Metastatic tumors	Lungs, breast, kidney, thyroid, prostate

Complications

The following complication may occur due to the obstruction of the ventricles occluding the outlet leading to ventricular enlargement, i.e. hydrocephalus.

Diagnostic studies

- Complete history and a comprehensive neurological examination to know in detail about patient's condition.
- MRI and PET allow for the detection of very small tumors and may provide more reliable diagnostic information.
- CT scan of brain is used to diagnose the location of the lesion.
- Cerebral angiography can be used to determine blood flow to the tumor and further localize the tumor.
- Histological studies are used to make the correct diagnosis of brain tumor. In most of the patients, tissue is obtained at the time surgery. Computer guided stereotactic biopsy is also an option if complete resection is not possible.

MANAGEMENT

Goals

- Identifying the tumor type and location
- Removing or decreasing tumor mass
- Preventing or managing increased ICP.

Surgical Therapy

- Surgical removal is the preferred treatment for brain tumors.
- Stereotactic surgical techniques are used to perform a biopsy and remove small brain tumors.
- The outcome of the surgery depends on the type, size and location of the tumor.
- Meningiomas and oligodendrogliomas can usually be completely removed, where the more invasive gliomas and medulla blastomas can be only partially removed.
- Surgery can reduce tumor mass, decreases ICP and provides relief of symptoms with an extension of survival time.

Radiation Therapy and Radiosurgery

- Radiation therapy is commonly used as a follow-up measure after surgery.
- Radiation therapy seeds can also be implanted into the brain.
- Cerebral edema and rapidly increasing ICP may be a complication of radiation therapy, but they can be managed with high doses of corticosteroid (dexamethasone, prednisolone).
- **Stereotactic radiotherapy** is a method of delivering a high concentrated dose of radiation precisely directed at a location within the brain.

Chemotherapy

1. A group of chemotherapeutic drugs called the nitrosoureas, e.g. carmustine (BCNU), lomustine (CCNU) are used to treat brain tumors, which crosses the blood brain barrier to enter the tumor cells.
2. Other drugs being used include methotrexate and procarbazine (matulane). One method used to deliver chemotherapeutic drugs directly to the CNS is intrathecal administration via Ommaya reservoir.
3. Temozolomide (temodar) is the first oral chemotherapeutic agent found to cross the blood brain barrier.

NURSING MANAGEMENT

Assessment

Subjective data

Medical history, intellectual abilities and educational level and history of nervous system infections and trauma should be asked.

Objective data

Complete neurological status including the LOC and content of consciousness, motor abilities, sensory perception, integrated function, etc. Determination of the presence of seizures, syncope, nausea and vomiting, and headaches or other pain is important in planning care for the patient.

Nursing Diagnosis

- Impaired tissue perfusion (cerebral) related to cerebral edema.
- Acute pain (headache) related to cerebral edema and increased ICP.
- Self-care deficits related to altered neuromuscular function secondary to tumor growth and cerebral edema.
- Anxiety related to diagnosis and treatment.
- High risk of seizures related to abnormal electrical activity of the brain.

Nursing Interventions

Planning/Goals

- Maintain normal ICP
- Achieve control of pain and discomfort
- Maximize neurologic functioning.

Maintain normal ICP

- Assess neurologic status and vital signs frequently and compare with baseline values.
- Elevate head of bed to 30 degrees.
- Change position slowly.
- Monitor intake and output.
- Monitor pulse oximetry and arterial blood gases.
- Administer steroids or osmotic diuretics as ordered.

Achieve control of pain and discomfort

- Assess the behavioral instability of a confused patient.
- Administer analgesic as ordered.
- Closely supervise the activity of the patient.
- Use side rails.
- Administer sedatives as ordered.

Maximize neurologic functioning

- Assess Glasgow coma scale score to identify the state of consciousness.
- Encourage open communication between patient, family and caregiver.
- Clear patient's doubts. Provide opportunities for expression and ventilation of feelings and issues.
- Encourage the patient to participate in self-care activities such as combing, brushing, dressing, etc.
- Administer antiseizure drugs as ordered.
- Establish an effective nurse patient relationship.

ALZHEIMER'S DISEASE

Definition

- Alzheimer's disease is a progressive neurologic disease of the brain leading to the irreversible loss of neurons and the loss of intellectual abilities, including memory and reasoning.
- Alzheimer's disease is also known as simply Alzheimer's, and Senile Dementia of the Alzheimer Type (SDAT).
- Alzheimer's disease is the most common form of dementia.

Incidence

About 4 million older Americans have Alzheimer's, a disease that usually develops in people age 65 or older. This number is expected to triple by the year 2050.

Causes and Risk Factors

Age

Affects people older than 65 rarely affects those younger than 40.

Heredity

Appears to be slightly higher if a first-degree relative—Parent, sister or brother has the disease. Three genetic mutations are known to cause early onset Alzheimer's. One form of the apolipoprotein E (APOE) gene increases the risk of developing late onset Alzheimer's.

Sex

Women are more likely to develop than men.

Lifestyle

High blood pressure, high cholesterol, poorly controlled diabetes is some risk factors.

Toxicity

Overexposure to certain trace metals or chemicals.

Pathophysiology

- Alzheimer's disease is named after Dr. Alois Alzheimer, a German neurologist.
- He examined the brain of a woman who had died after long years of progressive dementia.
- Her brain tissue showed abnormal clumps and irregular knots of brain cells.
- These clumps (plaques) and knots (tangles) are considered as hallmark of the disease.
- Plaques are made up of a normally harmless protein called beta-amyloid. Three genetic mutations—In amyloid precursor protein and presenilin1 (PS1) and presenilin 2 (PS2) proteins are known to cause a small number of early onset forms of Alzheimer's disease. These mutations result in the production of amyloid plaques.
- The internal support structure for brain neurons depends on the normal functioning of a protein called tau. In people with Alzheimer's threads of tau

protein undergo alterations that cause them to become twisted and this may damage the neurons causing them to die.

Clinical Manifestations

- Increasing and persistant forgetfulness
- Difficulties with abstract thinking
- Difficulty finding the right word
- Disorientation
- Loss of judgment
- Difficulty performing familiar tasks
- Personality changes.

Diagnostic Tests

Medical history

Collect detail history about general health and past medical problems.

Blood tests

To rule out any thyroid disorder or vitamin deficiency.

Mental status evaluation

These tests screen memory, problem solving abilities, attention spans, counting skills and language.

Neuropsychological testing

An extensive assessment of cognitive (thinking), attention spans, counting skills, language and memory skills. It can take several hours. These types of tests are extremely useful in detecting Alzheimer's as well as other dementias.

Brain scans

CT scan, MRI and PET scan are used to detect an increased risk of Alzheimer's in healthy people before symptoms begin.

Complications

In advanced Alzheimer's disease, people may lose all ability to care for themselves. This can make them more prone to additional health problems such as:

Pneumonia

Difficulty in swallowing food and liquids may lead to aspiration into lungs causing aspiration pneumonia.

Infections

When the patient becomes incontinent it may be necessary to place a urinary catheter. This increases the risk of urinary tract infections

Falls and their complications

Disorientation and wandering are common symptoms of Alzheimer's. Patients are likely to fall and fracture a bone or sustain a head injury.

Prevention

Healthy aging

Losing weight, exercising, controlling high blood pressure and cholesterol may prevent Alzheimer's.

Nonsteroidal anti-inflammatory drugs

Ibuprofen, naproxen sodium and indomethacin may reduce the risk of developing Alzheimer's.

Statins

Atorvastatin (Lipitor), Simvastatin (Zocor) are normally used to lower cholesterol levels also reduce the risk of Alzheimer's.

Selective estrogen receptor molecules (SERMs)

A SERM called raloxifene (Evista) is used to protect against the bone loss associated with osteoporosis. It also lowers the risk of developing mild cognitive impairment.

Vitamin E and gingko

Substances have been linked to improvements in cognitive abilities.

Mental fitness

Maintaining mental fitness may delay inset of dementia.

Management

- Alzheimer's is a terminal disease. This means it has no cure and will end in death.
- There are various medications which can help slow down the progression of the disease, and others that can improve the signs and symptoms, such as sleeplessness, wandering, depression, anxiety and agitation.

Cholinesterase Inhibitors

- Improve the levels of neurotransmitters in the brain. The medication contains a chemical that inhibits the cholinesterase enzyme from breaking down the neurotransmitter acetylcholine—resulting in an increase in both the neurotransmitter's level and duration of action.
- Cholinesterase inhibitors are prescribed to treat problems related to memory, thinking, language, judgment and other thought processes.

Examples of cholinesterase inhibitors include:
- Donepezil (Tablet Aricept)—Treat all stages.
- Galantamine (Razadyne)—Mild to moderate stages.
- Rivastigmine (Tablet Exelon)—Mild to moderate stages.

Memantine

Protects brain cells from damage caused by glutamate, a chemical messenger. It is used to treat moderate to severe stages of Alzheimer's. Memantine is prescribed along with a cholinesterase inhibitor.
- Examples include axura, akatinol, namenda, ebixa and abixa, and memox.
- Memantine is prescribed to improve memory, language, reason, attention, and the ability to carry out simple tasks.

ACE inhibitors

ACE inhibitors that affect the brain by crossing the blood-brain barrier may reduce inflammation that could contribute to the development of Alzheimer's disease.

Stem cells

Neural stem cells can rescue memory in mice with advanced Alzheimer's disease, raising hopes of a potential treatment for humans.

Insulin

Insulin could protect against damage to brain cells key to memory.

NURSING MANAGEMENT

Nursing Assessment

Subjective data

- **Past health history**: Repeated head trauma, stroke, exposure to metals, previous CNS infections , family history of dementia.
- **Medications**: Use of any drugs to decrease symptoms (e.g. tranquilizers, hypnotics, antidepressants, antipsychotics).

Objective data

- **General**: Agitation, out of the world looks.
- **Neurologic**
  - Early: Loss of recent memory, disori-

entation to date and time, flat affect, lack of spontaneity, impaired abstraction, cognition and judgment.
- Middle: Agitation; impaired ability to recognize close family and friends, loss of remote memory, confusion, apraxia, aphasia. Inability to do simple tasks.
- Late: Inability to do self care, incontinence; immobility; limb rigidity.

NURSING DIAGNOSIS

- Disturbed thought process related to effects of dementia as evidenced by loss of memory and other cognitive deficits.
- Self-care deficit (Bathing, dressing, toileting) related to memory deficit and neuromuscular impairment as evidenced by inability too independently and appropriately bathe, dress or toilet.
- Risk for injury related to impaired judgment, possible gait instability, muscleweaknessandsensoryperceptual deprivation alternation.

Nursing Interventions

Planning/Goals

- Maintain functional ability for as long as possible.
- Maintain safe environment with minimum of injuries.
- Have personal care met.
- Have dignity maintained.

Maintain functional ability for as long as possible

- Determine type and extent of cognitive deficits.
- Involve family members in planning, providing and evaluating care for the patient.
- Identify usual pattern of behavior for such activities as sleep, medication use, elimination, food intake, and self-care to maintain familiar routines.
- Give one simple direction at a time to decrease confusion and frustration.
- Stimulate memory by repeating patient's last expressed thought.
- Inform patient of person, place and time to promote memory and to reduce confusion.
- Monitor patient's ability for independent self care to plan appropriate interventions.
- Provide desired personal articles. (Toothbrush, comb, dress, soap, deodorant, etc.) that is needed for personal hygiene.
- Assist patient with toileting(providing urinal, bedpan and bedside commode).

Maintain safe environment with minimum of injuries

- Identify cognitive and physical deficits of the patient that may increase patient fall in a particular environment.
- Provide assistive devices (e.g. walker) to steady gait and provide ambulation support.
- Advice the significant others or the caregivers not to leave the patient alone.

EPILEPSY

Definition

- A common chronic neurological condition that is characterized by recurrent unprovoked epileptic seizures.
- Seizures are transient signs and or symptoms due to abnormal excessive or synchronous neuronal activity in the brain.

Incidence

Affects approximately 50 million people worldwide. It is high in underdeveloped countries.

Causes

During the first 6 months of life

- Severe birth injury.
- Congenital defects involving the central nervous system infections.
- Inborn errors of metabolism.

Patients between 2 and 30 years of age

- Birth injury
- Infection
- Trauma and genetic factors.

Patients between 20 and 30 years of age

- Structural lesions such as trauma, brain tumors or vascular disease.

Patients after 50 years of age

- Cerebrovascular lesions
- Metastatic brain tumors.

Pathophysiology

- A group of abnormal neurons seems to undergo spontaneous firing in recurring seizures. This firing spreads by physiologic pathways to involve adjacent or distant areas of the brain.
- If this abnormal activity spreads to involve the whole brain a generalized seizure occurs.
- Any stimulus that causes the cell membrane of the neuron to depolarize induces tendency to spontaneous firing.
- The area of the brain tissue from which the activity arises is found to have scar tissue (gliosis).
- This scarring is thought to interfere with the normal chemical and structural environment of the brain neurons, making them more likely to fire abnormally.

Classification

The epilepsy or seizure disorder is classified as:

Generalized seizure

- Characterized by bilateral synchronous epileptic damage in the brain from the onset of seizure.
- No warning or aura.
- Unconsciousness: Few seconds to minutes.
- It is divided into:

Tonic-clonic seizures

- Characterized by loss of consciousness and falling to the ground if the patient is upright.
- Stiffening of the body (tonic phase) for 10–20 sec.
- Jerking of the extremities (clonic phase) for another 30–40 second.
- Cyanosis, excessive salivation, tongue or cheek biting and incontinence.
- Patient may be tired, sleep for hours and no memory about the incident.

Typical absence seizures (petit mal)

- Occurs in children.
- May cease as the child matures or may evolve into another type of seizure.
- Manifestations include: Brief staring spell lasting for few seconds so often it is unnoticed, brief loss of consciousness.
- If not treated the seizures may occur 100 times a day.

Atypical absence seizures

- Characterized by a staring spell accompanied by brief warning, peculiar behavior during the seizure, or confusion after the seizure.

Myoclonic seizures

- Characterized by a sudden, excessive jerk of the body or extremities.
- The term akinetic (arrest of movement), atonic (loss of tone), and aslatic (loss of balance) are used to describe drop attacks or falling spells.

- It involves either a tonic episode or a paroxysmal loss of muscle tone and begins suddenly with person falling to the ground.

Partial seizures

- Begins in specific region of cortex as indicated by the EEG, e.g. If the discharging focus is located in the medial aspect of the postcentral gyrus, the patient may experience paresthesias and tingling or numbness in the leg on the side opposite of the focus.
- It is confined to one side of the brain and remains partial or focal in nature. May spread to involve the entire brain culminating in a generalized tonic clonic seizure.
- Any tonic-clonic seizure, preceded by an aura or warning is a partial seizure that generalizes secondarily.
- Secondary generalized seizure may result in a transient residual neurologic deficit postictally called as Todd's paralysis (focal weakness) that resolves after varying length of time.
- **Partial seizures are further divided into**:
  - **Simple partial seizures**: Symptoms that do not involve loss of consciousness, rarely last longer than 1 minute. Involves motor, sensory or autonomic phenomena or a combination of these. Terms used are focal motor, focal sensory and jacksonian.
  - **Complex partial seizures**: It involves variety of behavioral, emotional, affective and cognitive functions. Lasts longer than 1 minute and are frequently followed by a period of postictal confusion.
  - Manifestations of complex partial seizures is clouding of consciousness or a confused state without any motor or sensory components. (Termed as temporal lobe absence).
  - The most common type is psychomotor seizure (repetitive movements), e.g. counting out change, picking items from grocery shop, etc. Patient forgets the activity done during seizure.

Clinical Manifestations

- Depends on the type of seizure that may progress through several phases:

Prodromal phase

Signs or activity that precede a seizure.

The aural phase

Sensory warning.

The ictal phase

Full seizure

Postictal phase

Period of recover after seizure.

Complications

It is divided into:

Physical

- Status epilepticus is a state of continuous seizure activity or a condition in which seizures reoccur in rapid succession without return to consciousness between seizures.
- Permanent brain damage occurs.

Psychosocial stigma (social stigma)

- Patient with epilepsy may experience discrimination in employment and educational opportunities.
- Patient develops ineffective methods of coping.

Diagnostic Studies

- Health history: Collect birth and developmental history, any significant illness or injuries, family history, febrile

seizures, and comprehensive neurologic assessment.
- EEG: Determine the type of seizure and help to pinpoint the seizure focus.
- Magneto encephalography may be done in conjunction with the EEG: It has greater sensitivity in detecting small magnetic fields generated by neuronal activity.
- Complete blood counts, serum chemistries, studies of liver and kidney functions—To rule out any metabolic disorders.
- CT scan or MRI: To rule out any structural lesion in any new onset seizure.
- Cerebral angiography, single photon emission computer tomography (SPECT), magnetic resonance spectroscopy (MRS), MRA, and positron emission tomography (PET) may be used in selected clinical situation.

Management

Drug therapy

- Seizure disorders are primarily treated with antiseizure drugs.
- Therapy is aimed at preventing seizure but cure is not possible.
- Drugs act by stabilizing nerve cell membranes and preventing spread of the epileptic discharge.
- The goal of antiseizure drug therapy is to obtain maximum seizure control with minimum of toxic side effects.
- The primary drugs for treatment of generalized tonic-clonic and partial seizures are phenytoin (dilantin), carbamazepine (tegretol), phenobarbital and divalproex.
- The drugs for the treatment of absence and myoclonic seizures include ethosuximide (zarontin), divalproex (depakote) and clonazepam (klonopin).
- Felbamate (felbatol) is used to treat patients whose seizure disorders are refractory to other drugs.
- Treatment of status epilepticus: IV administration of antiseizure drugs. Drugs used are lorazepam (ativan) and dizepam (valium).

Surgical therapy

- Goal is to remove the epileptic focus or prevent spread of epileptic activity in the brain.
- Interventions include—Limbic resection, primarily temporal lobe resection, amygdalohippocampectom, neocortical resection, including extratemporal resection, and lesionectomies, hemispherectomies, multilobar resection and corpus collosum sections.

Other therapies

Vagal nerve stimulation and biofeedback.

NURSING MANAGEMENT

Nursing Assessment

Subjective data

- **Past health history**: Previous seizure, birth defects or injuries, CNS trauma or infections, stroke, metabolic disorders, fever, pregnancy.
- **Medications**: Compliance with antiseizure drugs, alcohol withdrawal, use and overdose of cocaine, amphetamines, lidocaine, penicillin, antidepressants.

History of headache, abdominal pain, muscle pain, mood and behavioral changes, anxiety depression, loss of self-esteem.

Objective data

- Precipitating factors include severe metabolic acidosis or alkalosis, hyperkalemia, dehydration.
- Soft tissue damage, cyanosis, diaphoresis (postictal).
- Abnormal respiratory rate, rhythm, abnormal breath sounds, Hypertension, tachycardia or bradycardia.

- Bowel incontinence, excessive salivation, incontinence.
- Neurological changes according to the type of seizures such as loss of consciousness, muscle tightening, then jerking, dilated pupils.
- Weakness, paralysis, ataxia (postictal).

Nursing Diagnosis

- Ineffective breathing pattern related to neuromuscular impairment secondary to prolonged tonic phase of seizure as evidenced by abnormal respiratory rate, rhythm, and/or depth.
- Risk for injury to seizure activity and subsequent impaired physical mobility secondary to postictal weakness.
- Ineffective coping related to perceived loss of control and denial of diagnosis as evidenced by verbalizations about not having seizure, noncompliant behavior.

GOAL/PLANNING OUTCOME

- Maintains a normal breathing pattern.
- Be free from injury during a seizure.
- Expresses acceptance of seizure disorder.

Nursing Interventions

Maintains a normal breathing pattern

- Ensure patient airway.
- Assess respiratory rate, rhythm and oxygen saturation level.
- Assist ventilation if patient does not breathe spontaneously after seizure.
- Anticipate need for intubation if gag reflex is absent.
- Do suction as needed.
- Give supplemental oxygen as ordered.

Be free from injury during a seizure

- Stay with the patient until seizure has passed.
- Protect patient from injury during seizure. Do not restrain. Pad side rails.
- Establish IV access.
- Anticipate administration of phenobarbital, phenytoin sodium (dilantin) or Benzodiazepine (diazepam, midazolam, lorazepam) to control seizures.
- Remove or loosen tight clothing.
- Monitor vital signs, level of consciousness, O_2 saturation, GCS scale, pupil size and reactivity.
- Reassure and orient the patient after seizure.
- Never force an airway if the patient clenched teeth.
- Give dextrose for hypoglycemia.

Expresses acceptance of seizure disorder

- Appraise patient's adjustment to changes in body image.
- Discuss alternative responses to situation.
- Provide information concerning diagnosis, treatment, and prognosis.
- Describe possible complications.
- Describe rationales behind management/treatment recommendations.

CEREBROVASCULAR ACCIDENT

Definition

- Stroke or "brain attack" is an acute CNS injury that results in neurologic signs and symptoms brought on by a reduction or absence of perfusion to a territory of the brain.
- The disruption in flow is from either an occlusion (ischemic) or rupture (hemorrhagic) of the blood vessel.

Incidence and Prevalence

a. Third leading cause of death in the USA
750,000+ people/year
175,000 die within one year (25%).
b. Leading cause of long-term disabilities
5.5 million survivors (USA)
15–30 % live with permanent disability.

Classification

There are two major types of stroke: Ischemic stroke and hemorrhagic stroke.

- Ischemic stroke occurs when a blood vessel that supplies to the brain is blocked by a blood clot. This may happen in two ways:
  a. A clot may form in an artery that is already very narrow. This is called a thrombotic stroke.
  b. A clot may dislodged from another place in the blood vessels of the brain, or from some other part of the body, and travel up to the brain. This is called cerebral embolism or embolic stroke.
- A hemorrhagic stroke occurs when a blood vessel in part of the brain becomes weak and bursts open, causing blood to leak into the brain. It can be divided into:
  – Intracerebral hemorrhage is bleeding within the brain caused by rupture of a blood vessel.
  – Subarachnoid hemorrhage (SAH) occurs when there is intracranial bleeding into the cerebrospinal fluid-filled space between the arachnoid and pia mater membranes on the surface of the brain. Other causes of SAH include arteriovenous malformations(AVM), trauma and drug abuse.

Risk Factors

Risk factors of the condition are given in Table 1.2.

Causes

Causes of both types of stroke are given in Table 1.3.

Table 1.2: Risk factors

Modifiable	Nonmodifiable
Hypertension Diabetes mellitus Heart disease A-fib Asymptomatic carotid stenosis Hyperlipidemia Obesity Oral contraceptive use Heavy alcohol use Physical inactivity Sickle cell disease Smoking Procedure precautions	Age 2/3 over 65 yrs Gender M>F (except very young and very old) Race Africans>Americans>Asian Heredity Family history Previous TIA/CVA

Table 1.3: Causes

Hemorrhagic stroke	Ischemic stroke
Chronic HTN Cerebral Amyloid Angiopathy Anticoagulation	Embolic stroke Atrial fibrillation Recent MI

Contd...

Contd...

Hemorrhagic stroke	Ischemic stroke
AVM Ruptured aneurysm (usually subarachnoid) Tumor Sympathomimetics Infection Trauma Transformation of ischemic stroke Physical exertion, pregnancy Postoperative	Endocarditis Cardiac tumors Patent foramen ovale Carotid/basilar artery stenosis Atherosclerotic lesions Vasculitis

Pathophysiology

- Brain requires a continuous supply of blood to provide the oxygen and glucose that neurons need to function.
- Short-term ischemia leads to temporary neurologic deficits or a transient ischemic attack(TIA).
- If the blood flow is not restored, brain tissue sustains irreversible damage or infarction within minutes.
- The extent to infarction depends on the location and size of the occluded artery and the adequacy of collateral circulation to the area.
- Ischemia alters cerebral metabolism.
- Cell death and permanent damage occurs within 3 to 10 minutes.
- Decreased cerebral perfusion is usually caused by occlusion of a cerebral artery or intracerebral hemorrhage.
- Occlusion produces ischemia in the brain tissue supplied by the affected artery and edema in the surrounding tissue.
- Cells in the center of the stroke area, die almost immediately after stroke onset referred as primary neuronal injury.
- A zone of hypo perfusion also exists around the infarcted zone called penumbra. The size of this zone depends on the amount of collateral circulation present.
- A cascade of biochemical changes occurs within minutes of cerebral ischemia.
- Neurotoxins, including oxygen-free radicals, nitric oxide, and glutamate are released. Local acidosis occurs. Membrane depolarization occurs.
- Resulting in influx of calcium and sodium. Cytotoxic edema and cell death occurs called as secondary neuronal injury.
- Area of edema after ischemia may lead to temporary neurologic deficits.

Clinical Manifestations

- Sudden numbness or weakness of face, arm or leg.
- Sudden confusion, trouble speaking or understanding.
- Sudden trouble with vision.
- Sudden trouble walking, dizziness, loss of balance or coordination.
- Sudden severe headache.
- Tachycardia or bradycardia.
- Respiratory distress.
- Seizures.
- Hypertension.
- Unequal pupils.
- Nausea and vomiting.
- Vertigo.
- Facial drooping on affected side.

- A stroke can have an effect on many body functions including motor activity, bladder and bowel elimination, intellectual function, spatial-perceptual alternations, personality, affect sensation, swallowing and communication.
  - **Motor function**: Akinesia, alterations in muscle tone, impairment of integration of movements, alteration in reflexes. Hemiplegia or paraplegia, hemiparesis or paraparesis.
  - **Communication**: Aphasia, dysphasia, dysarthria.
  - **Affect**: Depression, frustration, sudden crying.
  - **Intellectual function**: Impaired memory and judgment.
  - **Spatial-perceptual alterations**: Patient's incorrect perception of self and illness, patient's false perception of self in space, agnosia, the inability to recognize an object by sight, touch or hearing, apraxia, the inability to carry out learned sequential movements on command.
- **Elimination**: Voluntary urination, patient experiences frequency, urgency and incontinence. Constipation is associated with immobility, weak abdominal muscles, dehydration, diminished response to the defection reflex.

Diagnostic Tests

- **CT scan**: It indicates the size and location of the lesion and differentiates between ischemic and hemorrhagic stroke.
- **Computed tomographic angiography (CTA)**: Provides visualization of vasculature and can be performed at the same time with CT scan.
- **MRI**: It is used to determine the extent of brain injury.
- Positron emission tomography (PET) shows the metabolic activity of the brain and provides a depiction of the extent of tissue damage after a stroke.
- Cerebral angiography identifies cervical and cerebrovascular occlusion, atherosclerotic plaques and malformation of vessels.
- Transcranial Doppler (TCD) ultrasonography is a noninvasive study that measures the velocity of blood flow in the major cerebral arteries.
- Skull X-ray, brain scan, lumbar puncture, electroencephalogram (EEG) are currently used much less in the diagnosis of stroke.
- **Blood tests**: Complete blood counts, platelets, prothrombin time, activated partial thromboplastin time, electrolytes, blood glucose, renal and hepatic studies, lipid profile, and ABG analysis.

MANAGEMENT

Goals

- Preserving life
- Preventing further brain damage
- Reducing disability.

Medical Management

Acute care

- Ensure patent airway: Oxygen administration, artificial airway insertion, intubation, and mechanical ventilation is required.
- Do detail neurological assessment.
- Start an IV line with normal saline.
- Administer antihypertensive drug as ordered to maintain blood pressure.
- Administer diuretics drug such as mannitol and lasix to reduce cerebral edema and intracranial pressure.
- Obtain CT scan immediately.
- Elevate the head end if no symptoms of shock or injury are present.
- Institute seizure precautions.

Drug therapy

- Recombinant tissue plasminogen activator (tPA) is administered IV to reestablish blood flow through a blocked artery to prevent cell death in patients with ischemic stroke. It must be given within 3 hours of the onset of clinical signs of stroke.
- Acetylsalicylic acid(aspirin) is used within 48 hours of the stroke.
- Anticoagulants (Warfarin), platelet inhibitors (aspirin, ticlopidine, clopidogrel and dipyridamole) can be used to prevent further stroke.
- Calcium channel blockers (Nimodipine) are given to the patient with subarachnoid hemorrhage to decrease the effects of vasospasm and minimize cerebral damage.
- Acetaminophen or aspirin is used to treat hyperthermia.
- Antiseizure medications such as phenytoin sodium (dilantin) is administered if seizure occurs.

Surgical management

- Immediate evacuation of aneurysm – induced hematomas larger than 3cm.
- Use of endovascular techniques: Treatment of aneurysm involves clipping, wrapping or coiling the aneurysm to prevent rebleeding. In coiling procedure, a metal coil can be inserted into the lumen of the aneurysm via interventional neuroradiology. Guglielmi detachable coils (GDCs) provide immediate protection against hemorrhage by reducing the blood pulsations within the aneurysm.
- Surgical resection is done for arterio venous malformation(AVM).
- Mechanical embolus retrieval in cerebral ischemia (Merci) retriever is introduced inside the blocked artery of patients who experiences ischemic strokes.

NURSING MANAGEMENT

Objective Data

Altered level of consciousness, sluggish pupillary reaction, motor and sensory dysfunction, cranial nerve deficits (extraocular, eye movements ,facial droop, presence of ptosis, speech difficulties, and visual disturbance, headache and nuchal rigidity other neurologic deficits.

Nursing Diagnoses

- Ineffective tissue perfusion (cerebral) related to bleeding or vasospasm.
- Anxiety related to illness and/ or medically imposed restrictions (aneurysm precautions).
- Impaired physical mobility related to hemiparesis, loss of balance, and coordination, spasticity and brain injury.
- Acute pain related to hemiplegia and disuse.
- Self care deficits (bathing, hygiene, toileting, dressing, grooming and feeling), related stroke sequel.
- Disturbed sensory perception related to medically imposed restrictions.
- Disturbed thought process related to brain damage, confusion or inability to follow instructions.
- Impaired verbal communication related to brain damage.
- Risk for impaired skin integrity related hemiparesis, hemiplegia, or decreased mobility.
- Interrupted family process related to long-standing illness and caregiver burden.

Planning/ Goals

- Optimizing cerebral tissue perfusion.
- Relieving sensory deprivation and anxiety.

- Improving mobility and preventing joint deformities.
- Preventing shoulder pain.
- Enhancing self-care.
- Managing sensory perceptual difficulties.
- Improving thought process.
- Improving communication.
- Maintaining skin integrity.
- Improving family coping.

Nursing Interventions

Optimizing cerebral tissue perfusion

- Monitor the patient closely for neurologic deterioration resulting from recurrent bleeding, increased ICP or vasospasm.
- Monitor vital signs, level of consci-ousness, pupillary reaction, motor function, etc. hourly those are indicators for cerebral perfusion.
- Elevate head of the bed to 15 to 30 degrees to promote venous drainage.
- Promote immediate and absolute bed rest in a quiet, nonstressful environment, because activity, pain and anxiety elevate blood pressure, which increases risk of bleeding.
- Ask the patient/caregiver to avoid any activity that suddenly increase the blood pressure or obstructs venous return including Valsalva maneuver, straining, forceful sneezing, pushing oneself important in bed, acute flexion or rotation of the head and neck and cigarette smoking.
- Use thigh high elastic compression stockings to decrease the incidence of deep vein thrombosis.

Relieving sensory deprivation and anxiety

- Orient the patient everyday to reduce the patient's sense of isolation.
- Reassure the patient to relieve the patient fear and anxiety.

Improving mobility and preventing joint deformities

- Assess the muscle strengths and reflexes.
- Give correct posture to prevent contractures, use measures to relieve pressures, maintain good body alignment, and prevent compressive neuropathies.
- Provide prone position with pillow support to help prevent hip flexion.
- Provide passive range of motion exercises, 4 to 5 times a day to maintain joint mobility, regain motor control and prevent contractures.
- Start an active rehabilitation program as soon as the patient regains consciousness.

Preventing shoulder pain

- Assess the pain through pain intensity scale.
- Encourage the patient to do range of motion exercises.
- Administer analgesics as ordered.
- Antiseizure medication lamotrigine (Lamictal) is effective for poststroke pain.

Enhancing self-care

- Assess the activities of daily living patient can perform.
- Allow the patient to carry-out the activities such as combing hair, brushing teeth, eating, etc. by himself or with assistance.
- Provide assistive devices to facilitate.

Managing sensory perceptual difficulties

- Assess the sensory deficits of the patient.

- Keep visual stimulators (e.g. clock, calendar, TV) near the patient's bedside.
- Maintain eye contact and draw patient's attention to the affected side by encouraging the patient to move the head.
- Provide proper lighting, natural and artificial lighting in the room and eyeglasses to increase vision.

Improving thought process

- Assess the various cognitive, behavioral and emotional deficits related to brain damage.
- Review the results of neuropsychological testing, observes the patient's performance and progress.
- Encourage the patient, give positives hope and confidence.

Improving communication

- Assess the patient's ability to express him or herself, communication needs.
- Make the atmosphere conducive for communication.
- Provide encouragement and emotional support.
- Use communication board that includes pictures of common needs and phrases.
- Speak slowly to the patient and give one instruction at one time.

Maintaining skin integrity

- Assess the skin including bony prominences and dependent parts of the body.
- Provide water mattress/ air mattress to prevent pressure ulcer.
- Turn the patient in a regular schedule (preferably at least every 2 hours).
- Keep the patient's skin clean and dry.
- Give gentle back massage.
- Maintain adequate nutrition and hydration level.

Improving family coping

- Assess the family members' response towards patient's illness.
- Encourage family members to participate patient care.
- Use counseling and other support system that will help with the emotional and physical stress of caring for the patient.
- Make family members understand that rehabilitation of the hemiplegic patient requires months and progress may be slow.

2

Nursing Management of Patients with Disorders of Eye and Vision

NURSING ASSESSMENT OF PATIENT WITH EYE DISORDERS

Subjective Data

A complete ophthalmic history includes demographic data, exploration of chief complaint and related manifestations, review of system, etc.

Demographic data includes the age, and gender, incidence of cataracts, dry eye, retinal detachment, glaucoma.

Current health history: The four most common preventable causes of permanent vision loss in developed nations are—

- Amblyopia (reduced visual acuity that is not correctable with glasses in the absence of anatomic defects in the eye or visual pathways).
- Diabetic retinopathy.
- Age related maculopathy.
- Glaucoma.

Chief complaint

Change or loss of vision associated with headache or eyestrain. Past medical history related with diabetes mellitus rheumatoid arthritis, thyroid disorders, hypertension, multiple sclerosis and myasthenia gravis. If the client wear eye glasses or contact lenses, ask when the last eye examination done.

Surgical history includes corrective vision surgery such as laser assisted in situ keratomileusis (LASIK), radial keratotomy (RK), and cataract removal and glaucoma treatment or muscle correction.

Allergies to medications (eye drop) and other substances such as inhalants (dust, chemicals, or pollens) and environmental contact (cosmetics). Clinical manifestations eye redness, tearing and itching.

- Medications: Ask about use of over the counter eye drops, as those with antihistamines, and decongestants can dry the ocular surface.

Dietary habits

Use of herbal remedies and dietary supplements (vitamins).

Social history includes occupational hazards, leisure activities and hobbies and health management behavior.

Family history ocular disorders tends to be familial (strabismus, glaucoma, myopia, hyperopia), DM, retinoblastoma, retinitis, pigmentosa, and macular degeneration.

Objective Data

Ocular manifestations can be divided into three basic categories—Vision (refractive error, lid ptosis, clouding or interference in the cornea, lens or aqueous or vitreous space, malfunction of the retina, optic nerve or intracranial visual pathway).

External changes in appearance include growth or lesions, edema, ptosis and abnormal position.

Red eye the most common appearance

- Abnormal sensation reflex spasm of the ciliary muscle and iris sphincter that occurs with inflammation may produce browache and photophobia (sensitivity to light) or a constricted pupil.
- Physical examination of the eyes includes assessment of external structures via inspection and palpation.
- Eye position—Sunken or protruding eyes.
- Lids: Sagging of upper lids that cover part of pupil.
- Blink: Rapid, infrequent or asymmetrical blinking.
- Eyeball: Asymmetrical, hard or soft.
- Lacrimal apparatus: Swelling, edema, excessive moisture and regurgitation of fluid.
- Conjunctiva: Paleness or a bright red color.

Cornea surface irregularity and cloudiness (opacity)

- Anterior chamber: Shallow or deep chambers (3mm is normal) are abnormal.
- Iris: Cloudy or nontransparent, bulging or uneven coloring,
- Pupil: Light intolerance (photophobia), irregular or unequal pupils, pupils that do not react to light on accommodation.
- Direct ophthalmoscope uses a light source and reflective mirrors to provide a magnified image of the fundus and a detailed view of the disk and retinal vascular bed.
- Indirect ophthalmoscope provides a stereoscopic picture over a large area of the retina. The light source comes from a head mounted light. The indirect ophthalmoscope provides for a binocular visual inspection with depth perception and permits a wider field of view compared with the direct method.

Diagnostic Tests

Fundus photography

Special retinal cameras are used to document fine details of the fundus for study and future comparison and to identify changes in disk shape and color.

Exophthalmometry

It is designed to measure forward protrusion of the eye, record progression/regression of the prominence.

Ophthalmic radiography (X-ray, tomography, and CT)

Which are useful in evaluation of orbital and intracranial conditions and detection of foreign bodies.

MRI

It is multidimensional waves are obtained with repositioning client; used to image edema, areas of demyelination and vascular lesions.

Ultrasonography

It is used to determine refractive power of an intraocular lens in cataract surgery, used to evaluate lesions and their growth over time, or the presence of a foreign body.

Ophthalmodynamometry

It gives an approximate measurement of the relative pressures in the central retinal arteries and indirectly assess carotid arterial flow.

Electroretinography (ERG)

It measures the change in electrical potential of the eye caused by a diffuse flash of light through electrodes incorporated onto a contact lens that is placed directly on the eye.

GLAUCOMA

Definition

- **Glaucoma** is an eye disease in which the optic nerve is damaged in a characteristic pattern. This can permanently damage vision in the affected eye(s) and lead to blindness if left untreated.
  - It is normally associated with increased fluid pressure in the eye (aqueous humour). The term 'ocular hypertension' is used for people with consistently raised intraocular pressure (IOP) without any associated optic nerve damage.
  - Conversely, the term 'normal tension' or 'low tension' glaucoma is used for those with optic nerve damage and associated visual field loss, but normal or low IOP.

Incidence

- Glaucoma has been called the 'silent thief of sight' because the loss of vision often occurs gradually over a long period, and symptoms only occur when the disease is quite advanced.
- Once lost, vision cannot normally be recovered, so treatment is aimed at preventing further loss.
- Worldwide, glaucoma is the second-leading cause of blindness after cataracts.
- Glaucoma affects one in 200 people aged 50 and younger, and one in 10 over the age of 80.
- The word 'glaucoma' comes from the greek word meaning 'opacity of the crystalline lens'.

Etiology and Pathophysiology

- The etiology of glaucoma is related to the consequences of elevated IOP. A proper balance between the rate of aqueous production (referred to as inflow) and the rate of aqueous reabsorption (referred to as outflow) is essential to maintain the IOP within normal limits. When the rate of inflow is greater than the rate of outflow, IOP can rise above normal limits. If IOP remains elevated, permanent vision loss may occur.
- The nerve damage involves loss of retinal ganglion cells in a characteristic pattern. The many different subtypes of glaucoma can all be considered to be a type of optic neuropathy. Raised intraocular pressure (above 21 mmHg or 2.8 kPa) is the most important and only modifiable risk factor for glaucoma.
- However, some may have high eye pressure for years and never develop damage, while others can develop nerve damage at a relatively low pressure. Untreated glaucoma can lead to permanent damage of the optic nerve and resultant visual field loss, which over time can progress to blindness.

Types

Primary open angle glaucoma (POAG)

In POAG, the outflow of aqueous humor is decreased in the trabecular mesh work. In essence, the drainage channels become clogged, like a clogged kitchen sink.

Primary angle closure glaucoma (PACG)

The mechanism, reducing the outflow of aqueous is angle closure. Usually, this is caused from the lens bulging forward as a result of an age-related process. Angle closure may also occur as result of pupil dilation in the patient with anatomically narrow angles. Dilation causes peripheral iris bulging with the same outcome of covering the trabecular mesh work and blocking the outflow channels.

Secondary glaucoma

It is increased IOP results from other ocular or systematic conditions that may block the outflow channels in some way.

Secondary glaucoma may be associated with inflammatory process that blocks the outflow channels such as trauma and ocular neoplasm.

Clinical Manifestations

- POAG develops slowly and without symptoms. The patient with POAG reports no symptoms of pain or pressure. The patient usually does not have the gradual visual field loss until peripheral vision has been severely compromised. The patient with untreated glaucoma had 'tunnel vision' in which only a small center field can be seen, and all peripheral vision is absent.
- Acute primary acute angle glaucoma causes definite symptoms, including sudden excruciating pain in or around the eye. This is often accompanied by nausea and vomiting. Visual symptoms include seeing colored halos around lights, blurred vision and ocular redness. The acute rise in IOP may also cause corneal edema, giving the cornea a frosted appearance.

Diagnostic Tests

- IOP is usually elevated in Glaucoma. Normal IOP is 10 to 21 mm Hg. In open angle glaucoma IOP is usually between 22 and 32 mm Hg. In acute closure glaucoma IOP may be 50 mm Hg or high.
- **Acuity Test**: When visual fields perimetry may reveal subtle changes in the peripheral retina early in the disease process. A small, football-shaped defect that gradually progresses to a nasal and superior field defect in chronic open angle glaucoma. In acute angle glaucoma, central visual acuity will be reduced. The patient has corneal edema and the visual fields may be markedly decreased.
- **Ophthalmoscopy**: Direct or indirect visualization ophthalmoscopy detects the optic disk cupping. The optic disk becomes wider, deeper and paler (light gray or white). Optic disk cupping may be one of the first signs of chronic open angle glaucoma.

Management

- The modern goals of glaucoma management are—
  - To avoid glaucomatous damage and nerve damage.
  - To preserve visual field and total quality of life for patients, with minimal side effects.

Balance and postural control

- There is an important role of the visual system in balance and maintaining posture in human beings, glaucoma patients should consider themselves at greater risk of falls, and would be advised to take the necessary precautions to help prevent any accidents.

Medical management

- Intraocular pre-ssure can be lowered with medication, usually eye drops. Several different classes of medications are used to treat glaucoma, which are as follows:
- **Prostaglandin analogs**, such as latanoprost (Xalatan), bimatoprost (Lumigan) and travoprost (Travatan), increase uveoscleral outflow of aqueous humor. Bimatoprost also increases trabecular outflow.
- **Topical β-adrenergic receptor antagonists**, such as timolol, levobunolol (Betagan), and betaxolol, decrease aqueous humor production by the ciliary body.
- **α_2-adrenergic agonists**, such as brimonidine (Alphagan) and apraclonidine, work by a dual mechanism, decreasing aqueous humor production and increasing uveoscleral outflow.
- **Less-selective alpha agonists**, such as epinephrine, decrease aqueous humor production through vasoconstriction of ciliary body blood vessels, useful only in open-angle glaucoma.
- **Miotic agents (parasympathomimetics)**, such as pilocarpine, work by contraction of the ciliary muscle, tightening the trabecular meshwork and allowing increased outflow of the aqueous humor. Echothiophate, an acetylcholinesterase inhibitor, is used in chronic glaucoma.
- **Carbonic anhydrase inhibitors**, such as dorzolamide (Trusopt), brinzolamide (Azopt), and acetazolamide (Diamox), lower secretion of aqueous humor by inhibiting carbonic anhydrase in the ciliary body.
- **Physostigmine** is also used to treat glaucoma.

Surgical Management

Laser and conventional surgeries are performed to treat glaucoma. Surgery is the primary therapy for those with congenital glaucoma. Generally, these operations are a temporary solution, as there is not yet a cure for glaucoma.

Canaloplasty

- Canaloplasty is a nonpenetrating procedure using microcatheter technology. To perform a canaloplasty, an incision is made into the eye to gain access to the Schlemm's canal in a similar fashion to a viscocanalostomy.
- A microcatheter will circumnavigate the canal around the iris, enlarging the main drainage channel and its smaller collector channels through the injection of a sterile, gel-like material called viscoelastic. The catheter is then removed and a suture is placed within the canal and tightened.

Laser surgery

- Argon laser trabeculoplasty (ALT) may be used to treat open-angle glaucoma. A 50-µm argon laser spot is aimed at the trabecular meshwork to stimulate opening of the mesh to allow more outflow of aqueous fluid. Usually, half of the angle is treated at a time. Traditional laser trabeculoplasty uses a thermal argon laser in an argon laser trabeculoplasty procedure.
- **A newer type of laser trabeculoplasty** uses a 'cold' (nonthermal) laser to stimulate drainage in the trabecular meshwork. This newer procedure, selective laser trabeculoplasty (SLT), uses a 532-nm, frequency-doubled, Q-switched Nd:YAG laser, which selectively targets melanin pigment in the trabecular meshwork cells.
- **Nd:YAG laser peripheral iridotomy (LPI)** may be used in patients suscepti-

ble to or affected by angle closure glaucoma or pigment dispersion syndrome. During laser iridotomy, laser energy is used to make a small, full-thickness opening in the iris to equalize the pressure between the front and back of the iris, thus correcting any abnormal bulging of the iris. In people with narrow angles, this can uncover the trabecular meshwork. In some cases of intermittent or short-term angle closure, this may lower the eye pressure. Laser iridotomy reduces the risk of developing an attack of acute angle closure. In most cases, it also reduces the risk of developing chronic angle closure or of adhesions of the iris to the trabecular meshwork.
- **Diode laser cycloablation** lowers IOP by reducing aqueous secretion by destroying secretory ciliary epithelium.

Trabeculectomy
- The most common conventional surgery performed for glaucoma is the trabeculectomy. A partial thickness flap is made in the scleral wall of the eye, and a window opening is made under the flap to remove a portion of the trabecular meshwork.
- The scleral flap is then sutured loosely back in place to allow fluid to flow out of the eye through this opening, resulting in lowered intraocular pressure and the formation of a bleb or fluid bubble on the surface of the eye.

NURSING MANAGEMENT

Nursing Assessment

Subjective data

Collect data of age and race, family history of glaucoma, ocular surgery, infections, and trauma. Any history of allergic reaction to dyes or medications. Ask for any changes in vision, decreased visual acuity.

Objective data

Increased intraocular pressure, cupping or indentation of the optic nerve head(disc), and visual field defects.

Nursing Diagnoses

- Visual/Sensory perceptual alteration related to recent loss of vision.
- Anticipatory grieving related to loss of vision.
- Risk of ineffective therapeutic regimen related to complex medication schedule.

PLANNING OUTCOMES/GOALS

- Maintain functional vision as possible.
- Express grief, describing meaning of loss.
- Describe disease process and the regimen for disease control.

Nursing Interventions

Maintain functional vision as possible

- Assess the visual acuity and intraocular pressure.
- Reassure the patient that further vision loss can be prevented.
- Administer medications as ordered.
- Assist the patient with activities of daily living.
- Prepare the patient for surgical management if planned.

Express grief, describing meaning of loss

- Assess the causative and contributing factors that may delay the work of grieving and promote family cohesiveness.
- Encourage and give positive hope of success.
- Advice the family members to cooperate with the patient and assist him in all aspects of care.

- Advice the family members for selecting appropriate rehabilitation program for the patient.

Describe disease process and the regimen for disease control

- Assess the current level of knowledge and understanding with prescribed therapy.
- Advice and educate the patient to administer eye drops at right time and dose as ordered.
- Explain the patient and family members about the importance of the drug that is to decreased the intraocular pressure.
- Encourage him to comply with the treatment regimen.

CATARACT

Definition

A **cataract** is a clouding that develops in the crystalline lens of the eye or in its envelope (lens capsule), varying in degree from slight to complete opacity and obstructing the passage of light.

- Early in the development of age-related cataract, the power of the lens may be increased, causing near-sightedness (myopia), and the gradual yellowing and opacification of the lens may reduce the perception of blue colors.
- Cataracts typically progress slowly to cause vision loss, and are potentially blinding if untreated. The condition usually affects both eyes, but almost always one eye is affected earlier than the other.

Classification

- Cataracts may be partial or complete, stationary or progressive, or hard or soft.
- The various types of cataracts are nuclear, cortical, mature, and hypermature.
- Cataracts are also classified by their location, e.g. posterior (classically due to steroid use) and anterior (common (senile) cataract related to aging).

The following is a classification of the various types of cataracts. This is not comprehensive, and other unusual types may be noted.

Classified by etiology

- Age-related cataract
- Cortical senile cataract
  - Immature senile cataract (IMSC): Partially opaque lens, disc view hazy.
  - Mature senile cataract (MSC): Completely opaque lens, no disc view.
  - Hypermature senile cataract (HMSC): Liquefied cortical matter: Morgagnian cataract
- Senile nuclear cataract
  - Cataracta brunescens
  - Cataracta nigra
  - Cataracta rubra
- Congenital cataract
  - Sutural cataract
  - Lamellar cataract
  - Zonular cataract
  - Total cataract
- Secondary cataract
  - Drug-induced cataract (e.g. corticosteroids)
  - Traumatic cataract
    - Blunt trauma (capsule usually intact).
    - Penetrating trauma (capsular rupture and leakage of lens material—calls for an emergency surgery for extraction of lens and leaked material to minimize further damage).

Causes

Several factors can promote the formation of cataracts:

- Long-term exposure to ultraviolet light, exposure to ionizing radiation, secondary effects of diseases such as diabetes, hypertension and advanced age, or trauma (possibly much earlier); they are usually a result of denaturation of lens protein.

- Genetic factors are often a cause of congenital cataract, and positive family history may play a role in predisposing someone to cataracts at an earlier age, a phenomenon of 'anticipation' in presenile cataracts.
- Eye injury or physical trauma.
- Atopic or allergic conditions are also known to quicken the progression of cataracts, especially in children.
- Iodine deficiency.
- Drugs can induce cataract development, such as corticosteroids and the antipsychotic drug quetiapine.
- Bilateral cataracts in an infant due to congenital rubella syndrome.

Clinical Manifestations

- As a cataract becomes more opaque, clear vision is compromised.
- A loss of visual acuity is noted.
- Contrast sensitivity is also lost, so contours, shadows and color vision are less vivid.
- Veiling glare can be a problem, as light is scattered by the cataract into the eye.
- The affected eye will have an absent red reflex.
- A contrast sensitivity test should be performed, and if a loss is demonstrated, an eye specialist consultation is recommended.
- It may be advisable to seek medical opinion, particularly in high-risk groups such as diabetics, if a 'halo' is observed around street lights at night, especially if this phenomenon appears to be confined to one eye only.
- The symptoms of cataracts are very similar to the symptoms of ocular citrosis.

Prevention

- Wearing ultraviolet-protecting sunglasses may slow the development of cataracts.
- Regular intake of antioxidants (such as vitamins A, C and E) is helpful.
- Statins are known for their ability to lower lipids, they are also believed to have antioxidant qualities.
- Oxidative stress is believed to play a role in the development of nuclear cataracts, which are the most common type of age-related cataracts.

MANAGEMENT

Medical Management

- Topical treatment (eye drops) with the less well-known antioxidant N-acetylcarnosine has been shown to improve transmissivity and reduce glare sensitivity for patients with cataracts.
- Long-term (average five year) observation showed systematic application of azapentacene sodium polysulfonate (Quinax) slows down the progress of the disease.

Surgical Management

- Cataract surgery, using a temporal approach phacoemulsification probe (in right hand) and 'chopper' (in left hand) being done under operating microscope.
- The operation to remove cataracts can be performed at any stage of their development. There is no longer a reason to wait until a cataract is 'ripe' before removing it.
- All surgery involves some risk, it is usually worth waiting until there is some change in vision before removing the cataract.
- The risk of infective endophthalmitis following extraction is about 1 in 1000.

- The most effective and common treatment is to make an incision (capsulotomy) into the capsule of the cloudy lens to surgically remove it. Two types of eye surgery can be used to remove cataracts: extracapsular cataract—Extraction (ECCE) and intracapsular cataract extraction (ICCE).
- ECCE surgery consists of removing the lens, but leaving the majority of the lens capsule intact. High frequency sound waves (phacoemulsification) are sometimes used to break up the lens before extraction.
- Intracapsular (ICCE) surgery involves removing the lens and lens capsule, but it is rarely performed in modern practice.
- In either extra capsular surgery or intra capsular surgery, the cataractous lens is removed and replaced with a plastic lens (an intraocular lens implant) which stays in the eye permanently.
- Cataract operations are usually performed using a local anesthetic, and the patient is allowed to go home the same day.

Complications after cataract surgery

Endophthalmitis, posterior capsular opacification and retinal detachment.

Laser surgery

It involves cutting away a small circle-shaped area of the lens capsule, enough to allow light to pass directly through the eye to the retina. There are, as always, some risks, but serious side effects are very rare. High frequency ultrasound is also used for cataract surgery.

Nursing Management

Subjective data

Ask the patient about any predisposing factors such as trauma, systemic diseases, medications such as corticosteroids, and other ocular problems. Ask the patient to describe visual disturbances.

Objective data

Visual acuity (both distant and near) in each eye is documented. Observe for difficulties in carrying out activities of daily living.

Nursing Diagnosis

- Sensory/Perceptual alterations (visual) related to lens extraction and replacement.
- Risk for infection related to surgical procedure.

PLANNING OUTCOMES/GOALS

- Improve vision and adapt to changes in visual corrections.
- Minimize risk of infection.

Nursing Interventions

Improve vision and adapt to changes in visual corrections

- Assess the level of activity patient can perform by himself.
- Assist the patient or maintain as much independence as possible.
- Evaluate patient's lifestyle, abilities and home environment.
- Explain the need of surgery and help him with the perioperative events.
- Administer eye drops at right time and dose as ordered.
- Clarify his doubts and provide correct information about the disease process.

Minimize risk of infection

- Assess the condition of eye after surgery to assess for any local signs of infection.

- Maintain personal hygiene.
- Cover the eye with eye shield or eye pad to prevent from any further injury or foreign body.
- Administer eye drops as ordered.
- Encourage the patient to wear goggles to protect from excessive light glare.

RETINAL DETACHMENT

Definition

Retinal detachment is a disorder of the eye in which the retina peels away from its underlying layer of support tissue. Initial detachment may be localized, but without rapid treatment the entire retina may detach, leading to vision loss and blindness.

Types

- Rhegmatogenous retinal detachment (secondary to a tear in the retina) is characterized by retinal hole, liquid in the vitreous body with access to the hole, and subsequent fluid accumulation between retina and retinal pigment epithelium.
- Retinal breaks are divided into three types—holes, tears and dialyses. Holes form due to retinal atrophy especially within an area of lattice degeneration. Tears are due to vitreoretinal traction. Dialyses which are very peripheral and circumferential may be either tractional or atrophic, the atrophic form most often occurring as idiopathic dialysis of the young.
- Exudative, serous, or secondary retinal detachment—An exudative retinal detachment occurs due to inflammation, injury or vascular abnormalities that results in fluid accumulating underneath the retina without the presence of a hole, tear, or break.
- Tractional retinal detachment—a tractional retinal detachment occurs when fibrous or fibrovascular tissue, caused by an injury, inflammation or neovascularization, pulls the sensory retina from the retinal pigment epithelium.

Incidence

Occurs mainly in the adult eye. The overall incidence is 1in 15,000 people per year.

Risk Factors

- Age between 50 to 70 years
- Cataract extraction
- Degeneration of the retina
- Trauma
- Severe myopia
- Previous retinal detachment in the other eye
- Family history of retinal detachment.

Causes

- Retinal tears and holes usually occurs from spontaneous vitreous traction.
- Presence of abnormal adhesions between the retina and vitreous body secondary to diabetic retinopathy, injury or other ocular disorders.
- Atrophy of the vitreous body also results in a retinal tear.

Pathophysiology

- Spontaneous vitreous traction gives rise to retinal tears and holes.
- Retina is separated from its choriodal blood supply.
- A vascular necrosis occurs due to deprivation of oxygen and nutrients.

Clinical Manifestations

- A retinal detachment is commonly preceded by a posterior vitreous

detachment, which gives rise to these symptoms—
  - Flashes of light (photopsia)—Very brief in the extreme peripheral (outside of center) part of vision.
  - A sudden dramatic increase in the number of floaters.
  - A ring of floaters or hairs just to the temporal side of the central vision.
  - A slight feeling of heaviness in the eye.
- Although most posterior vitreous detachments do not progress to retinal detachments, those that do produce the following symptoms:
  - A dense shadow that starts in the peripheral vision and slowly progresses towards the central vision.
  - The impression that a veil or curtain was drawn over the field of vision.
  - Straight lines (scale, edge of the wall, road, etc.) that suddenly appear curved (positive Amsler grid test).
  - Central visual loss.

Diagnostic tests

- Direct and indirect ophthalmoscope: To identify the portion of the retina involved and the extent of the detachment.

Management

There are several methods of treating a detached retina, each of which depends on finding and closing the breaks that have formed in the retina. All three of the procedures follow the same three general principles:

- Find all retinal breaks
- Seal all retinal breaks
- Relieve present (and future) vitreoretinal traction.

Cryopexy and Laser Photocoagulation

- Cryotherapy (freezing) or laser photocoagulation are occasionally used alone to wall off a small area of retinal detachment so that the detachment does not spread.

Scleral Buckle Surgery

- Scleral buckle surgery is an established treatment in which the eye surgeon sews one or more silicone bands (bands, tyres) to the sclera (the white outer coat of the eyeball).
- The bands push the wall of the eye inward against the retinal hole, closing the break or reducing fluid flow through it and reducing the effect of vitreous traction thereby allowing the retina to re-attach.
- Cryotherapy (freezing) is applied around retinal breaks prior to placing the buckle. Often subretinal fluid is drained as part of the buckling procedure. The buckle remains in situ.

Pneumatic Retinopexy

- Method of repairing a retinal detachment in which a gas bubble (SF_6 or C_3F_8 gas) is injected into the eye after which laser or freezing treatment is applied to the retinal hole.
- The patient's head is then positioned so that the bubble rests against the retinal hole. Patients may have to keep their heads tilted for several days to keep the gas bubble in contact with the retinal hole.
- The surface tension of the air/water interface seals the hole in the retina, and allows the retinal pigment epithelium to pump the subretinal space dry and suck the retina back into place. This procedure is usually combined with cryopexy or laser photocoagulation.

Vitrectomy

It involves the removal of the vitreous gel and is usually combined with filling the eye with either a gas bubble (SF_6 or C_3F_8 gas) or silicon oil.

NURSING MANAGEMENT

Nursing Assessment

Subjective data

Ask the patient about visual disturbances and flashes of light.

Objective data

Visual field loss is present in the opposite quadrant of the actual detachment.

Nursing diagnosis

- Altered vision related to decreased retinal function as evidenced by flashes of light, visual disturbances.
- Anxiety related to prognosis, treatment of the disease condition.

PLANNING OUTCOMES/GOALS

- Maintain functional vision as possible.
- Decrease level of anxiety.

Nursing Interventions

Maintain functional vision as possible

- Assess the level of visual disturbances.
- Explain the patient about the preoperative preparation.
- Administer sedative as ordered.
- Observe the eye patch for any drainage in the postoperative period.
- Restrict activities if the air or gas bubble is injected.
- Maintain the head down and one side tilting position for several days.
- Monitor intraocular pressure for 24 hours in the postoperative period of scleral buckling procedure.
- Encourage the patient to resume regular diet and fluids as tolerated.
- Remove the eye patch on the first postoperative day and observe for any redness and swelling of lids and conjunctiva.
- Administer eye drops (antibiotic and steroid combination) to prevent infection and reduce swelling.
- Administer cycloplegic agents to dilate the pupils and relax ciliary muscle that decreases discomfort and prevents iris adhesions.
- Apply warm or cold compress to reduce discomfort.
- Instruct the patient to clean the eye with warm tap water using clean washcloth.
- Advice the patient to wear glasses during the daytime and eye shield during a nap (small sleep) or at night.
- Instruct the patient to avoid vigorous exercises and heavy weight lifting during the immediate postoperative period.
- If a gas or air bubble is injected, advise the patient to avoid travelling by air as the gas and air expand at high altitude.

Decrease level of anxiety

- Assess the level of anxiety of the patient.
- Explain the disease condition and the surgical outcome.
- Clear his doubts, listen attentively.
- Discuss the home care to the patient and the caregiver.

CONJUNCTIVITIS

Definition

Conjunctivitis is an inflammation of the conjunctiva (the outermost layer of the eye and the inner surface of the eyelids). It is most commonly due to an infection (usually viral, but sometimes bacterial) or an allergic reaction.

Classification

Classification can be either by cause or by extent of the inflamed area.

By Cause

Allergic conjunctivitis

Allergic conjunctivitis referes to eye inflammation resulting from an allergic reactions to substances like pollen or mold spores. The conjunctiva is susceptible to irritation from allergens, specially during hay fever season. Allergic conjunctivitis are of two types:

a. **Acute allergic conjunctivitis**—This is a short-term condition that is more common during allergy season.
b. **Chronic allergic conjunctivitis**—It is a response to allergens like food, dust and animal dander.

   Symptoms of allergic conjunctivitis include red, itchy, watery and burning eyes (Fig. 2.1).

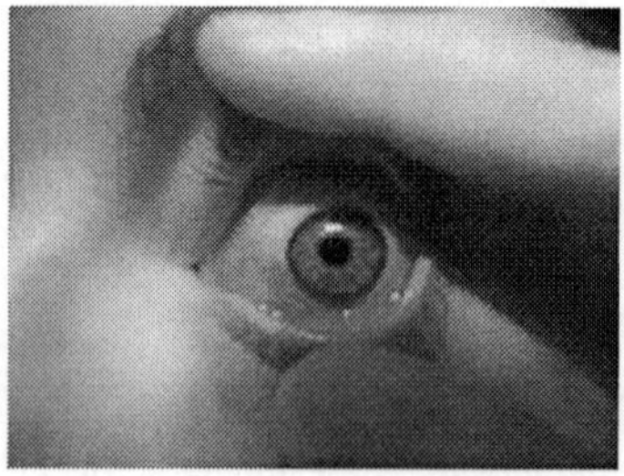

Fig. 2.1: An eye with allergic conjunctivitis

Bacterial conjunctivitis

Bacterial conjunctivitis causes the rapid onset of conjunctival redness, swelling of the eyelid, and mucopurulent discharge.

Symptoms develop first in one eye, but may spread to the other eye within 2 to 5 days.

Bacterial conjunctivitis due to common pyogenic (pus-producing) bacteria causes marked grittiness/irritation and a stringy, opaque, grayish or yellowish mucopurulent discharge that may cause the lids to stick together, especially after sleep. The more acute pyogenic infections can be painful.

Pathophysiology

- Bacteria such as *Chlamydia trachomatis* or *Moraxella* cause a nonexudative but persistent conjunctivitis without much redness (Fig. 2.3).
- Bacterial conjunctivitis may cause the production of membranes or pseudomembranes that cover the conjunctiva.
- Pseudomembranes consist of a combination of inflammatory cells and exudates, and are loosely adherent to the conjunctiva, while true membranes are more tightly adherent and cannot be easily peeled away.
- Cases of bacterial conjunctivitis that involve the production of membranes or pseudomembranes are associated with *Neisseria gonorrhoeae*, hemolytic streptococci, and *C. diphtheriae*.

Viral conjunctivitis

- Viral conjunctivitis is often associated with an infection of the upper respiratory tract, a common cold, and/or a sore throat.
- Symptoms include excessive watering and itching. The infection usually be-

gins with one eye, but may spread easily to the other.
- Viral conjunctivitis, commonly known as **pink eye**, shows a fine, diffuse pinkness of the conjunctiva.

Chemical conjunctivitis

- Chemical eye injury is due to either an acidic or alkali substance getting in the eye.
- Mild burns will produce conjunctivitis while more severe burns may cause the cornea to turn white.
- Irritant or toxic conjunctivitis show primarily marked redness.

By Extent of Involvement

- Blepharoconjunctivitis is the dual combination of conjunctivitis with blepharitis (inflammation of the eyelids).
- Keratoconjunctivitis is the combination of conjunctivitis and keratitis (corneal inflammation).

Clinical Manifestations

- Red eye (hyperemia)
- Swelling of conjunctiva (chemosis) and
- Watering (epiphora) of the eyes are symptoms common to all forms of conjunctivitis. However, the pupils should be normally reactive and the visual acuity normal.
- A purulent discharge suggests a bacterial infection. Bacteria can also cause it from feces, pet hair, or by smoke or other fumes (Fig. 2.2).
- Infection with *Neisseria gonorrhoeae* should be suspected if the discharge is particularly thick and copious.

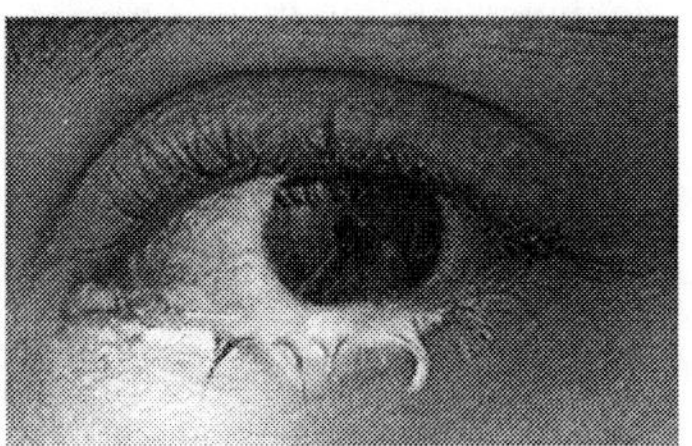

Fig. 2.2: An eye with bacterial conjunctivitis

- Itching (rubbing eyes) is the hallmark symptom of allergic conjunctivitis. Other symptoms include history of eczema, or asthma (Fig. 2.1).

Others

- Pain.
- blurring of vision.
- photophobia, should not be prominent in conjunctivitis.
- Fluctuating blurring is common, due to tearing and mucoid discharge. Mild photophobia is common.
- However, if any of these symptoms are prominent, it is important to exclude other diseases such as glaucoma, uveitis, keratitis and even meningitis or caroticocavernous fistula.
- Many people with conjunctivitis have trouble opening their eyes in the morning because of the dried mucus on their eyelids. There is often excess mucus over the eye after sleeping for an extended period.
- Episcleritis is an inflammatory condition that produces a similar appearance to conjunctivitis, but without discharge or tearing.

Diagnoses Tests

- **Culture and sensitivity tests**: Swabs for bacterial culture are necessary if the history and signs suggest bacterial

conjunctivitis, but there is no response to topical antibiotics.
- Conjunctival incisional biopsy is occasionally done when granulomatous diseases (e.g. sarcoidosis) or dysplasia are suspected.

Prevention

- Maintenance of hygiene and not rubbing the eyes by infected hands.
- Vaccination against adenovirus, *Hemophilus influenzae*, pneumococcus, and *Neisseria meningitidis* is also effective.

Management

Allergic conjunctivitis

- Pour cool water over the face with the head inclined downward constricts capillaries.
- Artificial tears sometimes relieve discomfort in mild cases.
- Nonsteroidal anti-inflammatory medications and antihistamines is administered.
- Persistent allergic conjunctivitis may also require topical steroid drops.

Bacterial conjunctivitis

- Bacterial conjunctivitis usually resolves without treatment.
- Antibiotics, eye drops, or ointment may be administered if no improvement is observed after three days.
- For acute cases, 3rd or 4th generation fluoroquinolones, sodium sulfacetamide, or trimethoprim/polymyxin may be used, typically for 7 to 10 days.
- Cases of meningococcal conjunctivitis can be treated with systemic penicillin, as long as the strain is sensitive to penicillin.
- Chlamydial eye infections (Fig. 2.3) are the world's leading cause of blindness, and these cases will not resolve without antibiotics. If the conjunctivitis is known to be caused by gonorrhea, then it may be treated with a one-time injection of ceftriaxone, followed by 2 to 3 weeks of oral tetracycline or erythromycin.

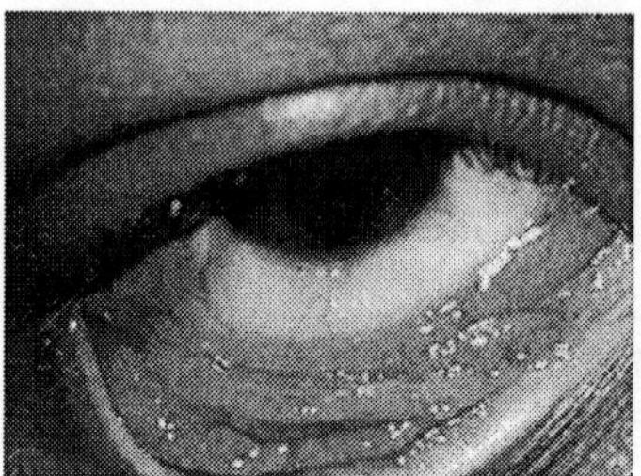

Fig. 2.3: An eye with chlamydial conjunctivitis

Viral

- The new treatment for viral eye infection involves a single treatment of iodine solution (Betadine 2.5%–5% concentration).
- After ocular anesthetization, the iodine solution's irritating nature to the eye, a series of drops are instilled in the patient's eye.
- It is generally advisable to avoid touching the eyes or sharing towels and washcloths in the case of viral conjunctivitis infection.

Chemical

- Eye irrigation with Ringer's lactate or saline solution.
- Avoid touching eye with bare hands.

3

Nursing Management of Patients with Disorders of Ear, Nose and Throat

NURSING ASSESSMENT OF PATIENT WITH EAR DISORDERS

Subjective Data

- Otologic history includes demographic data, current clinical manifestations, past history, family history, and psychological history.
- Demographic data relevant to otologic assessment includes the client's age. Hearing impairment may occur as consequences of the aging process.
- Current health history: Communication skills, reduction in physical, functional and social activities leading to isolation and depression. Hearing loss resulting in feelings of frustration, embarrassment and loneliness.
- Chief complaints: Nausea or vomiting, pain hearing loss, vertigo, tinnitus, drainage, infection.
- Past medical and surgical history: History of common childhood diseases—Complications of ear infections—Chronic otitis media, frequent upper respiratory tract infections, acute and chronic sinus infections. Any history of mastoidecomy,tympanolasty, stapedectomy.
- Allergies—Resulting in nasal stiffness and congestion.
- Medications: Damage the vestibulocochlear nerve (eight cranial nerve) with resulting hearing loss, tinnitus or disturbances in equilibrium. Aspirin is a common cause of tinnitus. Other drugs include aminoglycosides, analgesics, salicylates, quinine, chemotherapeutic agents and antiprotozoal agents.

Objective Data

- **External ear and canal**: Inspect and palpate the external ear. Auricle, periauricular area, and mastoid area are observed for symmetry of ears, color of skin, nodules, swellings, redness and lesions. The auricle and mastoid areas are then palpated for tenderness and nodules. Assess for sebaceous cyst, behind ears, tophi, impacted cerumen, discharge in canal, swellings of pinna, pain, scalingor lesions, enotosis.
- **External auditory canal and tympanum**: Inspect the canal opening for patency, palpate the tragus, and gently move the auricle to check for discomfort. Look for retracted eardrum (blockage of eustachian tube).Bulging red or blue eardrum, lack of landmark

(middle ear filled with fluid) and blood, pus. Perfortion of eardrum is present in chronic otitis media, mastoiditis.

- Observe the tympanic membrane for color, landmarks, contour and intactness. It is pearl gray, white or pink, shiny and translucent.
- Observe the ear canal for size, shape, color, amount and type of cerumen.

Diagnostic Studies

Tests for hearing acuity

1. Whispered and spoken voice provides gross screening information about the patient's ability to hear.
2. Tuning fork tests helps in differentiating conductive and sensorineural hearing loss. Tuning fork of 512 Hz is used for this test. Commonly used tets are Rinne test and Weber test.
   - Rinne test: It is positive when the patient reports that air conduction (AC) is heard longer than bone conduction (BC). It indicates normal hearing or sensorineural loss. If the patient hears the tuning fork better by bone conduction, the Rinne test is negative and indicates that a conductive hearing loss is present.
   - Weber test: An actual tuning fork is placed on the midline of the skull, the forehead or the teeth. If a patient has a conductive hearing loss in one ear, sound is heard louder in that ear. If a sensorineural loss is present, sound is louder in the unaffected ear.

     Results of tuning fork tests are subjective.
3. Audiometry is useful as a screening test for hearing acuity and as diagnostic tests for determining the degree and type for determining the degree and type of hearing loss. Audiometer procedure puretones at varying initiatives to which the patient can respond.
   - Screening audiometry is the testing of large numbers of persons with a fast, simple test to detect possible hearing problems.
   - Pure tone audiometry: A puretone audiometer produces pure tones at varied frequencies and intensities and is performed by an audiologists. Purpose is to determine the hearing range of the patient in terms of decibels and hertz.
4. Test for structure—
   - X-ray of the temporal bone, mastoid bone is done to rule out any structural abnormality.
   - CT scan and MRI is done to rule out any tumor of the temporal bone.
   - Arteriography is used to assess vascular abnormalities in the temporal bone.
5. Laboratory tests—
   - Complete blood count is necessary to assess any acute ear infections.
   - Ear drainage culture is done to identify an infecting organism.
   - Tests for presence of cerebrospinal fluid in the ear can rule out meningitis.
   - Biopsy of the abnormal tissue in the ear canal is done to rule out a malignancy or to identify unusual problems.

COMMON EAR INFECTIONS

Children are the vulnerable group for ear infections. Infections may be viral or bacterial. Different types of ear infection may be listed down as:

1. Otitis externa:
   - Bacterial infection.
   - Viral infections mainly from herpes simplex, herpes zoster, bullous myringitis.
   - Fungal otomycosis.
2. Tympanic membrane infections.

3. Otitis media
   - Acute suppurative otitis media
   - Chronic suppurative otitis media.
4. Mastoiditis.
5. Chlolesteatoma.

Otitis Externa

It primarily occurs in the external auditory canal or may be a manifestations of a generalized skin condition. It may be viral or fungal.

Bacterial infection

Etiology
- Genetic factors like narrow canal inherent tendency to eczema, excessive wax formation.
- Traumatic factors like match stick.
- Environmental factors heat, humidity, swimming, etc.

Viral infection

Etiology
Herpes Simplex occurs most commonly on the lips, however may be occasionally found involving external canal. The eruption consists of a crop of small vesicles, which dries up after a few days.

Herpes zoster involving the geniculate ganglion may give rise to skin lesions, with or without involvement of VII cranial nerve. The blister adherent crust which persist for a week.

Fungal infections

Fungal infection or otomycosis is quite a common cause of otitis externa in the tropical climate regions.

Etiology
- Humidity occurs due to water entering the ear as a result of swimming or during bath.
- Infections: *Candida albicans* and *Aspergillus niger* can cause.
- Antibiotic ear drops used over a long period lead to destruction of normally present bacteria resulting in growth of fungus.

Clinical manifestations

- Pain.
- Discharge from ear.
- Deafness.
- Itching.
- External canal appears congested edematous.
- Trismus.
- Tinnitus.

Tympanic Membrane Infections

Infections of the external ear canal can involve the surface of tympanic membrane. The infections of tympanic membrane are:

Tympanosclerosis

It is the result of repeated infection and trauma to the tympanic membrane. It consists of a deposit of collagen and calcium within middle ear that can harden around ossicles, causing a conductive hearing loss.

Bullous myringitis

It is characterized by formation of blebson in the tympanic membrane and the deep meatal skin. The color of blebs is purplish due to hemorrhagic effusion filling the vesicles.

Etiology—Above infections are mainly caused by:
- Bacterium *mycoplasma pneumoniae.*

Clinical manifestations—Holes or perforations of tympanic membrane can be caused by infections and accompanied by drainage.

Otitis Media

Otitis media is the most prevalent disorders of the middle ear. It is most common in children but does occur in adults.

Acute suppurative otitis media (ASOM)

When an infection is sudden in onset and short in duration, the diagnosis is acute suppurative otitis media.

Etiology—Organism like streptococcus, staphylococcus causes the infection. Disease condition like nasopharyngitis, rhinitis, sinusitis. Previous trauma or tympanotomy. The disease is rarely by blood-borne.

Chronic suppurative otitis media. (CSOM)

When an infection is repeated, usually causing drainage and perforation, then it is called chronic suppurative otitis media.

Etiology—Organisms like *Pseudomonas, Staphylococcus*, and *Klebsiella* are responsible for CSOM. Residue of an ASOM infection during childhood. Repeated infection from eustachian tube. Large size traumatic perforation.

Clinical manifestations

- Discharge is mucoid, copius, and non-foul smelling.
- Deafness.
- Ear ache.
- Fever.
- Radiography of mastoid shows cloudiness of aircells.
- Necrosis of bone covering facial nerve.

Mastoiditis

The mastoid system is a series of air cells contained within the temporal bone that communicate with middle ear.

Etiology

It results from an ASOM when there is lowered resistance in the patients. Virulence of organism is great. Drainage via Eustachian tube is poor. Improper inadequate antibiotics given.

Clinical manifestations

- Pain occurs again, as was present with acute otitis media.
- Ear discharge would increase in quantity.
- Tenderness is elicited over the mastoid antrum area.
- Sagging of the posterior superior bony canal wall.

Cholesteatoma

Cholesteatoma is a three dimensional epidermal and connective tissue structure, usually in the form of sac and frequently confirming to the architecture of various spaces of middle ear and mastoid.

Etiology

- CSOM
- Marginal perforation of the tympanic membrane.

Clinical manifestations

- Ear discharge is scanty, foul smelling and sometimes blood stained.
- Deafness may be unnoticed if a portion of the cholesteotoma may bridge gap in the ossicular chain.
- Erosion of surrounding structures leading to other problem like brain abscess, vertigo, etc.

PATHOPHYSIOLOGY

Otalgia or ear pain related to a problem in the ear is usually the result of an inflammatory process that can be caused by trauma or infection.

Inflammation causes chemical mediators to be released into the tissues and the chemotaxis of leukocytes to the damaged areas, resulting in tissues edema, pain, heat and redness.

This inflammatory process results in swelling of tissues that impinges on nerve ending and surrounding areas, causing otalgia.

Sometimes infection may erode into tissue and bone as in cholesteatoma and causes further inflammation and pain.

- Etiological factors
- Chemical mediators are released and inflammation occurs
- Resulting in tissue edema, pain, heat and redness
- Inflammatory process results in swelling of tissues
- That swelling impinges on nerve endings and surrounding areas
- Causing the otalgia or ear pain
- Masses such as tumors grow and press on nearby tissues and nerves
- Causing pain, discharge and other complication like deafness.

DIAGNOSTIC TESTS

Otitis Externa

Laboratory studies

Gram staining and culture of canal discharge is occasionally helpful, particularly in fungal infection.

Imaging studies

To look for sign of a bone infection next to ear canal, the CT scan of head, MRI and radionuclide scan may be performed.

Otitis Media

Laboratory studies

Culture and sensitivity of a specimen from a fresh perforation or a tympanocentesis.

Imaging studies

CT scan, MRI to detect intracranial complications.

Audiometry

For checking conductive hearing loss the test is done.

Tympanometry

It is helpful to identify presence or absence if middle ear effusion is present.

Mastoiditis

- The early diagnosis of mastoiditis is clinical based on medical history and physical examination.
- Complete blood count with differential, blood cultures, tympanocentesis, Gram stain , acid-fast staining is done.
- Audiography for assessing hearing loss.
- CT scan for showing fluid collection in middle ear and mastoid region, abscess formation, etc.

MANAGEMENT

Medical Management

Goals

- Promote healing
- Alleviate pain
- Restore normal function of ears.

Promote healing

- Ear irrigation: Ear is commonly irrigated to cleanse the external auditory canal or to remove debris, impacted wax, or foreign body. Periodic suctioning of ear canal helps to keep open, remove debris, and decrease bacterial counts.
- Antibiotics: Antibiotic ear drop to reduce infection.
- Corticosteroid: Hydrocortisone ear drops for few weeks.

- Antifungal agents: Nystatin ear drop is used to treat fungal infection.
- Burrow's solution or topical corticosteroid cream or lotions are also given.

Alleviate Pain—Analgesics are used to reduce pain, e.g. Acetaminophen, NSAIDs, opiods, ibuprofen.

SURGICAL MANAGEMENT

Myringotomy

A small incision is made in eardrum to allow fluid to drain and keep the eardrum from rupturing.

Myringoplasty

It is an operation specifically designed to close tympanic membrane defects with use of operating microsepsis.

Tympanoplasty

The purpose of tympanoplasty is to repair the perforated eardrum and sometimes the middle ear bones that consist of incus, malleus and stapes.

Ossiculoplasty

It is the surgical reconstruction of middle ear bone to restore hearing. Prosthetic made of materials such as teflon, stainless steel are used to reconnect the ossicles.

Mastoidectomy

It involves incision, drainage of surgical repair of the mastoid process.

NURSING MANAGEMENT

Nursing Assessment

Subjective data

When obtaining the history of the pain, ask the patient about, what events have triggered, the ear pain, paying special attention to a recent history of the following:

- Upper respiratory tract infection
- Travel by airplane
- Exposure to loud noise.

Objective data

Pain, discharge from ear, deafness, itching, external canal appears congested edematous, trismus, tinnitus, earache, fever, radiography of mastoid shows cloudiness of air cells, necrosis of bone covering facial nerve.

Nursing Diagnoses

- Risk for infection related to tissue destruction.
- Acute pain related to inflammation in the externa or middle ear or from referred pain in head and neck area.
- Disturbed perception (auditory) related to infection, discharge.
- Knowledge deficit related to the disease condition.
- Impaired verbal communication related to auditory impairment secondary to infection in ear.

PLANNING OUTCOMES/GOALS

- Minimize risk of infection
- Minimize pain
- Improve in auditory perception
- Increase knowledge level
- Improve verbal communication.

Nursing Interventions

Minimize risk of infection

- Monitor for redness swelling, pain as signs of infection.
- Administer antibiotics or other medications like antihistamines, decongestants, etc. steroid nasal spray
- Do ear irrigation.

- Teach the client to continue the prescribed doses.

Minimize pain

- Assess pain-by-pain rating scale.
- Give comfort using anesthetic ear solutions or systemic analgesics.
- Apply heat by warm compress.
- Give proper position.
- Provide soft diet and quiet environment.

Improve auditory perception

- Assess the client for the level of hearing loss.
- Administer antibiotics for decreasing infections.

Increase knowledge level

- Assess the knowledge level of the client regarding the disease process.
- Describe about the pathophysiology and clinical manifestation of the disease condition.
- Describe the reason behind each treatment approaches.
- Clarify patients doubt.

Improve verbal communication

- Assess the ability of the patient to communicate.
- Use nonverbal communication.
- Use communication board.
- Encourage him to talk.
- Advice the patient for rehabilitation.
- Provide hearing aids.

DEVIATED NASAL SEPTUM

Definition

A deviated nasal septum is a condition when there is a shift from the midline on center position (Fig. 3.1).

- It refers to the deformity of the partition of the nose that separates the two nostrils.

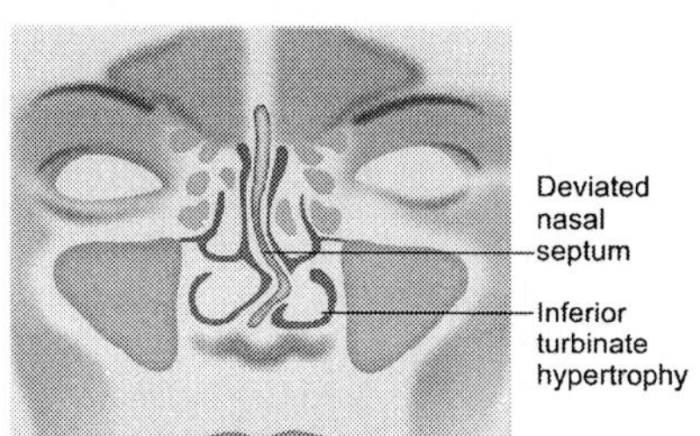

Fig. 3.1: Deviated nasal septum

- It occurs when the thin wall (Nasal septum) inside the nose is displaced to one side.
- In deviated nasal septum (DNS) the top of the cartilaginous ridge leans to the left or right causing obstruction of the affected nasal passage. It changes the velocity of the air altering normal nasal activities and resulting in dryness, crusting, nasal bleeding, and changes in the membranous lining of the nose.

Etiology

- Trauma to the nose commonly occurs during contact sports, active play on rough houses automobile accidents.
- Congenital disorder: Approximately 5% are birth defects or congenital disorder caused by compression of the nose during childbirth.

Pathophysiology

Deformity of the nasal septum may be classified into:

- Spur
- Deviation
- Dislocation.

Spur

These are sharp angulations seen in the nasal septum occurring at the junction of the vomer below with the septal cartilage and on ethmoid bone above.

Deviations

These are characterized by a more generalized bulge. They may be 'C' shaped and 'S' shaped and usually involve both cartilage and bone.

Cartilaginous deviations—In these patients' upper bony septum and the bony pyramid are central, but there is a dislocation or deviation of the cartilaginous septum and vault.

The C-deviation—There is displacement of the upper bony septum and the pyramid to one side and the whole of the cartilaginous septum and vault to the opposite side.

The S-deviation—The deviation of the middle-third is opposite to that of the upper and lower-thirds. With deviation of the nose, the dominant factor is the position of the nasal septum, hence the edge as straighten the septum and if this objective is not achieved, there is no hope of successful straightening of the external pyramid

Thickened septum—It may be congenital or trauma: Cottle has classified septal deviations:
- Simple deviation: There is a mild deviation of nasal septum, there is no nasal obstruction. This is a commonest condition encountered. It needs no treatment.
- Obstruction: There is more severe deviation of the nasal septum, which may touch the lateral wall of the nose, but no vasoconstriction the turbinates shrink away from the septum. Hence, surgery is not indicated even in these cases.
- Impaction: There is marked angulations of the septum with a spur which lies in contact with lateral nasal wall. The space is not increased even on vasoconstriction. Surgery is indicated for these patients.

Dislocations

In this the lower border of the septal cartilages displaced from its medial position and projects into one of the nostril.

Clinical Manifestations

The most common symptom of a deviated septum is nasal congestion, with one side of the nose being more congested than the other, along with difficulty breathing. Recurrent or repeated sinus infections can also be a sign of a deviated septum. Other symptoms include frequent:
- Nosebleeds
- Facial pain
- Headache
- Postnasal drip
- Loud breathing and snoring during sleep.

A deviated septum may also cause sleep apnea, a serious condition in which a person stops breathing during sleep.

Diagnostic Tests

- During a physical examination ask the patient about the symptoms — such as nosebleeds or nasal congestion — and ask whether he had any trauma to nose.
- Using a bright light and an instrument (nasal speculum) designed to spread open the nostrils; examine the inside of the nose. Based on this exam, the physician should be able to diagnose deviated septum and determine the seriousness of the condition.

Complications

Immediate after surgical intervention

- Hemorrhage

- Tear of flaps
- CSF rhinorrhea.

Delayed

- Hemorrhage
- Septal hematoma
- Septal abscess
- Septal perforation
- Adhesions.

Late

- Atrophic rhinitis
- Columellar retraction
- Flappy septum.

Others

- Facial pain
- Chronic sinus infection
- Postnasal drip or nasal congestion.

MANAGEMENT

Medical Management

Managing symptoms

Initial treatment of deviated septum may be directed at managing the symptoms of the condition, such as nasal congestion and postnasal drip.

- Decongestants: Decongestants are medications that reduce nasal congestion, helping to keep the airways on both sides of the nose open. Decongestants are available as a pill or as a nasal spray. Use nasal sprays with caution, however, frequent use can create dependency and cause symptoms to be worse (rebound).
- Antihistamines: Antihistamines are medications that help prevent many cold and allergy symptoms, including runny nose.
- Nasal steroid sprays: Prescription nasal corticosteroid sprays can reduce inflammation in the nasal passage and help prevent a runny nose.
- Analgesics: To reduce pain, relieve headache.
- Antibiotics: to eliminate a suspected infection.

Surgical Management

Corrective surgeries are used when the deviation is more severe and obstructs breathing and for more persistent, trouble some symptoms.

Septal surgeries are required for symptomatic deviation.

The surgeries are

- Septal reconstruction
- Rhinoplasty.

Surgical repair (septoplasty)—Septoplasty is the usual way to repair a deviated septum. During septoplasty, the nasal septum is repositioned in the center of your nose. This may require the surgeon to cut and remove parts of the septum before reinserting it in the proper position.

Reshaping the nose—In some cases, surgery to reshape the nose (rhinoplasty) is performed at the same time as septoplasty. Rhinoplasty involves readjusting the bone and cartilage of the nose to change its shape or size or both.

NURSING MANAGEMENT

Nursing Assessment

Subjective data

History of nosebleeds, facial pain, headache, drip, loud breathing and snoring during sleep.

Objective data

Assess for repeated sinus infections, nasal congestion, difficulty breathing.

Nursing Diagnoses

- Acute pain related to surgical procedure as evidenced by patient's facial expression, verbal report and through pain scale measurement.
- Activity intolerance related to pain, discomfort as evidenced by inability to perform activities of daily living, weakness and fatigue.
- Knowledge deficit related to awareness and prevention of complications.

PLANNING OUTCOMES/GOALS

- Minimize pain
- Improve activities of daily living
- Improve knowledge regarding awareness and prevention of complications.

Nursing Interventions

Minimize pain

- Assess the duration, intensity and radiation of pain through pain scale.
- Place the patient in a comfortable position.
- Check the surgical site for any excessive bleeding or drainage.
- Provide a noise-free environment to the patient.
- Administer analgesics as ordered.

Improve activities of daily living

- Assess the level of activity the patient can perform by himself.
- Allow the patient to perform brushing, combing, feeding once condition is stable.
- Plan activity and rest period.
- Provide a well-balanced diet when allowed after surgery.

Improve knowledge regarding awareness and prevention of complications

- Assess the knowledge and understanding regarding the disease condition.
- Explain the causative factors in details.
- Educate the patient regarding surgical procedure and its prognosis.
- Explain the patient about the prevention of complications.

4

Nursing Management of Patients with Disorders of Respiratory System

ASSESMENT OF PATIENTS WITH DISORDERS OF RESPIRATORY SYSTEM

Subjective Data

- **Dyspnea**: Its onset, duration, timing, associated with chest pain, cough or weakness, increases with exertion, stress, anxiety, allergies and decreases by upright position, medications, etc.
- **Cough**: Its onset, duration, dry, hacking, wheezy, associated with chest pain, fevers, sputum production, relieved by medications.
- **Hemoptysis**: Duration, amount, color, whether on anticoagulant therapy.
- **Wheezing**: Onset and duration, aggravating factors like exertion; emotional stress; allergies, relieving factors like medicine, associated cough and chest pain.
- Stridor, sleep apnea, changes in voice, hoarseness, etc.
- Sinus problems such as nosebleed, postnasal drips, nasal, facial or referred ear pain.
- **Chest pain**: Its location, duration, radiation, type of pain such as aching, burning, sharp, associated with nausea; cough; diaphoresis or weakness, aggravating factors, e.g. exertion; movement; breathing; coughing; allergies; and relieved by medications.
- Past history of asthma, COPD, pneumonia, tuberculosis, frequent respiratory infections.
- **Use of medications**: Prescribed or over the counter such as antihistamines, bronchodilators, cough suppressants, corticosteroids, antibiotics, oxygen inhalation, etc.
- Past history of hospitalization for respiratory problems, surgery, intubation, or any other respiratory therapy such as nebulization, humidifier, etc.
- History of activities of daily living, changes in activity tolerance, exercises, sleep disturbances due to respiratory problems.
- Family history of respiratory problems such as asthma, emphysema, cystic fibrosis, tuberculosis.
- History of recent travel to out of country.
- **Living conditions**: Overcrowding.
- **Habits of smoking**: Number of pack years, drinking alcohol.
- Urinary incontinence during paroxysms of coughing.
- Apprehension, irritability, changes in memory.

Objective Data

- **Vital signs**: Temperature, pulse, respiration, blood pressure and SpO_2 (oxygen saturation obtained by pulse oximetry).
- Nasal flaring or discharge, mass or perforation, dry nasal mucosa, nasal septum deviation, pursed lip breathing, tripod position (unable to lie down), tracheal deviation, splinting of chest, tachypnea, Kussmaul respiration, labored respiration, abdominal paradox, cyanosis, clubbing of fingers, barrel chest, pigeon chest on inspection.
- **On palpation**: Tenderness on nose, sinuses, swelling, crepitus, tracheal deviation, asymmetrical chest wall, presence of lump, masses, tenderness, altered tactile fremitus, increase or decrease in vibrations, altered chest movement.
- Hyperresonance or dullness on chest during percussion.
- On auscultation diminished breath sounds in certain areas or bronchovesicular and bronchial sounds in certain areas of peripheral lung fields or absent breath sounds. Fine crackles, coarse crackles, rhonchi, wheezes, stridor or pleural friction rub may also be present.

Diagnostic Studies

1. Blood Studies

- Hemoglobin percentage.
- *Hematocrit level*: Elevated in chronic hypoxemia.
- *Pulse oximetry*: A noninvasive method of assessing oxygenation. The pulse oximeter passes a beam of light through the tissue. Amount of light absorbed by the oxygen saturated hemoglobin is measured by a sensor attached to fingertip, toe or earlobe. Thus the pulse oximeter gives a reading of percentage of hemoglobin that is saturated with oxygen (SpO_2).
- *Arterial blood gas analysis (ABG)*: The test involves use of arterial blood through radial or femoral arterial puncture for measurement of oxygen concentration (PaO_2), carbon dioxide concentration ($PaCO_2$) and pH directly.

Arterial blood gas studies aid in assessing the ability of the lungs to provide adequate oxygen and remove carbon dioxide and the ability of the kidneys to reabsorb or excrete bicarbonate ions to maintain normal body pH.

2. Sputum studies

- Sputum test for acid-fast bacilli (AFB) such as *Mycobacterium tuberculosis*.
- Sputum test for culture and sensitivity to detect bacterial infections and select proper antibiotics.
- Sputum test for Gram staining is done to classify infecting organism as gram-positive or gram-negative. Result guides therapy till culture and sensitivity report is obtained.
- Sputum for cytology is done to detect abnormal cells in order to detect malignancy.

3. Biopsy

- Lung biopsy
- Pleural biopsy.

4. Radiology

- *Chest X-Ray*: Most commonly used test for assessing respiratory disorders. The test also assesses progress of the disease and the response to treatment.
- *Computed tomography (CT Scan)*: Uses radiation to examine cross section

of the body. The test is performed to evaluate areas of the chest that are not possible with X-ray such as mediastinum, hilum and pleura.
- *Magnetic resonance imaging (MRI)*: Uses strong magnetic field to obtain images that are difficult to obtain by CT scan. Particularly helpful in distinguishing vascular from nonvascular structures, images from lung apex or spine.
- *Ventilation-perfusion scan*: It is used to assess lung ventilation and lung perfusion. The test is useful in identifying pulmonary embolism, pulmonary infarcts, bronchiectasis and emphysema. A radioactive isotope is injected through intravenous route and scanning done to evaluate the pulmonary vasculature for the perfusion portion of the test. For ventilation portion of the test, the patient inhales a radioactive gas which outlines the alveoli and detected through scanning.
- *Positron emission tomography (PET Scan)*: It is useful in distinguishing malignant lung tumor from benign tumor. Intravenous radioactive glucose preparation is injected. Scanning detects increased uptake of radioactive glucose by the malignant lung cells.
- *Pulmonary angiogram*: It is the study of pulmonary vasculature after injection of a contrast medium to the pulmonary artery or right side of the heart. The test is conducted to locate obstruction or any other conditions such as thrombus or embolus.

5. *Endoscopic procedures*
   - *Bronchoscopy* is the visualization of bronchi by introducing a fiberoptic bronchoscope. Bronchoscopy is also used to obtain specimen for cytological test (biopsy) or by bronchoalveolar lavage.
   - *Mediastinoscopy* is visualization of the mediastinal structure after insertion of a endoscope. Test is performed for biopsy of lymph nodes of the mediastinum area.

6. *Pulmonary function test*
   - The test is used to evaluate lung function. With the help of a spirometer air movement is measured while the patient performs different respiratory maneuvers as directed by the technician.

7. *Thoracentesis*
   - Thoracentesis is aspiration of pleural fluid for diagnostic and therapeutic purpose. The procedure may also be conducted to instill medications in the pleural cavity.

BRONCHIECTASIS

Definition

Bronchiectasis, an extreme form of bronchitis is characterized by permanent, abnormal dilation of one or more lung bronchi.

Etiology

Congenital

- Cystic fibrosis
- Sinusitis
- Dextrocardia (heart located on right side)
- Alterations in ciliary activity (Kartagener's syndrome).

Acquired

- Pneumonia (complications of whooping cough in children)
- Measles
- Pulmonary tuberculosis
- Aspiration of foreign bodies, vomitus or material from the upper respiratory tract
- Bronchial tumor
- Immune disorders.

Pathophysiology

- Pulmonary infections initiate inflammatory process.
- Recurrent infections and inflammations cause destruction of the elastic and muscular structures of the bronchial wall.
- Bronchial walls get permanently distended and distorted. Mucociliary functions get disturbed.
- Infection and inflammation spreads to peribronchial tissue.
- Pockets of infection resembling lung abscess begin to form. These abscesses drain exudates freely in the bronchial lumen.
- Retention of secretions and subsequent obstruction cause alveoli distal to the obstruction to collapse (atelectasis).
- Inflammatory scarring and fibrosis replaces functioning lung tissue.

Clinical Manifestations

- Persistent or recurrent cough, purulent sputum production in large amount.
- Some patient may have hemoptysis.
- Exertional dyspnea.
- Loss of weight, anorexia.
- Lassitude, low grade fever.
- Fetid breath.
- Clubbing of the fingers.

Diagnostic Studies

1. Chest X-ray

Shows streaky infiltrates or normal.

2. Bronchoscopy

Identifies the source of secretions or hemoptysis and collects specimen for microbiological examination.

3. Sputum examination

Detects presence of active infections.

4. Complete blood count

It reveals anemia and leukocytosis from chronic infections.

5. CT scan

It confirms the diagnosis.

MANAGEMENT

Goals

1. To promote bronchial drainage to clear the affected portion of the lung of excessive secretions.
2. To prevent or control infection.

Medical Management

- Chest physiotherapy including percussion and postural drainage.
- Smoking cessation and to avoid air pollutants.
- Antibiotics according to sputum culture report.
- Bronchodilators.
- Mucolytics, expectorants and plenty of fluids.

Surgical Management

Lobectomy

Surgical resection of the affected lobe or segment (segmental resection) is performed when medical treatment is not effective.

Nursing Management

Goals

1. To promote drainage and removal of bronchial mucus.
2. To promote rest.
3. To maintain optimum nutrition.
4. To prevent complications.

Nursing Interventions

To promote drainage and removal of bronchial secretions

- Teach patient effective deep breathing and coughing exercises.
- Provide chest physiotherapy and postural drainage on the affected part of the lung.
- Administer prescribed antibiotics, bronchodilators and expectorants.
- Teach patient importance of adhering to prescribed regimen.
- Encourage patient to report if he/she experiences any side effects of drugs.
- Teach patient to report promptly if any significant clinical manifestations, e.g. increased sputum production, grossly bloody sputum, increasing dyspnea, fever, chills, and chest pain.

To promote rest

- Provide bed rest during the acute phase of illness.
- Permit activities gradually with periods of rest in between activities.

Promote nutritional status

- Provide small frequent nutritious foods.
- Provide oral care before each meal to remove dried sputum crusts and improve appetite.
- Provide 3 liters of fluid to liquefy secretions.
- Instruct patient to take low sodium fluid to prevent systemic fluid retention.

PNEUMONIA

Definition

Pneumonia (pneumonitis) is an acute inflammation of the lung parenchyma caused by a microbial agent.

Etiology

There are many causes of pneumonia, which include:

1. Microorganisms
   - Bacteria, e.g. *Streptococcus pneumoniae, Staphylococcus aureus,* Hemophilus influenzae, *Klebsiella pneumoniae, Legionella pneumophila,* mycoplasma, oral anaerobes.
   - Viruses, e.g. influenza virus, Fungi.
   - Parasites, e.g. protozoa, nematodes, platyhelminthis.
2. Aspiration of food, fluids or vomitus
3. Inhalation of toxic or caustic chemicals, smokes, dusts or gasses.

Risk Factors

- Children and persons with advanced age.
- A history of smoking.
- Upper respiratory infection.
- Tracheal intubation.
- Prolonged immobility.
- Immunosuppressive therapy.
- A nonfunctional immune system.

- Malnutrition.
- Dehydration.
- Chronic disease states, e.g. diabetes, heart disease, chronic lung disease, renal disease and cancer.
- Exposure to air pollution.
- Altered consciousness, alcoholism, head injury, seizures, anesthetic drug overdose, stroke.
- Inhalation or aspiration of noxious substances.
- Aspiration of foreign or gastric material.

Types of Pneumonia

Several systems are used to classify pneumonias:

1. According to causative organism, e.g. pneumococcal pneumonia, viral pneumonia.
2. On the basis of location and radiologic appearance:
   - *Lobar pneumonia*: One or more entire lobes are involved.
   - *Bronchopneumonia*: It involves the terminal bronchioles and alveoli.
   - Interstitial (reticular) pneumonia: It involves inflammatory responses within lung tissue surrounding the air spaces or vascular structures rather than the air passages themselves.
   - *Alveolar or acinar pneumonia*: There is fluid accumulation in lung's distal air spaces.
   - *Necrotizing pneumonia*: It causes death of a portion of lung tissue surrounded by viable tissue.
3. On the basis of where it is acquired
   - *Community acquired pneumonia (CAP)*: Lower respiratory tract infection of the lung parenchyma with onset in the community or during the first 2 days of hospitalization.
   - *Hospital acquired pneumonia / Nosocomial pneumonia*: Pneumonia occurring 48 hours or longer after hospital admission and not incubating at the time of hospitalization.
4. Pneumonia in the immunocompromised host or *opportunistic pneumonia*: Patients with compromised immune system, commonly, acquired pneumonia from organisms of low virulence, e.g. pneumocystis carinii pneumonia, fungal pneumonia and mycobacterium tuberculosis.
5. *Aspiration pneumonia*: Refers to the sequela occurring from abnormal entry of secretions or substances into the lower airway. It usually follows aspiration of material from the mouth or stomach into the trachea and subsequently the lungs.

Pathophysiology

The pathology of all types of pneumonia is similar. There are four characteristic stages of the disease process:

1. Congestion
   - Initiation of inflammatory pulmonary response to the offending organism or agent takes place.
   - Growth of microorganisms in the serous fluid leads to spread of infection.
   - Interference with lung function by overwhelming growth of organisms occurs.
2. Red hepatization
   - Massive dilatation of the capillaries takes place.
   - Alveoli are filled with organisms, neutrophils, red blood cells and fibrin.
   - Lung appears red and granular (similar to the liver).
3. Gray hepatization
   - Blood flow decreases.
   - Infiltration of leukocytes (neutrophil and macrophages) causes phagocytosis in alveoli.
   - Fibrin and lukocytes deposit on pleural surfaces.

4. Resolution
   - Exudate breakdown and processed by the macrophages.
   - Removal of degenerated neutrophils, fibrin and bacteria from the alveoli starts.
   - Restoration of normal lung tissue begins.
   - Gas exchange ability of the person returns to normal.

Clinical Manifestations

- Any or all of the following manifestations generally mark the onset of all pneumonias:
  - Fever, chills, sweat
  - Pleuritic chest pain
  - Cough productive of purulent sputum
  - Hemoptysis
  - Dspnea
  - Headache
  - Fatigue
  - Altered mental states and dehydration—May be the prominent finding in the elderlies or debilitated patients.
- On examination:
  - Bronchial breath sounds over areas of consolidation
  - Dullness to percussion
  - Increased fremitus
  - Crackles
  - Unequal chest wall expansion, if a large area of the lung is involved.

Complications

Individual with chronic diseases or other risk factors may develop the following complications:

1. Pleurisy
2. Pleural effusion
3. Atelectasis
4. Delayed resolution
5. Lung abscess
6. Empyema
7. Pericarditis
8. Arthritis
9. Meningitis
10. Endocarditis
11. Shock
12. Respiratory failure.

Diagnostic Studies

1. History and physical examination.
2. Chest X-ray shows areas of consolidation and provides information about the location and extent of pneumonia.
3. Gram stain of sputum identifies organisms.
4. Sputum culture and sensitivity—For definitive diagnosis or when drug resistant pathogen is suspected.
5. Pulse oximetry or arterial blood Gas analysis—To assess the need for supplemental oxygen.
6. Complete blood count and differential.
7. Routine blood chemistries if indicated.
8. Blood and urine cultures to assess systemic spread (if indicated).

Collaborative Therapy

1. Antibiotic: Broad spectrum antibiotic or specific antibiotic when the offending organism has been identified.
2. Increased fluid intake (at least 3 liters per day).
3. Limited activity and rest during the acute febrile period.
4. Antipyretics, e.g. aspirin or acetaminophen—To control fever.
5. Analgesics—To relieve the chest pain.
6. Oxygen therapy in high concentration to all hypoxemic patients.
7. Bronchodilators
8. Physiotherapy—Chest physiotherapy which includes percussion, vibration and postural drainage; assisted coughing and tracheal suctioning to maintain airway patency.

NURSING MANAGEMENT

Assessment

Subjective data

Chest pain, pain with breathing, sore throat, headache, fever, anorexia, nausea, vomiting, chills, dyspnea, cough, fatigue, weakness, previous lung cancer, COPD, diabetes, debilitating disease, malnutrition, AIDS, unconsciousness, exposure to chemical toxins, dust or allergens, use of antibiotic, chemotherapy, corticosteroids, immunosuppressants, recent abdominal or thoracic surgery, tube feeding, endotracheal intubation, recent upper respiratory tract infection, smoking, alcoholism.

Objective data

Fever, restlessness or lethargy, splinting of affected area, tachypnea, asymmetric chest movements, nasal flaring, use of accessory muscles, grunting, crackles, pleural friction rub, dullness on percussion over consolidated area, increased tactile fremitus on palpation, pink rusty, purulent, green, yellow or white sputum, tachycardia, changes in mental status (confusion, delirium).

Possible findings

Leukocytosis, abnormal ABGs; positive sputum Gram stain and culture; patchy or diffuse infiltrates, abscesses, pleural effusion, or pneumothorax on chest X-ray.

Nursing Diagnoses

1. Ineffective breathing pattern related to inflammation and pain as manifested by rapid respirations, dyspnea, tachypnea, nasal flaring, and altered chest excursion.
2. Ineffective airway clearance related to thick secretions as manifested by ineffective cough or thick tenacious sputum, abnormal breath sounds, dyspnea.
3. Acute pain related to inflammation as manifested by pleuritic chest pain, pleural friction rub, shallow respirations, decreased breath sounds.
4. Imbalanced nutrition: Less than body requirements related to increased metabolism, fatigue, and anorexia as manifested by weight loss and patient's complain of foul taste in mouth.
5. Activity intolerance related to hypoxia and weakness as manifested by fatigue, unwillingness to exert self, dyspnea, increased pulse and respiration, dizziness on exertion.
6. Ineffective therapeutic regimen management related to knowledge deficit about the disease process, treatment regimen and preventive health measures as evidenced by frequent questioning about illness, management, self care at home.

GOALS

1. Normal breathing pattern
2. Patent airway
3. Control of pain
4. Improving nutritional status
5. Activity tolerance
6. Adherence to treatment protocol and preventive strategies.

Nursing Interventions

Normal breathing pattern

- Monitor respiratory and oxygenation status to provide baseline asessment.
- Auscultate breath sounds, noting areas of decreased or absent sounds, ventilation and presence of adventitious sounds.
- Position to minimize respiratory efforts to reduce oxygen needs.

- Initiate and maintain supplemental oxygen as prescribed to improve respiratory status.
- Administer drugs, e.g. bronchodilators that promote airway patency and gas exchange.

Patent airway

- Monitor rate, rhythm, depth and effort of respiration to provide baseline assessment.
- Auscultate breath sounds, noting areas of decreased or absent ventilation and presence of adventitious sounds for ongoing evaluation of patient's response to therapy.
- Assist patient to a sitting position with head slightly flexed, shoulders relaxed and knees flexed to improve respiratory status.
- Encourage use of incentive spirometry as appropriate to aid in lung expansion and prevent atelectasis.
- Promote systemic fluid hydration as appropriate to help liquefy secretions.

Control of pain

- Assess pain, its location, onset, duration, frequency, quality, intensity and precipitating factors to know baseline status of pain.
- Encourage patient to monitor own pain and to intervene appropriately to allow independence and prepare for discharge.
- Teach the use of nonpharmacologic techniques before, after and during painful activities along with other pain relief measures to relieve pain and reduce the need for analgesia.
- Initiate pain control measures before pain becomes severe because mild to moderate pain is controlled more quickly.
- Medicate before an activity to increase participation, but evaluate the hazards of sedation to minimize pain that will be experienced.

Maintain nutritional status

- Weigh patient at specified interval to assess status of weight.
- Monitor food and fluid ingested and calculate daily caloric intake to assess if meeting patient's need.
- Determine food preferences with consideration of cultural and religious preferences to provide appropriate intake.
- Provide oxygen therapy via nasal canula during mealtime to maintain oxygen status. Position of patient in high Fowler's position to help relieve dyspnea.
- Provide patient with high-protein, high caloric soft foods and fluids, as appropriate to meet nutritional needs.

Activity tolerance

- Determine patient's physical limitations to establish patient's needs and capabilities.
- Monitor cardiorespiratory and oxygen response to activity, e.g. heart rate, pulse rate, pulse oximetry status, etc.
- Plan activities for the periods when patient has the most energy and alternate rest and activity periods.
- Encourage afternoon naps, if appropriate, to reduce stress and promote rest.

Adherence to treatment protocol and preventive strategies

- Determine the patient's current level of knowledge about the disease process, management and preventive strategies to obtain information on patient's teaching needs.

- Explain the pathophysiology of the disease, details of antibiotics treatment their action, dose, duration, so that patient understands the importance of appropriate antibiotic therapy.
- Discuss with patient:
  1. The importance of breathing exercises to clear the lungs and to promote full lung expansion.
  2. Gradual increase of activity.
  3. Importance of follow-up X-ray and physical examination.
  4. To stop smoking as smoking reduces tracheobronchial ciliary action.
  5. To avoid fatigue, sudden changes in temperature and excessive alcohol intake—which lower resistance to pneumonia.
  6. Importance of adequate nutrition and rest to prevent recurrent attacks of pneumonia.
  7. To avoid contact with person with upper respiratory infections and to get prompt treatment if upper respiratory tract infection occurs.

Prevention of Pneumonia

Teaching individuals

- To practice good health habits, e.g. proper diet, hygiene, adequate rest, and regular exercise, which maintain natural resistance to infecting organisms.
- To avoid contact with persons with upper respiratory tract infections.
- To get prompt treatment with supportive measures (rest, fluids) if upper respiratory tract infections occur.
- To obtain medical treatment if upper respiratory tract infection persists for more than 7 days.

In hospital nurse should

- Identify individual at risk for pneumonia (patient with long-term illnesses, debilitated, old).
- Take measures to prevent pneumonia, e.g.
  - Position unconscious patient to prevent aspiration (side lying).
  - Turning and positioning unconscious patient every 2 hours to discourage pooling of secretions.
  - Take appropriate measures to prevent aspiration in tube fed patients.
  - Assist patient with difficulty in swallowing (stroke patient) in eating, drinking and taking medications.
  - Assist postoperative patient in frequent turning, deep breathing.
  - Avoid overmedicating with narcotics and sedatives to postoperative patient.
  - Adhere to principles of medical asepsis and infection control measures to reduce the possibility of nosocomial infection.

ASTHMA

Definition

Asthma is defined as the common chronic inflammatory disease of the airways characterized by variable and recurring symptoms, reversible airflow obstruction, and bronchospasm.

Incidence

- Asthma is a common disease and its incidence is increasing.
- It can occur at any age and is the most common respiratory disease of childhood.

Etiology

- Exact mechanisms that cause asthma are unknown.
- The disease runs in families, which suggests that it is an inherited disorder.

- Environmental factors and other inciting factors (asthma triggers) interact with inherited factors to produce disease and its exacerbations.

Some Environmental Factors and Asthma Triggers are

Animal danders, house dust mites, pollens, cockroaches, exhaust fumes, perfumes, cigarette smoke, upper respiratory infections viz. sinusitis, exposure to cold, dry air, stress, certain foods viz. shrimp, food additives, beer, wine, dried fruits, drugs viz. aspirin, NSAIDs, occupational exposure to certain chemicals or plastics, mineral salts, etc. exercise, hormones or menses, gastroesophageal reflux disease.

Pathophysiology

- When a person with asthma is exposed to extrinsic allergens, irritants or any other factors, e.g. stress, cold air or exercise, immunoglobulin E (IgE) is stimulated.
- IgE antibodies attach to mast cells and basophils of bronchial walls releasing inflammatory mediators, e.g. histamine, bradykinins, prostaglandins, leukotrienes and slow releasing substance of anaphylaxis (SRS-A).
- These inflammatory mediators dilate the capillaries of the bronchial wall in order to dilute and wash away the allergen and cause edema of the bronchial wall and increased mucus secretion.
- These mediators also constrict the airways to prevent further entry of more allergen.
- In late phase these inflammatory mediators attract other inflammatory cells creating a self-sustaining cycle of inflammation and obstruction resulting in hyperresponsiveness of airways.
- Hyperresponsiveness of airways later on gives rise to subsequent episodes in response not only to specific allergens but also to other inciting factors, e.g. breathing cold air or physical exertion.

Clinical Manifestations

- Manifestations of asthma are variable.
- Onset may be abrupt or gradual.
- Asthma attacks often occur at night and may last for a few minutes to several hours.
- The patient may remain asymptomatic in between attacks with normal or nearly normal lung function.
- Some patients may develop an irreversible airway disease leading to a state of continuous asthma with chronic debility and impaired lung function.

The characteristic clinical manifestations of asthma attack are:

- *Wheezing*: Initially during expiration, later during inspiration and expiration.
- *Cough*: It may be the only symptom in some patients. Cough may be nonproductive. Secretions may be thick, tenacious, gelatinous mucus.
- Dyspnea and feelings of suffocation, chest tightness.
- Person shows marked respiratory effort, e.g. nasal flaring, pursed-lip breathing and use of accessory muscles. He sits upright or slightly bends forward, looks anxious.
- Respiratory rate increases to more than 30 per minute.
- Restlessness, increased anxiety, inappropriate behavior, increased pulse and blood pressure and pulsus paradoxus (a drop in systolic pressure during the inspiratory cycle greater than 10 mm Hg) may be evident due to hypoxemia.
- Hyperresonance on percussion of lungs.

- Inspiratory or expiratory wheezing on auscultation. Diminished or absent breath sounds or silent chest may be found in severe disease.
- On auscultation inspiratory or expiratory wheezing is detected. Diminished or absent breath sounds or silent chest may be found in severe disease.

Classification of Asthma

- According to the severity asthma may be classified as:
  - *Severe persistent*: Continual symptoms with limited physical ability.
  - *Moderate persistent*: Daily symptoms with exacerbations at least twice weekly, which affect activity.
  - *Mild persistent*: Symptoms more frequent than twice weekly but less than once a day. Exacerbations may affect activity.
  - *Mild intermittent*: Symptoms no more frequent than twice daily. Patient remains asymptomatic between exacerbations. Exacerbations brief, intensity may vary.
- Other types of asthma are:
  - *Extrinsic or atopic asthma*: It is caused by environmental allergen.
  - *Intrinsic or nonatopic asthma*: It is not caused by allergen.
  - *Exercise-induced asthma*: It occurs with strenuous physical exercise, e.g. asthma found in athletes.
  - *Occupational asthma*: It is caused by exposure to certain substances in the workplace.
  - *Cough variant asthma*: A persistent cough caused by asthma.
  - *Chronic severe corticosteroid-dependent asthma*: It requires continued treatment with oral corticosteroids.

Complications

- Severe acute asthma may result in:

1. Rib fractures
2. Pneumothorax
3. Pneumomediastinum
4. Atelectasis
5. Pneumonia
6. Status asthmaticus.

- Status asthmaticus:
  - A severe, life-threatening complication of asthma.
  - Acute episode of bronchospasms with increased intensity occurs.
  - Severe bronchospasms increase work of breathing leading to corpulmonale.
  - Hypoxia and acidosis develops.
  - Untreated status asthmaticus leads to respiratory or cardiac arrest.

Diagnostic Studies

1. Spirometry (pulmonary function test) reveals:
   - Decreased peak expiratory flow rate (PEFR).
   - Decreased forced expiratory volume in 1 second (FEV1).
   - Decreased forced vital capacity (FVC).
   - 12% to 15% improvement in FEV1 after administration of inhaled bronchodilator indicates reversible airflow obstruction, i.e. asthma.
2. Sputum and blood test reveals:
   - Eosinophilia
   - Elevation of IgE.
3. Chest X-ray during acute attack shows-hyperinflation and other complications of asthma.
4. ABGs:
   - In mild cases: Respiratory alkalosis with arterial oxygen pressure (PaO_2) near normal.
   - In severe cases: Hypercapnia and respiratory and metabolic acidosis.

5. Pulse oximetry: It indicates low oxygen saturation.

Medical Management

Goals

1. Prevention of chronic asthma and its exacerbation.
2. No limitations of normal activity.
3. Maintenance of normal lung function.
4. Minimal or no side effects from use of medications.

Management of Asthma

Patient education

It is the cornerstone of asthma management and involves teaching about—

- Nature of the disease.
- Practical skill necessary to manage asthma successfully.
- Difference between reliever and preventer medications.
- Use of inhaler, peak flow meter.
- Avoidance of precipitating factor.

Drug therapy

- Two general classes of medications are used:

Quick relief medications (reliever)

- Bronchodilators such as—(1) short-acting β_2 adrenergic agonists (albuterol, metaproterenol, pirbuterol, etc.) given by metered-dose inhaler or by nebulizer. (2) inhaled anticholinergics (ipratropium).
- Anti-inflammatory drugs such as corticosteroids may be given in systemic form to get rapid relief of symptoms.

Long-acting control medications (preventer)

Anti-inflammatory drugs

- Corticosteroids used as inhaled form initially or given orally.
- Mast cell stabilizers, e.g. cromolyn and nedocromil are mild to moderate anti-inflammatory drugs, act by suppressing the release of bronchoconstrictive substances during antigen-antibody reaction, used more commonly in children, to prevent exercise-induced asthma and in unavoidable exposure to known triggers.
- Leukotriene modifiers (inhibitors), e.g. montelukast, zafirlukast, zileuton mediate the actions of leukotrienes that are activated during antigen-antibody reaction. Administered orally, they are found to be effective in long-term control of asthma, well-tolerated and have low adverse effects.
- Monoclonal antibody to IgE, e.g. Omalizumab administered subcutaneously every 2 to 4 weeks may be given in moderate to severe allergic asthma that are not cured with inhaled corticosteroids.

Bronchodilators

- Long-acting β_2 adrenergic agonists e.g. bitolterol, formoterol, salmeterol used as metered-dose inhaler to dilate the airways. These are not used for immediate relief but mainly for night time asthma.
- Anticholinergic agents, e.g. ipratropium, tiotropium block the broncho-constricting effects of the parasympathetic nervous system. When used in combination with β_2 adrenergic agonists provide added benefits to the patient.
- Methylxanthines preparations, e.g. theophyllin, aminophyllin are less effective than β_2 adrenergic agonists. They are used when other agents are not effective. Administered orally.

Stepwise approach is used in the management of asthma with drugs. Drug therapy is **stepped up or stepped down** as required:

- Step 1: Occasional use of inhaled short-acting β_2 adrenoreceptor agonists, e.g. salbutamol is used by inhalation as required for the relief of mild symptoms.

  If patient is able to lead an active normal life free from nocturnal and exercise induced asthmatic symptoms he continues with step 1 treatment.

  If patient uses β_2 adrenoreceptor agonist more than once daily he moves to step 2.
- Step 2: Regular inhaled anti-inflammatory agents (inhaled corticosteroids), e.g. beclomethasone dispropionate, budesonide in low dose (800 microgram) and inhaled short-acting β_2 adrenoreceptor agonists as required is used by the patient.
- If no relief patient moves to step 3.
- Step 3: High dose inhaled corticosteroids (800 – 2000 microgram/day) or low dose inhaled corticosteroids (800 microgram) plus a long-acting β_2 adrenoreceptor agonists, e.g. formoterol fumarate 6 microgram 12 hourly or salmeterol 50 microgram 12 hourly is given.
- If no relief patient moves to step 4.
- Step 4: High dose inhaled corticosteroids and regular bronchodilators are given to the patients in addition to other step 3 drugs.
- Step 5: Addition of regular oral corticosteroid therapy together with step 4 treatment is given in step 5 treatment.

Oral corticosteroids, e.g. prednisolone tablets are prescribed in the lowest amount necessary to control symptoms as a single dose in the morning.

- Step down approach: In step down drug treatment, treatment regimen is so selected that disease control is achieved rapidly. If there has been good symptomatic relief for 3 to 6 months, a step down should be made.

Management of Acute Severe Asthma

- Measure FEV1 or PEFR
- Initiate pulse oximetry
- Oxygen inhalation at high concentration usually at 60%
- Administer β2 adrenergic agonists e.g. salbutamol 2.5 to 5 mg or terbutaline 5 to 10 mg by nebulizer every 20 minutes to 4 hours as necessary
- Systemic corticosteroids—oral prednisolone 30 to 60 mg or hydrocortisone 200 mg IV (if the patient cannot swallow or is vomiting) is administered initially and is continued until the patient is breathing comfortably, wheezing disappears and pulmonary function study results are near baseline values.
- Mechanical ventilation may be initiated in a few patients.

NURSING MANAGEMENT

Nursing Assesment

Subjective data

Dyspnea, cough, sputum, chest tightness, feelings of suffocation, interrupted sleep, insomnia, fatigue, decreased exercise tolerance, anxiety, fear, stress in work environment or in home, emotional distress, exposure to allergens, weather changes, exercise, previous asthma attacks, allergic rhinitis, use of aspirin, beta adrenergic blockers, bronchodilators, corticosteroids, allergies or asthma in family members.

Objective data

Increased respiratory effort with use of accessory muscles, tachypnea, upright position, restlessness or exhaustion, cyanosis, diaphoresis, confusion, prolonged expiration, wheezing, crackles, diminished or absent breath sounds, rhonchi on auscultation, hyperresonance on percussion, thick white tenacious sputum,tachycardia, pulsus paradoxus, hypertension, hypotension.

Possible findings

Abnormal ABGs during attacks, decreased oxygen saturation, serum and sputum eosinophilia, increased serum IgE, positive skin test for allergies, chest X-ray showing hyperinflation with attacks, abnormal pulmonary function tests that improve between attacks or with bronchodiators.

Nursing Diagnoses

1. Ineffective breathing pattern related to impaired exhalation and anxiety as evidenced by tachypnea, dyspnea, apprehension and hypoxemia.
2. Ineffective airway clearance related to increased production of secretions and bronchospasms as manifested by ineffective cough, inability to raise secretions and increased inspiratory and expiratory wheezes and rhonchi.
3. Impaired gas exchange related to air trapping as manifested by adventitious breath sounds, cyanosis, nonproductive cough and below normal oxygen saturation.
4. Anxiety related to difficulty in breathing and fear of suffocation as manifested by restlessness; elevated pulse, respiratory rate and blood pressure.
5. Ineffective therapeutic regimen management related to lack of knowledge about asthma and its treatment as manifested by frequent questioning regarding all aspects of long-term management.

GOALS

1. Improved breathing pattern
2. Effective airway clearance
3. Adequate gas exchange
4. Reduction of anxiety
5. Asthma control.

Nursing Interventions

Improved breathing pattern

- Assess patient frequently, respiratory rate and depth.
- Assess breathing pattern, shortness of breath, pursed lip breathing, nasal flaring, use of accessory muscles, or a prolonged expiratory phase.
- Place patient in Fowler's position.
- Administer oxygen as ordered.
- Monitor ABGs and oxygen saturation levels to detect effectiveness of treatment.
- Compare pulmonary function test result with normal values.

Effective airway clearance

- Monitor color and consistency of the sputum.
- Assist the patient to cough effectively.
- Encourage oral fluids to thin the secretions and to replace fluids lost through rapid respiration.
- Provide chest physiotherapy, frequent position changes.
- Administer expectorants as advised.
- Give frequent oral care every 2 to 4 hours to remove the taste of the secretions.

Adequate gas exchange

- Assess lung sounds every hour to determine adequacy of gas exchange.

- Assess skin and mucous membrane color for cyanosis.
- Monitor pulse oximetry for oxygen saturation level.
- Administer oxygen as ordered.

Reduction of anxiety

- Assess level of anxiety.
- Identify precipitating factors of anxiety.
- Use calm, reassuring approach to provide reassurance.
- Stay with patient to provide safety and reduce fear.
- Encourage verbalization of feelings, perceptions, and fears.
- Instruct patient on the use of relaxation techniques to relieve muscle tension and to promote ease of respiration.

Asthma control

- Assess patient's current level of knowledge related to the disease process.
- Instruct the patient on measures to prevent/minimize side effects of treatment for the disease to plan for future problems.
- Evaluate the patient's ability to self-administer medications to assess competence and correct usage.
- Instruct the patient on the purpose, action, dosages and duration of each medication (e.g. inhalers, spacers) to ensure proper use.
- Instruct the family and significant others to ensure knowledgeable help when the patient is in need.

CHRONIC OBSTRUCTIVE PULMONARY DISEASE (COPD)

Definition

Chronic obstructive pulmonary disease is a disease state characterized by the presence of airflow obstruction caused by chronic bronchitis or emphysema.

- The airflow obstruction:
  - Is usually progressive.
  - It may be accompanied by airway hyperreactivity.
  - Is usually irreversible or may be partially reversible.

Chronic bronchitis is the presence of chronic productive cough for 3 months in each of two successive years in a patient in whom other causes of chronic cough have been ruled out.

Emphysema is a disorder where there is an abnormal permanent enlargement of the airspaces distal to the terminal bronchioles, accompanied by destruction of their walls.

Incidence

- It is the 4th leading cause of death in America.
- It is the 6th leading cause of death and 12th leading cause of morbidity worldwide.

Etiology and Risk Factors

- Specific cause not yet understood. Major risk factors are:
  1. Cigarette smoking: The leading risk factor for COPD development is believed to be the effects of several irritants found in cigarette smoke, e.g.
     - Stimulation of excess mucus production and coughing.
     - Destruction of ciliary function in the respiratory tract.
     - Inflammation and damage of bronchiolar and alveolar walls.
  2. Chronic respiratory infections including sinusitis.
  3. Aging.

4. Heredity and genetic predisposition—A genetic abnormality, deficiency of α_1 antitrypsin, an enzyme inhibitor that normally counteracts the destruction of lung tissue by certain other enzymes.

Pathophysiology

A combination of emphysema and chronic bronchitis is commonly found in a person with COPD, often with one condition predominating.

Chronic bronchitis

- Smoking impairs lung's mucocilliary defenses:
  - Increases susceptibility to infection
  - Irritates goblet cells and mucus glands, causing an increased accumulation of mucus.
- When infection develops bronchial walls become inflamed and thickened, mucous production increases.
- Thick mucous and inflamed edematous bronchi obstruct the airways.
- The airways collapse and air is trapped in the distal portion of the lungs resulting into reduced alveolar ventilation.
- Abnormal ventilation/perfusion ratio develops. PaO_2 level decreases. $PaCO_2$ may rise. As a compensatory mechanism polycythemia occurs.

Emphysema

- Recurrent infectious processes lead to increased production and stimulation of neutrophils and macrophages. These cells release proteolytic enzymes (proteases and elastases) that can destroy alveolar tissue.
- In healthy person there is a balance between the proteolytic enzymes and antiproteases in the lungs. In smokers increased number of neutrophils and macrophages releases increased amounts of proteolytic enzymes so that normal antiproteases' action fails to combat alveolar destruction. In addition smoking also inactivates alpha antitrypsin (AAT). AAT inhibits the action of proteolytic enzymes. So lower level of AAT results in insufficient activation and subsequent destruction of alveolar tissue.
- Destruction of alveolar walls (septa), partial collapse of airway and loss of elastic recoil cause difficult respiration.
- As the alveoli and septa collapse, pockets of air form between the alveolar spaces, which are called blebs and when within the lung parenchyma, called bullae.
- This process leads to increased ventilatory dead spaces leading to decreased functional lung tissue that do not participate in gas or blood exchange.
- In the early stage of the disease patient compensates this deficit in ventilation by increasing the rate of respiration and thus does not develop hypoxemia at rest but later on fails to do so resulting into acidosis and hypercapnia.

Clinical Manifestations

Patients with COPD have manifestations of both chronic bronchitis and emphysema.

- Patient with COPD who has chronic bronchitis as the major disease has:
  - Productive cough
  - Dyspnea with exertion
  - Wheezing
  - Shortness of breath
  - Prolonged expiration
  - Frequent respiratory infections.
- With progress of disease:
  - Cough with large amount of sputum.
  - Hypoxemia and hypercapnia.
  - Patient leans over a table with shoulder girdle raised.

- Gait and walking pace changes to take frequent rest periods to breath.
- Patient develops bluish red color of skin due to cyanosis and polycythemia, which develops to combat hypoxemia.

- Manifestations of emphysema:
  - Dyspnea on exertion which gradually progresses to dyspnea at rest.
  - Minimal coughing with no sputum or small amounts of mucoid sputum.
  - Barrel chest due to enlarged anteroposterior diameter of the chest.
  - Effective abdominal breathing decreased, person becomes more of a chest breather.
  - Hyperresonance sound of chest on percussion.
  - X-ray chest shows hyperinflation and flattened diaphragm.
  - ABGs are normal until late in the disease.
  - Hypoxemia during exercise may develop but hypercapnia usually does not develop until late in the disease.
  - Secondary chronic bronchitis may develop in the late stage.

Complications

1. Cor pulmonale.
2. Acute exacerbation of chronic obstructive pulmonary disease.
3. Acute respiratory failure.
4. Peptic ulcer and gastroesophageal Reflux disease.
5. Pneumonia.
6. Depression or anxiety.

Diagnostic Studies

1. History and physical examination.
2. Chest X-ray—It may be normal in the early stage.
   - Hyperinflation, flattened diaphragm in the late stage.
3. Pulmonary function tests
   - Confirm and assess the severity of COPD.
   - Reveal FEV1/FVC<70%.
   - Reduced FEV1 determines the severity of lung disease.
4. Sputum test detects offending organism.
5. ABGs—Monitored in the later stages of COPD find
   - Normal or only slightly decreased PaO_2 and a normal $PaCO_2$ in early stages.
   - Low PaO_2, elevated $PaCO_2$, decreased pH and increased bicarbonate levels in the later stages.
6. Exercise testing with pulse oximetry-evaluates how much desaturation of O_2 occurs with exercise.
7. ECG—It may be normal or may show signs of right ventricular failure.
8. Echocardiogram—It evaluates right ventricular or left ventricular function.

Collaborative Care

- The primary goals of care for the COPD patient are:

A. To improve ventilation.
B. To facilitate the removal of bronchial secretions.
C. To prevent complications.
D. To slow the progression of clinical manifestations.
E. To promote health maintenance and patient management of the disease.

Improve ventilation

1. Bronchodilators are the mainstay in the treatment of COPD.
   a. β_2 agonists such as albuterol, metaproterenol are frequently used.
      They act on the β_2 adrenoreceptors in the smooth muscles of the airways and cause bronchodilation.

Parenteral, oral and inhalation forms are available.

Inhalation route such as metered-dose inhaler or nebulization is preferred because it produces greater bronchodilation and less side effects.

Side effects are tachycardia, tremor, nervousness and nausea.

b. Anticholinergic agents such as ipratropium bromide (atrovent, duolin) another type of bronchodilator.

They are more effective than β_2 adrenergic agonists in the patient with emphysematous COPD.

They act by blocking the cholinergic receptors located in the larger airways, resulting in bronchodilation.

Inhaled forms are preferred and they have minimal side effects.

Side effects include dry mouth, nervousness, dizziness, fatigue, and headache.

These drugs are best taken on a regular basis.

c. Methylxanthines such as theophylline, aminophylline may be used in parenteral or oral form to treat acute exacerbations.

In patients with COPD they act as a mild bronchodilator but they improve the contractility of the diaphragm and decrease diaphragmatic fatigue.

2. Corticosteroids are used in the acute management of patients with COPD exacerbation.

Exact mechanism of action in COPD is poorly understood.

They are administered either orally or parenterally.

3. Oxygen is used when the patient has severe exertional or resting hypoxemia (PaO_2 <40 mm Hg).

A low level of oxygen (1–3 L) is administered to raise the PaO_2 to at least 60 mm Hg.

Oxygen is administered cautiously in these patients. Because of long-standing hypercapnia, the respiratory drive in these patients is triggered by low oxygen levels rather than increased carbon dioxide levels. If high levels of oxygen are administered to these patients, their respiratory drive will not be triggered resulting in carbon dioxide retention.

Remove bronchial secretions

- Postural drainage and chest physiotherapy is prescribed to move secretions from the small to the large airways from which they can be expelled.
- Hospitalized patients may be treated with nebulized bronchodilators and positive end expiratory pressure devices to increase the diameter of the airways thus helping in removal of bronchial secretions.

Promote exercises

- Aerobic exercises are prescribed to strengthen respiratory muscles and to increase cardiovascular fitness to function more effectively.
- Breathing exercises such as diaphragmatic breathing and pursed-lip breathing are taught to the patient.
- Discourage rapid, shallow and panic breathing.

Control complications

- Diuretics and digitalis are used to treat edema and corpulmonale.
- Phlebotomy may be used to reduce blood volume and cardiac workload in patient with hematocrit level > 60%.

Improve general health

- Stop smoking.
- Avoid exposure to known allergens.
- Avoid high altitudes.
- Use supplemental oxygen during air travel.

Nutritional therapy

- Provide 5 to 6 small, frequent meals.
- Liquid, blenderized, grated or pureed foods are preferred.
- High calorie, high protein foods to be given to patient with emphysema.
- Deliver oxygen by nasal canula during meal time.
- Administer at least 3 liters of fluid if not contraindicated due to other medical conditions such as heart failure.

NURSING MANAGEMENT

Nursing Assessment

Subjective data

Repeated respiratory infections, anorexia, weight loss or gain, fatigue, inability to perform ADLs, palpitations, progressive dyspnea, wheezing, repeated cough, sputum production, edema in feet, insomnia, orthopnea, paroxysmal nocturnal dyspnea, long-time exposure to irritants, pollutants, smoking (duration, number—pack years). Use and duration of oxygen use, bronchodilators, corticosteroids, anticholinergics, OTC drugs, herbs, etc. previous hospitalizations. Family history of respiratory disease.

Objective data

Rapid shallow breathing, inability to speak, pursed lip breathing, wheezing, rhonchi, crackles, use of accessory muscles, hyperresonance or dull chest sounds on percussion. Debility/obesity, restlessness, depression, sitting up position, cyanosis or pallor, poor skin turgor, clubbing of nails, peripheral edema. Tachycardia, arrhythmia, jugular vein distension, edema in feet. Ascites, hepatomegaly, muscle atrophy, barrel chest.

Possible findings

Abnormal ABGs, polycythemia, pulmonary function test detects low FEV1/FVC, low FEV1, chest X-ray shows flattened diaphragm and hyperinflation, ECG reveals arrhythmias.

Nursing Diagnoses

1. Impaired gas exchange related to decreased ventilation as manifested by restlessness, anxiety, low PaO_2 value, elevated $PaCO_2$ value and low oxygen saturation at rest.
2. Ineffective airway clearance related to excessive secretions and ineffective cough as manifested by ineffective or absence cough, presence of abnormal breath sounds or absence breath sounds.
3. Anxiety related to acute breathing difficulty and fear of suffocation manifested by patient's behavior and verbal expression.
4. Activity intolerance related to inadequate oxygenation and dyspnea as manifested by increasing dyspnea, tachycardia, tachypnea, and reduced oxygen saturation on exertion.
5. Imbalanced nutrition—Less than body requirements related to reduced appetite, lowered energy level, dyspnea, gastric distention, sputum production and depression as manifested by weight loss, lack of interest in foods and low serum albumin level.

6. Disturbed sleep pattern related to anxiety, dyspnea and disturbing environmental stimuli.
7. Risk for infection related to decreased pulmonary function, ineffective airway clearance, possible corticosteroid therapy and lack of knowledge regarding manifestations of infections and preventive measures.
8. Knowledge deficit regarding home care manifested by frequent questioning about all aspect of home care and the.apeutic regimen.

GOALS

1. Maintenance of gas exchange within normal range for patient.
2. Improved airway clearance.
3. Reduction of anxiety.
4. Improved activity tolerance.
5. Improvement of nutritional status.
6. Improved sleep pattern.
7. Prevention of infection.
8. Adherence of therapeutic program and home care.

Nursing Interventions

Maintenance of gas exchange within normal range for patient

- Place patient in fowler position with support to upper extremity.
- Administer and teach appropriate use of bronchodilators to open the airways.
- Administer oxygen if needed to increase oxygen saturation.
- Teach patient pursed-lip breathing to prolong expiratory phase and slow rate.
- Teach sign, symptoms and consequences of hypercapnia such as confusion, somnolence, irritability, diaphoresis, etc. so that problem can be recognized early and treatment initiated.
- Teach patient to avoid drugs like sedatives, tranquilizers etc. as they further depress respirations.

Improved airway clearance

- Help patient in sitting up position to maximize ventilation.
- Position in semi Fowler position to facilitate cough and prevent aspiration.
- Administer adequate fluid (2–3 liters) to liquefy secretions for adequate expectoration.
- Humidify room air to prevent drying of secretions.
- Teach and supervise effective cough techniques to minimize airway collapse and aid in proper coughing.
- Provide chest physiotherapy such as positioning, percussion and vibration when indicated to use effect of gravity in removing secretions.
- Coordinate timing of inhaled bronchodilator administration, chest physiotherapy and coughing to facilitate expectoration of retained secretions.

Reduction of anxiety

- Remain with the patient during acute episode of breathing difficulties and provide care in a calm and efficient manner.
- Provide a calm and quiet environment to promote relaxation.
- During acute episode, open doors and windows and limit number of people in the room to lessen the patient's perception of suffocation.
- Encourage the use of breathing retraining and relaxation techniques.
- Give sedatives and tranquilizers with extreme caution if prescribed.

Improved activity tolerance

- Monitor the severity of dyspnea and oxygen saturation with and following activity.
- Stop or slow any activity that leads to a significant change in respiratory rate, pulse rate and mental status.
- Maintain supplemental oxygen therapy as needed during activity.
- Schedule active exercise after respiratory therapy or medication such as bronchodilator.
- Assist patient in scheduling a gradual increase in daily activities and exercise.
- Advise the patient to avoid conditions that increase oxygen demand such as extremes of temperature, excess body weight and stress.
- Teach patient energy conservation techniques, such as spacing activities throughout the day, frequent rest periods between activities.
- Teach patient use of pursed-lip and diaphragmatic breathing techniques during activities.

Improvement of nutritional status

- Assist the patient with mouth care before and after meals and as needed.
- Provide small, frequent meals that are high in calories and protein and avoid gas forming foods such as beans and cabbage.
- Provide high calorie high protein supplemental liquids.
- Give oxygen via nasal canula during meal to the hypoxic patient.
- Plan periods of rest after food intake.
- Monitor patient's food intake, weight and serum albumin, hemoglobin level.

Improved sleep pattern

- Identify patient's usual sleep pattern to provide baseline data.
- Identify causes of discomfort and wakefulness.
- Promote relaxation by providing a darkened quiet environment, ensuring adequate room ventilation, and following bedtime routines.
- Schedule care activities to allow periods of uninterrupted sleep.
- Avoid use of sedatives.

Instruct patient measures to promote sleep

- Practice of physical exercise during the day and non stimulating activities in the evening
- Avoid stimulants such as caffeine, alcoholic beverages.
- Maintain a consistent bedtime and a regular bedtime routine
- Eat a high protein snack before bedtime
- Use relaxation techniques such as meditation, massage, warm bath, and warm beverage.

Prevention of infection

- Teach patient to wash hands after contact with potentially infectious materials.
- Teach patient and family how to care for and clean respiratory equipment used at home.
- Teach patient and family manifestations of pulmonary infections such as change in color or volume of sputum, fever, chills, malaise, productive cough, confusion and increasing dyspnea.
- Teach patient self-care and when to call a physician when infection occurs.

Adherence of therapeutic program and homecare

- Help patient understand short and long term goals.
- Teach patient about disease, medications and therapeutic procedures, and how and when to contact physician.

- Teach patient pulmonary hygiene and to stop smoking.
- Refer patient to antismoking clinic if necessary.

PULMONARY TUBERCULOSIS

Definition

Tuberculosis (TB) is an infectious disease caused by *Mycobacterium tuberculosis* that primarily affects the lung parenchyma. But it also may be transmitted to the larynx, meninges, kidneys, bones, lymph glands and disseminated throughout the body.

Incidence

TB is the most common infectious disease. 19% to 43 % of the world's population is infected.

Etiology

Mycobacterium tuberculosis is a gram-positive acid-fast bacillus. It spreads from one person to other via air-borne droplets produced by individuals with pulmonary or laryngeal TB during coughing, sneezing, singing or speaking.

Risk Factors

- Close contact with someone who has active TB.
- Immuno compromised states, e.g. HIV infection, cancer, transplanted organs and prolonged high dose corticosteroid therapy.
- Substance abuse (IV drug users, alcoholics).
- Persons with inadequate healthcare.
- Preexisting medical conditions or special treatments, e.g. diabetes, chronic renal failure, malnutrition, hemodialysis, gastrectomy, etc.
- Institutionalization, e.g. psychiatric institutions, prisons
- Living in overcrowded, substandard housing.
- Healthcare worker performing high risk activities, e.g. bronchoscopy, suctioning, coughing procedures, intubation, etc.

Pathophysiology

Primary infection

The first time a person is infected with TB, the disease is said to be primary infection. Primary TB infections are usually located in the apices of the lungs or near the pleura of the lower lobe. The following sequence of events is typically observed during primary infection:

- After inhalation of *Mycobacterium tuberculosis* by a susceptible person, bacilli reach the alveoli and begin multiplication with no initial resistance from the host.
- Body's immune system is activated and initiates inflammatory reactions. A small area of bronchopneumonia develops in the lung tissue.
- Although phagocytes (neutrophils and macrophages) engulf many of the bacteria but they continue to survive within phagocytes until development of hypersensitivity and immunity. The live bacilli may be carried to other parts of the body by blood and lymph system. Thus the infection although small spreads rapidly.
- Eventually cellular immunity develops, which limits further multiplication and spread of infection. A characteristic tissue reaction called granuloma results.
- Granulomas, new tissue masses of live and dead bacilli are surrounded by neutrophils and macrophages forming a protective fibrous wall around the granulomas.

- The central portion of the granulomas called a Gohn tubercle may undergo a process of necrotic degeneration which produces cavities filled with a cheese-like mass of tubercle bacilli, dead white blood cells and necrotic lung tissue. This process is known as caseous necrosis. Later this material liquefies and drains into the tracheobronchial tree and may be coughed up leaving air-filled cavities which is detected on X-ray.
- Primary lesions heal by resolution, fibrosis and calcification. The granulomas become more fibrous and form a collagenous scar around the Gohn tubercle. A Gohn complex is formed consisting of Gohn tubercle and regional lymph nodes. Calcified Gohn complexes are seen on chest X-ray.
- Primary TB infections cause the body to develop an allergic reaction to tubercle bacilli or their proteins. This cell mediated immune response appears in the form of sensitive T cells and is detected as a positive reaction to a tuberculine skin test. This sensitivity reaction appears in all body cells 2 to 6 weeks after the primary reaction and is maintained as long as living bacilli remain in the body. This acquired immunity usually inhibits further growth of bacilli and the development of active infection. At this point bacilli remain dormant.
- If the initial immune response is not adequate, control of the organisms is not maintained and clinical disease results.

Secondary infection

- Dormant but living organisms persist for years.
- Reactivation of TB can occur if the host's defense mechanisms become impaired and progresses to a clinical form of active TB.
- In addition to progressive primary disease reinfection may also lead to active TB or secondary infection.

Clinical Manifestations

Onset of manifestations is usually gradual. Manifestations may be classified as systemic and pulmonary.

- Systemic manifestations
  - Fatigue, malaise
  - Anorexia, weight loss
  - Low grade fever, night sweats.
- Pulmonary manifestations
  - Cough, which is frequent, produces mucoid or mucopurulent sputum.
  - Hemoptysis usually associated with advanced disease.
- Some patients may develop acute symptoms, e.g.
  - High fever and chills
  - Generalized flu-like symptoms
  - Pleuritic pain
  - Productive cough.
- Some patients may be asymptomatic in early stage and diagnosed only during routine clinical examination.

Complications

1. Miliary Tuberculosis or hematogenous tuberculosis occurs when a necrotic Gohn complex erodes through a blood vessel spreading large number of organisms to all body organs through circulation. Patient may develop acute symptoms, e.g. fever, dyspnea and cyanosis or chronically ill with systemic manifestations, e.g. weight loss, fever, gastrointestinal disturbances, hepatomegally, splenomegally and generalized lymphadenopathy.
2. Pleural effusion is caused by release of caseous material into pleural space. Bacteria containing material produces inflammatory reaction with exudates of protein-rich fluid.

3. Empyema (less common) may occur from large numbers of organisms spilling in to the pleural space following rupture of a cavity.
4. Tuberculosis pneumonia—Acute pneumonia may result when large numbers of bacteria are discharged from the liquefied necrotic lesion into the lungs or lymph nodes.
5. Other organ involvement—Although the lungs are the primary site of tuberculosis infection, after initial invasion, bacilli can spread to other body organs via blood and lymphs. Meninges, bone, joints, kidneys, adrenal glands, lymph nodes and male and female genital tracts may also be involved.

Diagnostic Studies

- **Tuberculin skin test**: Positive reaction indicates the presence of tuberculosis infection but it does not show whether the infection is dormant or active causing a clinical illness.
- Chest X-ray reveals multinodular lymph node involvement with cavitations in the upper lobes of the lungs. Calcification of lung lesion suggests old primary infection.
- Bacteriologic studies—
  1. Sputum smear for acid-fast bacilli—Positive result usually confirms active disease. Three different sputum specimens are usually examined on three consecutive mornings.
  2. Sputum culture —It is the most accurate means of diagnosis. Positive culture for mycobacterium tuberculosis confirms active disease. But 6 to 8 weeks time is required for the bacilli to grow in the culture medium, which is a major disadvantage.

Management

Most patients are treated on an outpatient basis. Hospitalization may be required for:
- Diagnostic evaluation.
- Severely ill or debilitated person.
- Person experiencing severe drug reaction.
- Treatment failures.

Drug therapy

Drug therapy is the main modality of TB treatment and is used to:
- Treat an individual with clinical disease or active disease.
- To prevent disease in an infected person or latent tuberculosis infection.

Drug therapy for TB consists of a combination of at least four antitubercular drugs given for 6 to 9 months. Drugs are used in combination to: 1) increase the therapeutic effectiveness and 2) decrease the development of resistance strains of M. tuberculosis.

Antitubercular drugs are bacteriocidal and bacteriostatic. 13 antitubercular drugs are available. Among them 6 are considered to be essential, e.g.

1. Isoniazide (INH)	Bacteriocidal
2. Rifampicin (RMP)	,,
3. Pyrazinamide (Z)	,,
4. Streptomycin (S)	,,
5. Ethambutol (E)	Bacteriostatic
6. Thioacetazone	,,

NURSING MANAGEMENT

Assessment

Subjective data

Tuberculosis in the family, afternoon temperature elevation, anorexia, weight loss, night sweats, fatigue, productive cough, pleuritic chest pain, living in crowded environments, substance abuse, lack of knowledge regarding disease, treatment and prevention of transmission to others.

Objective data

Diminished breath sounds, bronchial sounds, crackles, fremitus, dullness on percussion, enlarged, painful lymph nodes.

Nursing Diagnoses

1. Ineffective airway clearance related to copious tracheobronchial secretions.
2. Noncompliance related to lack of knowledge of disease process, lack of motivation and long-term nature of treatment.
3. Ineffective health maintenance related to lack of knowledge about the disease process and therapeutic regimen.
4. Activity intolerance related to fatigue, decreased nutritional status and fever.
5. Risk of complications e.g. malnutrition, side effects of medications, e.g. hepatitis, neurological changes, skin rash, gastrointestinal upset, multidrug resistance, etc.

GOALS

1. Promoting airway clearance.
2. Compliance of therapeutic regimen.
3. Maintenance of health by acquisition of knowledge about the disease and therapeutic regimen.
4. Increased activity tolerance and promoting adequate nutrition.
5. Absence of complications.

Nursing Interventions

Promoting airway clearance

- Monitor rate, rhythm, depth of respiration, coughing effort, and sputum production.
- Auscultate lungs for presence of adventitious sounds.
- Encourage patient deep breathing to aid in lung expansion, prevent Atelectasis and induce coughing.
- Promote fluid intake to liquefy secretions.
- Assist patient correct positioning for postural drainage to facilitate airway drainage.

Complying with therapeutic regimen

- Make the patient understand that TB is a communicable disease and that taking medications is the most effective way of preventing transmission.
- Instruct the patient to take the drugs regularly as prescribed to prevent drug resistance and relapse.
- Refer patient to public health department for DOT (direct observation treatment) if noncompliance is suspected.

Maintenance of health by acquisition of knowledge about the disease and therapeutic regimen

- Teach patient regarding disease process, therapeutic regimen and health maintenance and examination of contacts.
- Teach patient about the disease process and drug therapy for prescribed duration, importance of good nutrition, hygienic measures, e.g. mouth care, covering mouth and nose while coughing and sneezing, proper disposal of sputum and hand washing.

Increased activity tolerance and promoting adequate nutrition

- Determine patient's physical limitation to establish patient's needs.
- Plan activities for periods when patient has maximum energy. Alternate rest and activity periods.
- Provide small frequent nutritious diet.
- Provide mouth care before and after each meal to stimulate appetite.

Absence of complications

- Malnutrition
  - Collaborate with dietitian, physician, and social worker, family and patient to identify strategies to ensure an adequate nutritional intake and availability of nutritional foods.

Side effects of medication therapy

- Instruct the patient to take the medication either on an empty stomach or 1 hour before meals to promote absorption.
- Monitor side effects of TB medication, e.g. hepatitis, hearing loss, neuritis, etc.
- Monitor serum creatinine level, liver enzyme, etc. to detect medication related changes in liver and kidney function.
- Monitor sputum for AFB report to evaluate the effectiveness of treatment regimen and adherence to therapy.
- Provide supplemental vitamins as prescribed.

Multi drug resistance

- Monitor patient's clinical status, e.g. body temperature, respiratory status.
- Report deterioration of clinical status promptly to the physician.
- Instruct patient to continue medicine strictly and continuously as advised.
- Explain the risk of drug resistance if the medication regimen is not followed as advised.
- Spread of TB infection (miliary tuberculosis)
  - Monitor vital signs of patient including body temperature, respiratory status, cough.
  - Assess anemia, debility, enlarged spleen, leucopenia, changes in renal function and cognitive function.
- Report physician patient's deteriorating condition promptly.

PLEURAL EFFUSION

Definition

Pleural effusion is an accumulation of fluid in the pleural space.

Etiology

Normally pleural fluid continually seeps into the pleural space from the capillaries lining the parietal pleura and is reabsorbed by the visceral pleural capillaries and lymphatic system.

Any condition that interferes with secretion or drainage of pleural fluid leads to pleural effusion.

Causes of pleural effusion are grouped into four major categories:

1. Conditions that increase systemic hydrostatic pressure, e.g. heart failure.
2. Conditions that reduce capillary oncotic pressure, found in chronic liver or renal failure.
3. Conditions that increase capillary permeability, e.g. infections or trauma.
4. Conditions that impair lymphatic functions, e.g. lymphatic obstruction by tumor.

Types

Depending on the protein content of the effusion, pleural effusion is classified as:

Transudative

- Transudates are substances that have passed through a membrane or tissue surface.
- Occur primarily in conditions in which there is protein loss and low protein content, e.g. hypoalbuminemia, cirrhosis, nephrosis, or increased hydrostatic pressure, e.g. heart failure.

Exudative

- Exudates are substances that have escaped from blood vessels.
- Contain an accumulation of cells, have a high specific gravity and a high lactate dehydrogenase (LDH) level.
- Occur in response to malignancies, infections or inflammatory processes, which increase capillary permeability.

Clinical Manifestations

Clinical manifestations depend on the amount of fluid present and the severity of lung compression.

Small effusion

- It may remain asymptomatic
- It may be discovered on chest X-ray.

Large effusion

- Decreased movement of the chest wall on the affected side (lung expansion restricted).
- Progressive dyspnea, primarily on exertion.
- Dry nonproductive cough due to bronchial irritation or mediastinal shift.
- Pleuritic pain due to underlying disease
- Dullness on percussion.
- Absent or decreased breath sounds over the affected area.
- Tracheal deviation away from the affected side may be noted.

Diagnostic Studies

- Physical examination
- Chest X-ray
- Chest CT scan.
- Thoracentesis and examination of pleural fluid helps to establish diagnosis such as:
  - Whether transudate or exudate (helps establish a specific diagnosis).
  - Presence of red blood cells, white blood cells, malignant cells, bacteria, glucose content, pH and LDH.
  - Hemorrhagic pleural fluid (may be due to tumor, trauma or pulmonary embolous with infarction).
  - Chylous or thick white pleural fluid (after lymphatic obstruction or trauma to the thoracic duct).
  - Rich in cholesterol (tuberculosis or rheumatoid arthritis).
  - High WBC count and purulent (empyema).

Management

Objectives

- To discover the underlying cause.
- To prevent reaccumulation of fluid.
- To relieve discomfort and dyspnea.

Objectives are achieved by

1. Treatment of underlying cause, e.g. heart failure, cirrhosis, pneumonia etc.
2. Thoracentesis to remove fluid, to obtain specimen for analysis and to relieve dyspnea.

Recurrent pleural effusion (malignancy induced effusion) is treated by

1. Chemical pleurodesis: The procedure involves instillation of a sclerosing substance (doxycycline, bleomycin or talc) into the pleural space via a chest tube to create an inflammatory response that causes the pleura to adhere and sclerose to each other. After instillation of the sclerosing agent the chest tube is clamped and the patient is assisted to take various positions to spread the agent uniformly throughout the pleural space.
2. Pleurectomy (pleural stripping): In this procedure surgical stripping of the parietal pleura away from the visceral pleura is done in order to produce an intense inflammatory reaction that promotes adhesion formation between the two layers during healing.

Nursing Management

1. Nursing care related to the underlying cause of the pleural effusion is specific to the underlying disease (discussed in different sections).
2. Care of a patient with a chest tube (discussed in page 93–95).
3. Implementation of the medical regimen:
   - Prepare patient for the medical regimen prescribed, e.g. thoracentesis, pleurodesis or pleurectomy.
   - Help patient in assuming desired position during and after the procedure.
   - Provide emotional support throughout the procedure.
   - Monitor the functioning of the chest tube drainage and water seal system if any.
   - Monitor respiratory rate and ventilation pattern of the patient.
   - Encourage deep breathing, change of position and ambulation to promote drainage.
4. Relief of pain:
   - Assess pain
   - Assist patient in assuming positions that are least painful
   - Administer analgesics as prescribed and as needed.

LUNG CANCER

Definition

Lung cancer is the malignancy in the epithelium of the respiratory tract.

Incidence

It is the leading cause of cancer deaths worldwide.

Incidence is more in male but the incidence in female is rising steadily.

Disease affects persons mostly in sixth or seventh decade of life.

Etiology and Risk Factors

- Cigarette smoke is the most important factor for lung cancer. Lung cancer is 10 times more in cigarette smokers than in nonsmokers. Persons exposed to passive smoking also are at increased risk compared to nonsmokers.
- Environmental and occupational inhaled carcinogens, e.g. asbestos, radon, nickel, iron, iron oxides, uranium, polycyclic aromatic hydrocarbons, arsenic and automobile fumes are the most important cause for nonsmokers.
- Genetic predisposition seems to play certain causative factor since incidence of lung cancer in close relatives has been found to be 2 to 3 times more.
- Dietary Factors—Smokers who eat a diet low in fruits and vegetables are at increased risk of lung cancers. The actual ingredients in diets rich in fruits and vegetables are yet to be determined.
- Underlying lung disease, e.g. pulmonary tuberculosis is also a causative factor.

Types and Characteristics of Lung Cancer

Nonsmall cell lung cancer (NSCLC)

Squamous cell carcinoma

- Arises from bronchial epithelium.
- Produces earlier symptoms as it causes bronchial obstruction.
- Spreads locally by direct extension, less tendency to metastasize.
- Surgical resection is usually attempted.
- Life expectancy is better than small cell lung cancer.

Adenocarcinoma

- Arises from bronchial mucous gland.
- Usually remain asymptomatic until widespread metastasis.
- Surgical resection is often attempted.

- Cancer does not respond to chemotherapy.

Large cell carcinoma
- Arises from peripheral bronchus.
- Causes cavitation.
- Highly metastatic.
- Surgery usually not attempted due to high rate of metastasis.
- Tumor may be radiosensitive but often recurs.

Small cell lung cancer (SCLC) (oat cell)

- Arises in the major bronchii and spread by infiltration along the bronchial wall.
- Most malignant form of lung cancer
- Metastasizes early
- Frequently associated with endocrine disturbances
- Causes bronchial obstruction and pneumonia
- Has poorest prognosis.

Pathophysiology

Tumor cells grow and invade surrounding lung tissue.

Cancerous lung tissue cannot exchange oxygen and carbon dioxide.

Tumor invades airways causing obstruction in the flow of air.

Certain lung cancers produce hormones, enzymes and antigens producing systemic manifestations called paraneoplastic syndrome.

Clinical Manifestations

Manifestations develop gradually. Most of the time patient remains asymptomatic until disease is advanced. Manifestations depend upon type of primary lung cancer, its location and size of the tumor, degree of bronchial obstruction and presence of metastasis.

Early manifestations

- Persistent dry cough initially, later with sputum production, sputum may also be blood tinged.
- Chest pain may be localized, unilateral, and mild to severe.
- Dyspnea.
- Auscultatory wheeze.

Late manifestations

- Nonspecific systemic symptoms, e.g. anorexia, nausea, vomiting, fatigue and weight loss.
- Hoarseness due to laryngeal nerve involvement.
- Dysphagia.
- Symptoms of pleural or pericardial effusion.
- Palpable lymph node in the neck and axilla.
- Head and neck edema due to superior vena cava obstruction.

Diagnostic Studies

- Chest X-ray shows obstructive feature of tumor, e.g. atelectasis or pneumonia, evidence of metastasis to the ribs or vertebra, pleural effusion.
- Sputum for cytologic study may show malignant cells.
- Bronchoscopy provides direct visualization when the lesion is endobronchial or near an airway and allows collection of specimen for histopathological studies.
- CT Scan is the most effective noninvasive technique. Location and extent of masses in the chest is evaluated.
- MRI provides high quality image of lung and mediastinum and detects extent of invasion.
- Mediastinoscopy and video assisted thoracoscopy detect the presence of tumor extrapleurally. Done for staging.

- Positron emission tomography is an useful tool for early diagnosis.
- Fine needle aspiration obtains tissue sample for histopathological examination.
- Lung scan assesses overall pulmonary status.

Management

Surgical therapy

- Lobectomy (removal of one or more lobes) or pneumonectomy (removal of one entire lung).
- Is the only hope for cure
- Done in early stage of disease when the tumor is localized and is resectable.
- Usually attempted in squamous cell carcinoma and adenocarcinoma.

Radiation therapy

- Used as a curative measure in a patient with resectable tumor but who is considered a poor surgical risk.
- Results in improved survival when used in combination with surgery and chemotherapy.
- Used as a palliative measure to relieve distressing symptoms of cough, hemoptysis, bronchial obstruction and superior venacava syndrome.

Chemotherapy

- Used in nonresectable tumors or as adjuvant therapy to surgery in NSCLC.
- Has strong response rate in SCLC but majority of patients still die from the disease.
- A variety of drugs and multidrug regimens are used.
- The drugs include etoposide, carboplatin, cisplatin, paclitaxel, vinorelbine, cyclophosphamide, ifosfamide, docetaxel, topotecan and irinotecan.

NURSING MANAGEMENT

Assessment

Subjective data

History of smoking, exposure to second hand smoke, environmental pollutants, air-borne carcinogen, lung cancer in family, frequent respiratory infections, use of cough medicines or other respiratory medications, anorexia, nausea, vomiting, dysphagia (late manifestation), weight loss, fatigue, persistent cough, dyspnea, hemoptysis (late manifestation), chest pain or tightness, shoulder and arm pain, headache, bone pain (late manifestation).

Objective data

Fever, neck and axillary lymphadenopathy, wheezing, hoarseness, stridor, pleural effusion, pericardial effusion, cardiac tamponade, pathologic fracture, jaundice (liver metastasis), edema of face and neck (superior vena cava syndrome), clubbing of fingers.

Possible findings

Lesion seen on chest X-ray, CT scan, positive sputum for cytologic studies, biopsy specimen positive for malignancy.

Nursing Diagnoses

1. Ineffective airway clearance related to increased tracheobronchial secretions and presence of tumor.
2. Anxiety related to lack of knowledge of diagnosis or unknown prognosis and treatments.
3. Acute pain related to presence of tumor on surrounding structures.
4. Imbalanced nutrition less than body requirements related to increased metabolic demands, increased secretions, weakness and anorexia.

5. Ineffective health maintenance related to lack of knowledge about the disease process and therapeutic regimen.
6. Ineffective breathing pattern related to decreased lung capacity.

GOALS

1. Promoting airway clearance
2. Establish effective breathing patterns and tissue oxygenation
3. Relief of pain
4. Developing a realistic attitude towards treatment and prognosis.

Interventions

Promoting airway clearance

- Place patient in Fowler's position to help in chest expansion, and facilitate cough.
- Ensure oral intake of 2 to 3 liters of fluid per day to liquefy secretions.
- Teach deep breathing and effective cough techniques to aid in proper coughing and removing secretions.
- Provide chest physiotherapy, suctioning when indicated in removing secretions
- Administer bronchodilators as prescribed to promote bronchial dilation.

Establish effective breathing patterns and tissue oxygenation

- Monitor respiratory and oxygenation status to determine the need for intervention.
- Help patient in assuming positions that promote lung expansion.
- Administer supplemental oxygen as indicated to promote tissue oxygenation.
- Teach patient energy conservation and airway clearance techniques to relieve dyspnea and fatigue.

Relief of pain

- Assess pain and discomfort using a pain scale.
- Assess other factors contributing to patient's pain, e.g. fatigue, fear, anger, etc.
- Administer analgesics to promote optimum pain relief as prescribed by the physician.
- Encourage strategies of pain relief if any that patient has used successfully in previous pain experience.
- Teach patient nonpharmacologic pain relief strategies, e.g. distraction, imagery, relaxation, cutaneous stimulation, etc.

Developing a realistic attitude towards treatment and prognosis

- Encourage verbalization of fears, concerns and questions regarding disease, treatment and future implications.
- Encourage active participation of patient in care and treatment decisions.
- Teach patient possible side effects of treatment and strategies to manage them.

CHEST TRAUMA

The chest is a large, exposed portion of the body that is vulnerable to impact injuries. Because it houses the heart, lungs and great vessels, trauma to the chest frequently produces life-threatening disruptions of cardiopulmonary functions.

Types

1. Blunt chest trauma results when the chest wall is subjected to severe sudden compression or positive pressure.
2. Penetrating chest trauma occurs when a foreign object penetrates the chest wall.

Causes

Causes of blunt chest trauma are

- Automobile crashes resulting in deceleration injuries.
- Pedestrian accident.
- Fall.
- Assault with blunt objects.
- Blows to the chest.
- Crush injury.
- Explosion.

Causes of penetrating chest trauma are

- Gunshot
- Knife, stick, arrow, other missiles.

Pathophysiology

Injuries to the chest are often life-threatening and result in one or more of the following pathophysiologic mechanisms:

a. Hypoxemia resulting from disruption in the airway, injury to the lung parenchyma, fractured ribs, injury to respiratory muscles, massive hemorrhage, collapsed lung and pneumothorax due to open chest wound.
b. Hypovolemia resulting from massive fluid loss from injured great vessels, cardiac rupture, and hemothorax.
c. Cardiac failure from cardiac tamponade, cardiac contusion, increased intrathoracic pressure.

These pathophysiologic mechanisms may lead to impaired ventilation perfusion giving rise to acute respiratory failure (ARF), hypovolemic shock and even death of patient.

Assessment

Initial assessment is directed toward identifying and treating immediate life-threatening condition. Any individual with chest trauma should be considered to have a serious injury unless it is proved otherwise.

Assessment of airway patency, adequacy of breathing and circulation is of primary concern.

- A quick history to be obtained from the injured person or witnesses regarding:
  - When the injury occurred
  - Mechanism of injury
  - Level of responsiveness
  - Specific injuries
  - Pain
  - Estimated blood loss
  - Recent drug or alcohol use
  - Significant medical history
  - Prehospital treatment.
- A quick (1 minute) assessment is performed for:
  - Shortness of breath and cyanosis
  - Skin color and temperature
  - Wound size and location
  - Paradoxical chest movement
  - Distended neck veins
  - Tracheal deviation
  - Respiratory stridor
  - Bilateral breath sounds
  - Use of accessory muscles
  - Subcutaneous emphysema
  - Sucking chest wounds
  - Heart sounds
  - Dysrhythmias.

Diagnostic Tests

- Chest X-ray
- Complete blood count
- Clotting studies
- Type and cross match
- Electrolytes
- Arterial blood gas analysis
- ECG
- CT scan.

COLLABORATIVE CARE

Goals

- To evaluate the condition of the patient
- To initiate aggressive resuscitation.

Emergency Management

1. Ensure patent airway.
2. Administer oxygen.
3. Establish IV access with two large bore catheters. Begin fluid resuscitation as appropriate.
4. Remove clothing to assess injury.
5. Cover sucking chest wound with non-porous dressing taped securely from all sides.
6. Stabilize impaled objects with bulky dressings. Do not remove.
7. Assess for other significant injuries and treat accordingly.
8. Stabilize flail rib segment with hand followed by application of large pieces of tape horizontally across the flail segment.
9. Place patient in semi-Fowler's position or position patient on the injured side if breathing is easier, after cervical spine injury has been ruled out.
10. Monitor vital signs, level of consciousness, oxygen saturation, cardiac rhythm, respiratory status and urinary output.
11. Anticipate intubation for respiratory distress.
12. Release dressing if tension pneumothorax develops after sucking chest wound is covered.

Drug Therapy

- Volume expanders, e.g. crystalloids, blood and blood products.
- Antibiotics.
- Analgesics, e.g. morphine, meperidine.
- Sedatives, e.g. lorazepam, diazepam, midazolam.
- Anesthetics, e.g. lidocaine.

SPECIFIC CHEST INJURIES

Fractured Ribs

Rib fractures are common chest injuries, particularly in the elderly. Ribs 5 through 10 are most commonly affected.

Etiology

- A fall
- A blow to the chest
- Impact of the chest against a steering wheel during rapid deceleration.

Pathology

- Pain due to fractured rib.
- Patient splints his chest wall, takes shallow breaths and coughs ineffectively to reduce pain.
- Shallow breathing and ineffective cough leads to accumulation of secretions in the bronchi.
- Accumulation of secretions obstructs bronchi and obstructed bronchi become the sites of infections leading to atelectasis and pneumonia.
- Bone splinters from fractured ribs may give rise to pneumothorax and hemothorax.

Clinical manifestations

- Localized pain and tenderness on inspiration and palpation
- Shallow respiration
- Tendency to hold the chest protectively or to breath shallowly
- Bruising or surface markings at the injured site
- Clicking sensation during inspiration
- Bright red sputum if the lung has been punctured by bone splinters.

Management

Goal is to decrease pain so that the patient can breathe adequately to promote good chest expansion and is achieved by:

- Analgesics
- Injections of local anesthetics at fracture site if pain is severe and impairs ventilation
- Intercostals nerve block may also be used if pain is severe
- Splinting or application of chest binder is controversial since they reduce lung expansion.

Flail Chest

Flail chest results when two or more adjacent ribs are fractured at two or more sites causing instability of the chest wall. The chest wall cannot provide the bony structure necessary to maintain bellows action and ventilation.

Pathophysiology

- Flail section looses bony or cartilaginous connections with the rest of the rib cage, moves independently of the chest wall during ventilation.
- Independent movement of the flail chest results in paradoxical motion, i.e. flail segment and underlying tissue are sucked in during inspiration and blown out during expiration.
- This abnormal movement results in inadequate tidal volume and ineffective cough.
- Hypoventilation and hypoxia thus produced leads to respiratory failure.
- Paradoxical movement of the mediastinal structures affect circulatory dynamics producing elevated venous pressure, impaired filling of the right side of the heart and decreased arterial pressure.

Clinical manifestations

- Asymmetric and uncoordinated movement of the thorax
- Rapid, shallow and labored breathing
- Breath sounds are absent or decreased on the affected side
- Crepitus is felt at fracture site
- Hypercapnia and hypoxia
- Tachycardia and hypotension.

Management

In mild to moderate flail chest injury

- Pulmonary physiotherapy which includes clearing secretions, coughing and deep breathing to aid in the expansion of lung.
- Humidified oxygen inhalation.
- Analgesics or intercostals nerve block to control pain.
- Monitoring fluid intake and appropriate fluid replacement.

In severe flail chest injury

- Endotacheal intubation and ventilatory support
- Monitoring by serial chest X-rays, ABGs, pulse oximetry and bedside pulmonary monitoring
- Analgesics or intercostal nerve block to control pain.

PNEUMOTHORAX

Pneumothorax is the presence of air in the pleural space that prohibits complete lung expansion.

It may be closed or open.

Closed Pneumothorax

It has no associated external wound. Air may escape into the pleural space from a puncture or tear in an intrapleural respiratory structure. Spontaneous pneumothorax is the most common form.

Causes

- Injury to the lungs from mechanical ventilator.
- Injury to the lungs from broken ribs.
- Injury to the lungs from insertion of a subclavian catheter.
- Ruptured blebs or bullae in a patient with chronic obstructive pulmonary disease.

Clinical manifestations

- Tachypnea, dyspnea.
- Sudden sharp pain on the affected side with chest movement, breathing or coughing.
- Asymmetric chest expansion, diminished or absent breath sounds on the affected side.
- Restlessness, anxiety, tachycardia.

In severe emphysema patient will also exhibit

- Distended neck veins
- Point of maximal impulse shift
- Subcutaneous emphysema
- Tracheal deviation toward the unaffected side
- Progressive cyanosis.

Management

A chest tube is inserted into the pleural space via the fourth intercostal space at midaxillary or anterior axillary line and then it is connected to the closed chest drainage.

Thoracotomy is performed to explore the chest surgically and repair the site of origin of pneumothorax or hemothorax (blood in the pleural space).

Open Pneumothorax

It occurs when air enters the pleural space through an opening in the chest wall viz. stab or gunshot wounds and surgical thoracotomies. A penetrating chest wound is often referred to as sucking chest wound.

Clinical manifestations

- Obvious injury at affected side.
- Sucking noise on inspiration.
- Subcutaneous emphysema in upper chest and neck.
- Signs of reduced venous return, i.e. neck vein distention, tachycardia.

Management

Cover the wound immediately with anything available in hand.

Assess for tension pneumothorax and mediastinal shift.

Insert chest tube attached with closed drainage to remove air from pleural space and allow lung to expand if collapsed.

TENSION PNEUMOTHORAX

Tension pneumothorax is a pneumothorax with rapid accumulation of air in the pleural space causing severely high intrapleural pressures with resultant tension on the heart and great vessels.

Pathophysiology

- It may result from either an open or a closed pneumothorax.
- In an open chest wound a flap may act as a one-way valve, thus air can enter on respiration but cannot come out.
- The intrathoracic pressure increases, the lung collapses, and the mediastinum shifts towards the unaffected side.
- Mediastinal shift may cause compression of the lung opposite the pneumothorax; compression, traction, torsion or kinking of the great vessels, seriously decreasing the return of blood to the

heart. This ultimately reduces cardiac output and blood pressure.
- If tension pneumothorax is not promptly treated patient may die due to circulatory and respiratory collapse.

Clinical Manifestations

- Marked severe dyspnea, tachypnea.
- Subcutaneous emphysema in the neck and upper chest.
- Progressive cyanosis.
- Acute chest pain on the affected side, a feeling of tightness or pressure within the chest.
- Asymmetrical chest wall movement.
- Diminished or absent breath sounds on the affected side.
- Tachycardia, extreme restlessness and agitation.
- Neck vein distension, severe hypotension leading to shock, muffled heart sound.
- Laryngeal and tracheal deviation or shift to the unaffected side.
- A point of maximal impact shift laterally or medially.

Management

Immediately convert a tension pneumothorax into an open pneumothorax by

1. Insertion of a large bore chest tube on the affected side at the 5th intercostal space anterior to the midaxillary line and connecting it to water seal drainage.
2. Insertion of a 18 gauze needle into the pleural space of the affected side at the level of the second intercostal space at the midclavicular line, if delay in chest tube insertion.

HEMOTHORAX

Hemothorax is an accumulation of blood in the intrapleural space. It is frequently found in association with open pneumothorax and is then called as hemopneumothorax.

Causes

- Chest trauma
- Lung malignancy
- Complications of anticoagulant therapy
- Pulmonary embolus
- Tearing of pleural adhesions.

Clinical Manifestations

Patient may be asymptomatic if small amount of blood (<300ml) in pleural space. In severe condition patient will have:
- Respiratory distress.
- Tachycardia, hypotension, shock.
- Mediastinal shift.
- Dullnes to percussion on the affected side.

Management

1. Aspiration of blood from pleural space by inserting a 16 gauze needle into 5th or 6th intercostal space, when the patient is in severe distress.
2. Closed chest drainage.
3. Exploratory thoracotomy if large amount of drainage (> 1500 mL) or continued large amount of drainage (200ml/hour) is present.

CARDIAC TAMPONADE

Cardiac tamponade is the compression of the heart as a result of fluid or blood within the pericardial sac.

Cause

Blunt or penetrating trauma to the chest.

Pathophysiology

- Normally the pericardial sac contains <50 mL fluid.
- An increase in fluid within the sac raises the pressure and compresses heart.
- This results in increased right and left ventricular end-diastolic pressures; decreased venous return; inability of the ventricles to distend adequately.

Clinical Manifestations

- Feelings of fullness or pressure or pain within the chest
- Anxiety and feelings of faintness due to decreased cardiac output
- Dyspnea, shortness of breath
- Tachycardia, hypotension,
- Distended neck veins from rising venous pressure
- Muffled or soft heart sounds
- Pulsus paradoxus (a large fall in blood pressure during inspiration when the pulse may be impalpable).

Management

Pericardiocentesis with proper hemodynamic monitoring.

SUBCUTANEOUS EMPHYSEMA

Subcutaneous emphysema occurs when the lungs and air passages are injured; air enters the tissue planes and passes for some distance under the skin at neck, chest, producing a crackling sensation when palpated.

It is not a serious complication.

Subcutaneous air is spontaneously absorbed if the underlying air leak is treated or stops spontaneously.

In severe condition a tracheostomy may be required if airway patency is threatened.

CLOSED CHEST DRAINAGE

Closed chest drainage means that the chest drainage system is closed to atmospheric pressure. It is performed using a glass bottle water-seal apparatus (one, two or three bottle set up) with or without controlled mechanical suction.

Purposes

1. To foster and permit the drainage of air, blood or serosanguineous fluid from the pleural space and to prevent the reflux of atmospheric air into the pleural space.
2. To help expand the remaining lung tissue by re-establishing normal negative pressure in the pleural space.
3. To prevent mediastinal shift and lung tissue collapse by equalizing pressures on both sides of the thoracic cavity.

Principles

Gravity

Air and fluid flow from a higher level to a lower level. Therefore chest drainage apparatus should always be kept below the level of the person's chest.

Water-seal

A water-seal drainage system must be airtight between the pleural space and the water-seal. Any air leak is an entry for atmospheric pressure into the pleural space, which will create positive pressure and collapse the lung. But there must be an air vent to provide an escape route for air passing through the water-seal from the pleural space (Fig. 4.1).

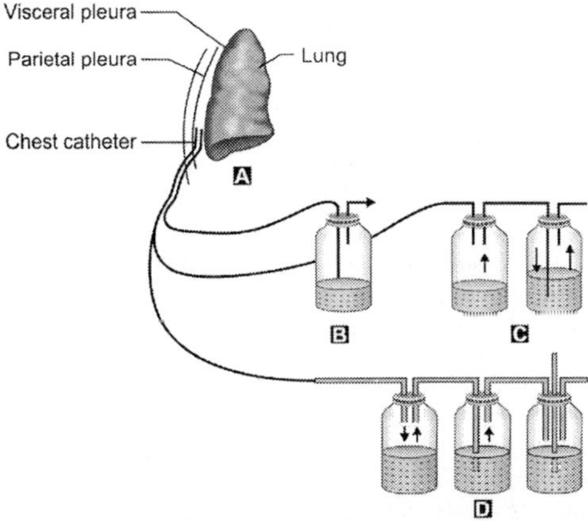

Fig. 4.1: Chest drainage system. (A) Placement of chest catheter; (B) One bottle system; (C) Two bottle system; (D) Three bottle system

Suction

Suction is a pull force. With suction air travels from the person's pleural cavity via the water-seal, through the air vent, into the suction chamber and then to the suction source. Suction may be applied to a two or three bottle water-seal system.

Insertion of Chest Catheters

Usually two catheters are placed in the chest. The upper or anterior tube is placed in the second intercostal space to permit escape of air. The lower or posterior tube is placed in eighth or ninth intercostal space in the midaxillary line to drain off blood and serosanguineous fluid.

Nurses' responsibilities when the patient is with chest drainage

1. Assessing chest drainage:
   a. Measure and document the amount and nature of drainage.
2. Assessment of water-seal functioning by observing the water-seal for:
   a. Rising fluid level in the water-seal compartment with inspiration and falling with expiration (tidalling).
   b. Intermittent bubbling in the water-seal compartment. Continuous bubbling during both inspiration and expiration indicates that air is leaking into the drainage system or pleural cavity.
3. Assessing functioning of suction apparatus.
4. Promoting chest drainage:
   a. The drainage bottle should be placed lower than the patient's chest.
   b. The drainage bottles are placed in a box or rack or taped securely to the floor so they will not be knocked over.
   c. If required the chest tubes may be double-clamped, very briefly during momentary movement of the apparatus above the level of the patient's chest.

d. The patient should not lie on (compress or kink) the catheter or tubing.
e. Drainage tubing should not be too short or too long.
f. Patency of the drainage system and the fluid collection in the drainage bottle should be checked frequently.
g. Routine milking or stripping chest tube should be avoided. But if required to remove air fluid or blood clots, milking is safer procedure than stripping.
h. Proper functioning of the system should always be ensured.

5. Preventing infection by observing strict aseptic technique, proper hand washing and not using chest catheter longer than 5 to 7 days.
6. Promoting activity with chest catheters:
   a. The patient with chest catheters should be encouraged to cough and take deep breaths; sit in bed; get in and out of bed if not otherwise contraindicated.
7. Clamping chest drainage tubing:
   a. Two clamps for each catheter should always be available at the bedside of the patient
   b. Chest drainage should never be clamped without an order to do so and except on emergency.
8. Potential emergencies:
   a. If water-seal bottle is accidentally elevated above the level of the patient's chest, the bottle should be immediately lowered and physician should be informed.
   b. If apparatus is broken accidentally—The chest catheters should immediately be clamped and the exposed end of the catheter to be connected to another chest drainage apparatus.
   c. If chest tube is accidentally removed the insertion site should be covered with sterile petroleum gauze and the physician be informed and to observe the patient for respiratory distress.

Removal of the Chest Catheters

Indications

- Evacuation of intrapleural air and fluid is completed and lung has expanded as evidenced by cessation of fluctuation in the long tube of the water-seal bottle.
- Chest auscultation, chest percussion and chest X-ray study confirm lung expansion.

Procedures for removal of chest catheters

- Discontinue suction and place patient on gravity drainage for a period of time before removal of the tubes.
- Administer pain medication as ordered before the tubes are removed.
- Remove suture, apply petroleum jelly gauze dressing at the site.
- Ask the patient to take a deep breath, exhale and bear down (Valsava maneuver) and then remove the tube.
- Cover site with an airtight dressing.
- Observe patient for respiratory distress which may signify a recurrent or new pneumothorax.

5

Nursing Management of Patients with Disorders of Cardiovascular System

NURSING ASSESSMENT OF PATIENT WITH CARDIOVASCULAR DISORDERS

A careful health history and physical examination should aid the nurse in differentiating symptoms that reflect a CVS problem from of other body system.

- Clues to cardiovascular problems:
  - Fatigue
  - Fluid retention
  - Irregular heart beat
  - Dyspnea
  - Pain
  - Tenderness in calf of leg
  - Syncope, near syncope
  - Altered neurologic function
  - Leg pain
- Past health history:
  - Ask patient about a
  - History of chest pain
  - SOB
  - Alcoholism and /or tobacco use
  - Anemia
  - Rheumatic fever
  - Streptococcal sore throat
  - Phlebitis
  - Intermittent claudication
  - Edema and varicosities
  - Obtain history of medication use—Aspirin, antidepressants, antipsychotics, anticancer agents corticosteroid, etc.
  - History of surgery or other treatments—specific treatments, past surgeries or hospital admission related cardiovascular problems.

Physical Examination

Vital signs

BP and HR's should be measured while the patient is lying, sitting and standing.

Peripheral Vascular System

Inspection: Skin for color, hair distribution and venous pattern. Extremities should be inspected for edema, thrombophelibitis, clubbing of the nail beds, cyanosis, etc.

Increased jugular venous pressure—Distension of the jugular neck vein and increased right atrial pressure (RAP)

Palpation

- Bilateral upper and lower extremities for temperature, moisture, pulses and edema.
- Palpate for thrill and rigidity.
- Measure capillary refill.

Auscultation

An artery that has a narrowed or bulging wall create turbulent blood flow—buzzing or humming termed as a bruit.

- **Thorax**: Inspection and palpation—Locate angle of Louis.

Locate and auscultate

- Aortic area: 2nd ICS right of the sternum.
- Pulmonic area: 2nd ICS left of the sternum.
- Tricuspid area: 5th left ICS close to the sternum.
- Mitral area: Left MCL at the level of the fifth ICS.

Murmurs are sounds produced by turbulent blood flow through the heart or the walls of larger arteries.

Pericardial friction rub

These are high pitched, scratchy sounds that may be transient or intermittent and may last several hours to days. They are caused by friction that occurs when inflamed surfaces of the pericardium, known are pericarditis, move against each other. Friction rubs are usually heart beat at the apex, with the patient's upright and leaning forward, and following expiration.

Diagnostic Tests

Blood tests

Blood for CKMB, cardiac markers such as troponins, myoglobins, CRP, homocysteine. These are the enzymes that are released into the circulation when the myocardial cells are injured. These biomedical markers are useful in the diagnosis of myocardial injury and necrosis.

Blood for Sr. Lipids

Cholesterol, triglycerides, phospholipids. They circulate in the blood bound to protein. Thus, they are often referred to as lipoproteins (LDL, HDL or VLDL). An elevation in LDL level has a strong and direct association with CAD.

Radiologic studies

- Chest X-ray: It shows cardiac contour, heart size, and configuration and anatomic changes in individual chambers.
- ECG: Basic PQRS and T wave forms are used to assess cardiac function. Deviations from normal sinus rhythm can indicate abnormalities in heart function.
- Holter monitoring: Continuous ambulatory ECG can provide diagnostic information over a greater period of time than a standard resting ECG.
- TMT(stress test): It used to evaluate the cardiovascular response to physical response.
- Echocardiogram: It uses ultrasound waves to record the movement of the structures of the heart .
- Positron emission tomography (PET): It is highly sensitive in distinguishing viable and nonviable myocardial tissue.
- MRI: It allows detection and localization of areas of MI in a 3D view.
- Cardiac catherization: It is a common outpatient procedure. It provides a means of obtaining information about CAD, congenital heart disease, valvular heart disease and ventricular function. It is used to measure intracardiac pressures and O_2 levels in various parts of the heart, as well as cardiac output and ejection fraction.
- Coronary angiography: Study involves injection of radioopaque contrast media directly into coronary arteries by the left heart catheterization. Used to evaluate patency of coronary arteries and collateral circulation.
- Peripheral arteriography and venography: It involves injection of radi-

oopaque contrast media into either arteries or veins. Serial X-rays taken to detect and visualize any atherosclerotic plaques, occlusion, aneurysm or traumatic injury.
- Hemodynamic monitoring: Arterial blood pressure, pulmonary artery pressure, pulmonary artery wedge pressure, and cardiac output is done to evaluate cardiovascular status and response to treatment.

RHEUMATIC FEVER AND HEART DISEASE

Definition

- Rheumatic fever is an inflammatory disease of the heart, mainly involving all layers (endocardium, myocardium and pericardium).
- The resulting damage of the heart from rheumatic fever is termed as rheumatic heart disease, a chronic condition characterized by scarring and deformity of the heart valves.
- Acute rheumatic fever is a complication of upto 3% of sporadic upper respiratory infections caused by group a β-hemolytic streptococci.

Etiology

Rheumatic fever occurs as a delayed sequela (usually after 2 to 3 weeks of a group A beta hemolytic streptococcal infection of the upper respiratory system, usually a pharyngeal infections.

Predisposing Factors

- Socioeconomic factors
- Malnutrition
- Overcrowding
- Familial factors
- Presence of an altered immune response.

Risk Factors

- Prosthetic cardiac valves
- History of bacterial endocarditis
- Aortic valve disease
- Mitral regurgitation
- Patent ductus arteriosus
- Ventricular septal defect
- Hypertropic cardiomyopathy
- Atrial septal defect.

Pathophysiology

- Injury is caused by an inflammatory or sensitive reaction to streptococci.
- Leukocytes accumulate in the affected tissues and form nodules which eventually are replaced by scar tissue.
- The layers (myocardium and pericardium) are affected by the inflammatory process.
- Rheumatic myocarditis develops which temporarily weakens the contractile power of the heart.
- The pericardium is affected and rheumatic pericarditis occurs during acute illness.
- Myocardial and pericardial involvement usually resolves without serious complications.
- Rheumatic endocarditis results in permanent and crippling adverse effects.
- Tiny transclucent vegetations or growth seen along the margins of the heart valves.
- Gradually the leaflets of the valves become thick, preventing them from closing completely.
- Blood flows backward through the valve, resulting in valvular regurgitation.
- Most common site of valvular regurgitation is mitral valve.
- Inflammed margins of the valve leaflets become adherent or the chordii tendinea fuse, resulting in valvular stenosis, a narrowed or stenotic valvular orifice.

Clinical Manifestations

- The diagnosis of ARF is suggested by a clustering of signs and symptoms as well as from laboratory findings.
- Criteria were established by T.D.Jones in 1944, revised by the American Heart Association in 1965, and updated in 1992 to provide a logical basis for diagnosis.
- The presence of 2 major criteria or one major and two minor criteria indicates a high probability of ARF.

Major criteria

1. Carditis: It is the most important manifestations of ARF with three signs: An organic heart murmur or murmurs of mitral or aortic regurgitation, or mitral stenosis. Cardiac enlargement and CHF occurring secondary to myocarditis and pericarditis resulting in distant heart sounds, chest pain, a pericardial friction rub or signs of effusion.
2. Polyarthritis: It is the inflammatory process affects the synovial membranes of the joints, causing swelling, heat, redness tenderness, and limitation of motion. The arthritis is migratory affecting one joint and then moving to another. The larger joints are most frequently affected particularly the knees, ankles, elbows and wrists.
3. Chorea (Sydenham's chorea): It is the major CNS manifestation of ARF characterized by weakness, ataxia and choreic movement that is spontaneous, rapid and purposeless, which tends to intensify with voluntary activity.
4. Erythema marginatum: It is the bright pink map-like macular lesions occurs mainly on the trunk or inner aspects of the upper arm and thigh but never on the face. It is usually transitory (lasting for a few hours) may recur intermittently for months and is exacerbated by heat, e.g. (warm bath).
5. Subcutaneous nodules: These are firm, small hard painless swellings found most commonly over bony prominences (e.g. knees, elbows, spine, and scapula).

Minor criteria

- Previous occurrence of rheumatic fever or RHD.
- Arthralgia.
- Prolonged PR interval.
- Lab findings: Increased ESR, increased WBC, increased CRP.

Diagnostic Tests

1. History and physical examination: History of sore throat within 5 weeks is a first symptom. Fever, headache, weight loss, fatigue, malaise, diaphoresis and pallor.
2. Lab findings: Increased ESR and CRP(C-reactive protein), Throat culture shows the presence of group A beta hemolytic streptococcal infection.
3. ECG: Sinus tachycardia, sinus bradycardia, first degree heart block, atrial fibrillation or atrial flutter.

MANAGEMENT

Medical Management

Goals

To identify and eradicate the causative organism and prevent additional complications such as rheumatic fever and rheumatic endocarditis.

- Inj penicillin IM administered as one time dose or oral penicillin is given. Penicillin eliminates residual group A beta hemolytic streptococci remaining in the tonsils and pharynx and prevents the spread of organism to close contacts.

- Erythromycin or cephalosporin may be administed for patients who are allergic to penicillin.
- Salicylates (aspirin) and corticosteroids (prednisone) are the two anti-inflammatory most widely used in the management of ARF. Both are effective in controlling the fever and joint manifestations.
- Prophylactic IM dose of penicillin is given every 3 to 4 weeks to prevent recurrence.

NURSING MANAGEMENT

Nursing Diagnosis

- Hyperthermia related infection of cardiac tissue as manifested by temperature elevation, diaphoresis, chills, headache, malaise tachycardia, and tachypnea.
- Decreased cardiac output related to valvular insufficiency and fluid overload as manifested by heart murmers,S3, tachycardia, diminished peripheral pulses, adventitious breath sounds, decreased urine output, restlessness.
- Activity intolerance related to generalized weakness and alteration in oxygen transport secondary to valvular dysfunction as manifested by fatigue, malaise, weakness, dyspnea, increased or decreased R/R and BP changes.
- Ineffective health maintenance related to lack of knowledge about disease and treatment process as manifested by nonperformance of desired prescribed health behavior, verbalization of misconceptions about desired or prescribed health behavior request for information.

Planning/Goals

- Maintenance of normal temperature, pulse (60 –100 beats/min) and respirations (12–20 breaths/min).
- Sufficient cardiac output to maintain mean arterial BP less than equal to 60 mmHg and urine output > 0.5 mL/kg/hr.
- Completion of activities of daily living with no to minimal fatigue or physiologic distress.
- Increased understanding of disease process and self-care management.

NURSING INTERVENTIONS

- Maintenance of normal temperature, pulse (60–100 beats/min)and respirations(12–20 breaths /min)
  - Monitor temperature to determine effectiveness of therapy.
  - Administer antipyretics and or sedatives as ordered to reduce fever and assist in sleep.
  - Reduce physical activity to decrease cardiac workload.
  - Administer antibiotics to treat the causative agent.
  - Monitor blood cultures and WBC count to evaluate patient's response to treatment.
- Sufficient cardiac output to maintain mean arterial BP less than equal to 60 mmHg and urine output > 0.5 mL/kg/hr
  - Ausculate heart sounds, rate and rhythm to detect a change in the character of the cardiac murmur and the presence of extra diastolic sounds.
  - Monitor for new onset of murmers, which could indicate infective endocarditis.
  - Assess breath sounds to identify pulmonary congestion and fluid overload.
  - Provide oxygen therapy to increase oxygen to the myocardium.
  - Administer diuretics, inotropic therapy, and other medications as

ordered to promote diuresis and strengthen myocardial contractility.
- Assess urine output to monitor renal function and evaluate fluid status.

• Completion of activities of daily living with no to minimal fatigue or physiologic distress.
  - Monitor vital signs during activity to evaluate cardiac response.
  - Monitor for signs of activity intolerance (e.g. tachycardia, hypertension, and diaphoresis, SOB to plan or alter activities.
  - Teach patient to check pulse rate and instruct patient to reduce activity if pulse increases more than or equal to 20 beats /min and to not increase activity if resting pulse > 20 beats / min because these signs indicate excessive cardiac effort.
  - Plan rest periods between activities to reduce cardiac workload.
  - Increased understanding of disease process and self-care management.
  - Assess patient's knowledge about disease and treatment process to identify teaching needs.
  - Discuss symptoms of recurrent infection so that health care provider can be notified and treatment initiated promptly.
  - Explain need to avoid persons with infections.
  - Encourage early treatment of common infections such as cold and flu to reduce the risk of recurrent infection so health care provider can be notified and treatment initiated promptly.
  - Explain need to report endocarditis history to the health care provider or dentist performing invasive procedures such as dental or gingival therapy, diagnostic tests, or medical and surgical procedures so prophylactic antibiotic therapy can be initiated to prevent the possibility of infection.
  - Discuss names of prescribed medications, dosages, time of administration, purpose and side effects to promote safe medication therapy.

MYOCARDITIS

Definition

Myocarditis is a focal or diffuse inflammation of the myocardium.

Causes

• The followings are the some of the causative organism:
  - Viruses (mainly Coxsackievirus type A and B), bacteria, fungi, radiation therapy and pharmacological and chemical factors.
  - It may be idiopathic with unknown cause. Myocarditis is often associated with acute pericarditis when it is caused by Coxsackie virus B.

Pathophysiology

• Entry of causative organism.
• Infection of the myocardium.
• Invasion through myocytes and causing cellular damage and necrosis.
• Activation of immune response, cytokines and oxygen-free radicals are released.
• Progression of the infection, leading to an autoimmune response, activating further destruction of myocytes.
• Results in cardiac dysfunction.
• Development of dilated cardiomyopathy.

Clinical Manifestations

- Ranging from mild to severe heart disease or sudden cardiac death (SCD).
- Fever, fatigue, malaise, myalgias, pharyngitis, dyspnea, lymphadenopathy, nausea, vomiting.
- Early manifestation occurs within 7 to 10 days after viral infection. These include pleuritic chest pain with pericardial friction rub and effusion because myocarditis is often associated with pericarditis.
- Late signs: Development of heart failure and may include an S3 heart sounds. Crackles, jugular venous distension, syncope, peripheral edema and angina.

Diagnostic Tests

- ECG: Dysrhythmias and conduction disturbances are present.
- Lab test: Mild to moderate leukocytosis.
- Atypical lymphocytes.
- Increased ESR, CRP.
- Elevated myocardial markers: Troponin.
- Elevated viral titers (Virus is generally only present in tissue and fluid samples during the intial 8–10 days of illness).
- Histologic examination: Confirmation of myocarditis is done through endomyocardial biopsy (EMB). This technique involves removing several small pieces of myocardial tissue percutaneously form the right ventricles with a special instrument called a bioptome and microscopically examining the samples. A biopsy done during the intial 6 weeks of acute illness is most diagnostic because this is the period in which lymphocytic infiltration and myocyte damage indicative of myocarditis are present.
- ECHO, nuclear scans and MRI to evaluate cardiac function.

Management

1. Digoxin (lanoxin) is often used to treat ventricular failure because it improves myocardial contractility and reduces ventricular rate.
2. Diuretics may be used to reduce fluid volume and increase preload.
3. If hypotension is not present, IV nitroprusside (nitropress), amrinone (Inocor) and milrinone (primacor) are used to reduce afterload and improve CO by increase systemic arterial resistance.
4. Based on the infections immune theory of myocarditis, immunosuppressive therapy with agents such as prednisalone. Azathioprine, cyclosporine has been used to reduce myocardial inflammation and to prevent irreversible myocardial damage.
5. Intravenous immunoglobulin (IVIG) is being used as an experimental basis to treat myocarditis—Improve left ventricular function and improves survival.
6. Antiviral agents—Ribavirin (virazole)—alfa interferon.
7. Oxygen therapy, bed rest, and restricted activity are important for the patients with myocarditis.
8. If complication of dilated CMP occurs—heart transplant is only the treatment.

NURSING MANAGEMENT

Nursing Assessment

Subjective data

History of infection related to virus, bacteria, recent surgery, intravascular procedures, recent dental and GI procedures (endoscopy or colonoscopy). Feeling of fatigue, malaise, myalgias, nausea are the usual complaints of the patient.

Objective data

Fever, dyspnea, chills, pharyngitis, lymphadenopathy, vomiting, pleuritic chest pain with pericardial friction rub and effusion, S3 heart sound,crackles, jugular venous distension, syncope, peripheral edema and angina.

Nursing Diagnoses

- Decreased cardiac output related to inflammatory changes of the heart muscles as evidenced by S3 heart sounds, crackles, jugular vein distension.
- Anxiety related to the prognosis of the disease and fear of death as evidenced by asking questions repeatedly, anxious look, restless.

Planning Outcomes/Goals

- Maintain adequate cardiac output.
- Reduce level of anxiety.

NURSING INTERVENTIONS

- Maintain adequate cardiac output
  - Monitor and document hemodynamic parameters such as arterial blood pressure, central venous pressure, pulmonary artery pressure, etc.
  - Use of semi–Fowler's position.
  - Planning of activity and rest period.
  - Provision for a quiet environment.
  - Administer prescribed medicine such as digoxin, lasix, etc.
- Reduce level of anxiety
  - Assessing level of anxiety.
  - Give psychological support.
  - Encourage the patient to ventilate his thoughts and feelings.
  - Provide divertional therapy to reduce anxiety such as music, newspaper, magazines,TV.
  - Keep patient and family informed about the therapeutic measures.

AORTIC ANEURYSM

Definition

- Aneurysms are outpouching or dilations of the arterial wall and are common problems involving the aorta.

Etiology and Pathophysiology

- Aortic aneurysm may involve the aortic arch thoracic aorta, or abdominal aorta.
- The growth rate of aneurysm is unpredictable, but the larger the aneurysm, the greater the risk or rupture.
- The exact cause of aneurysm is unknown.
- The most commonly accepted etiology of aneurysm is atherosclerosis.
- It is unknown that atherosclerotic plaque deposit beneath the intima (the innermost layer of the arterial wall).
- This plaque formation is thought to cause degenerative changes in the media (middle layer of the arterial wall) leading to loss of elasticity, weakening and eventual dilatation of aorta.

Classification

- **True aneurysm**: A true aneurysm is one in which the wall of the artery forms the aneurysm with at least one vessel layer still intact.
- True aneurysm can further subdivided into fusiform and saccular dilatations. A fusiform aneurysm is circumference and relatively uniform in shape. A saccular aneurysm is pounched with a narrow neck connecting the bulge to one side of the arterial wall.
- **False aneurysm**: A false aneurysm or pseudo aneurysm is not an aneurysm, but a disruption of all layers of the

arterial wall resulting in bleeding that is contained by surrounding structures.

Causes

- Trauma from infection, or after peripheral artery, bypasses graft surgery at the site of the graft to artery anastomosis.

Clinical Manifestations

- Thoracic aorta aneurysms are usually asymptomatic.
- Deep diffuse chest pain.
- Hoarseness of voice, as a result of pressure on the recurrent laryngeal nerve.
- Dysphagia.
- Distended neck veins.
- Edema of the head and arms.
- Abdominal aorta aneurysms are most often asymptomatic.

Symptoms

Mimic pain associated with any abdominal or back disorder.

Diagnostic Tests

- Routine physical examination.
- Chest X–ray: Mediastinal silhouette, any abnormal widening of the thoracic aorta.
- ECG: To rule out of evidence of myocardial infarction (MI).
- CT scan: To identify the presence of thrombus in the aneurysm.
- MRI: To diagnose and assess the location and severity of aneurysm.
- Angiography: Anatomic mapping of the aortic system by contrast imaging.

Complications

If rupture occurs posteriorly into the retroperitoneal space, bleeding may lead to tamponade.

Collaborative Care

Goal

To prevent rupture of the aneurysm. Early detection and prompt treatment is important.

Surgical therapy

1. Incising the diseased segment of the aorta. Patient often has severe back pain, or Flank ecchymosis (Grey Turner's sign).
2. Removing intraluminal thrombus or plaque.
3. Inserting a synthetic graft (Dacron or polytetrafluoro ethylene), which is sutured to the normal aorta proximal and distal to the aneurysm.

NURSING MANAGEMENT

Nursing Assessment

Patient should be monitored for indication of the rupture of the aneurysm:

Objective data

Diaphoresis, paleness, weakness, tachycardia, hypotension, abdominal, back, groin, or per umbilical pain, changes in sensorium, or a pulsating abdominal mass.

Nursing Diagnosis

- Ineffective tissue perfusion (peripheral and/or renal) related graft thrombosis, embolism ,prolonged aortic cross clamping, hypotension and blood loss or manifestated by absent or diminished, peripheral pulses, altered skin color, decreased urine output, altered ability to move extremities.
- Risk for infection related presence of prosthetic vascular graft and invasive lines.

PLANNING OUTCOMES/GOALS

- Maintain adequate tissue perfusion
- Minimize the risk of infection.

Nursing Interventions

Maintain adequate tissue perfusion

- Assess for dimished or absent peripheral pulses in the extremities.
- Compare extremities for warmth, capillary refill and color.
- Administer IV fluids.
- Maintain a warm environment to prevent temperature induced vasoconstriction.
- Administer anticoagulants/antiplatelet agents.
- Monitor urine output, daily weights, BUN and creatinine (signs of altered renal perfusion and renal failure).

Minimize the risk of infection

- Monitor for signs of infection.
- Administer broad spectrum antibiotic as ordered to maintain adequate blood levels of the drug.
- Use aseptic technique in caring for incising and any indwelling IV line tubing or catheter to maintain adequate blood levels of the drug.
- Use aseptic technique in caring for incision or catheter because these sites are potential portals of entry for infection.

SHOCK

Definition

Shock is defined as the failure of the circulatory system to maintain adequate perfusion of vital organs or shock is defined as a condition in which systemic blood pressure is inadequate to deliver oxygen to vital organs.

Shock affects all body system.

It may develop rapidly or slowly depending on the underlying causes.

Classification

Classification depending on its cause is given in Table 5.1.

Table 5.1: Classification and causes of shock

Types	Causes
• Hypovolemic shock	Hemorrhage from trauma, surgery, GI bleeding, vomiting, diarrhea, excessive diuresis.
• Cardiogenic shock	Myocardial infarction, cardiomyopathy, pericardialtamponade, dysrhythmias, stenosis or regurgitation, ventricular septal defect.
• Neurogenic shock	Spinal cord injury, spinal anesthesia, CNS depression.
• Anaphylactic shock	Contrast media, blood/blood products, drugs, insect bites, anesthetic agents, food additives, vaccines.
• Septic shock	Infection (urinary tract, respiratory tract, invasive lines, indwelling catheters)At risk patients are immunocompromised state, malnourished, debilitating patients, chronic kidney disease, older adults.

Pathophysiology

The pathophysiology of shock depends mainly on three major components of the circulatory system: Blood pressure, the cardiac pump and the vasculature which must respond effectively to complex, neural and hormonal feedback system to maintain adequate blood pressure and ultimately profuse body tissues.

1. Blood pressure is regulated through a complex interaction of neural, chemical and hormonal feedback system affected both cardiac output and peripheral resistance. This equation is given as MAP = CO × PVR, CO is determined by SV × HR (amount of blood ejected from systole) PVR = Diameter of the arterioles.
   - Tissue and organ perfusion depend on mean arterial pressure. MAP should exceed 80 mmHg to supply oxygen and nutrients to the body tissues which needed to sustain life.
2. Blood pressure is again regulated by baroreceptors which are situated in carotid sinus and aortic arch. These pressure receptors convey messages to the sympathetic nerves center which is situated in the medulla of the brain. When BP drops, catecholamines releases from the adrenal medulla of the adrenal gland. This increase HR, vasoconstriction thus restoring BP. Chemoreceptors which are also located in the aortic arch and carotid arteries, thus to restore BP in the same by vasoconstriction and increase HR and increase respiratory rate.
3. Kidneys: Kidneys regulate BP by releasing renin, an enzyme needed for the conversion of angiotension I to angiotension II, which is a potent vasoconstrictor. This effect directly leads to the release of aldosterone from the adrenal cortex, which promotes the retention of sodium and water. This increase concentration of sodium in the blood stimulates the release of antidiuretic hormone by the pituitary gland. ADH causes the kidneys to retain water further in an effort to raise blood volume and blood pressure.

Stages of Shock

There are three stages of shock.

Compensatory stage

- The patient's blood pressure remains' within normal limit.
- Increase heart rate, vasoconstriction and increase contractility of the heart tries to maintain the cardiac output.
- This results from the stimulation of the sympathetic nervous system and subsequent release of catecholamines.
- The patient is in the often described in the stage of 'fight or flight response'.

Progressive stage

- In the progressive stage, the mechanism that regulates blood pressure can no longer compensate and the MAP falls below normal limits; first the overworked heart becomes ischemic.
- This leads to failure of the heart even if the underlying cause of shock is not of cardiac origin.
- Second the auto regulatory function of the microcirculation fails to respond to the numerous biochemical mediators released by the cells, resulting in increased capillary permeability with areas of arteriolar and venous constriction further compromising cellular perfusion.

Irreversible stage

- The irreversible (or refractory) stage represents the point when the body is no longer having the energy to fight as because the organ damage is so severe, complete renal and liver failure is present.

- Complete metabolic acidosis occurs due to anaerobic metabolism. ATP stored depleted, ultimately multiple organ failure occurs and then leads to death.

Patients experiencing an anterior wall myocardial infarction are at greatest risk of developing cardiogenic shock because of the extensive damage to the left ventricles caused by occlusion of the anterior descending coronary artery.

- Decreased cardiac contractility.
- Decreased stroke volume and cardiac output.
- Decreased systemic tissue perfusion.
- Pulmonary congestion.
- Decreased coronary artery perfusion.

CARDIOGENIC SHOCK

Clinical Manifestations

- Respiratory distress.
- Diaphoresis.
- Cool, clammy extremities in addition to the typical signs and symptoms of acute MI.
- Orthopnea, dyspnea and oliguria.
- Altered mental status from cerebral hypoperfusion.

Physical Examinations Findings

- Auscultations: S3 gallop, pulmonary rales.
- BP: Hypotension.
- Pulse: Tachycardia, patient is prone to develop ventricular and supra ventricular arrhythmias.

Laboratory Investigations

- Arterial blood gas analysis.
- Chest X-ray: Showing pulmonary congestion.
- Blood for complete blood count and blood chemistry.
- ECG: Extensive ECG abnormalities consistent with massive infarction, severe diffusion is ischemia, extensive ST segment depression are common.

Diagnostic Tests

Cardiac catheterization

To identify RV infarction, acute mitral regurgitation and ventricular septal rupture that contributes to the shock state.

Echocardiography

It helps determine the extent of myocardial necrosis and identify complications of MI that contribute to cardiogenic shock.

MANAGEMENT

Major Goals of Management

Goals

1. Restoration of sinus rhythm.
2. Maintenance of adequate oxygenation and ventilation.
3. Correction of electrolyte abnormalities.
4. Correction of acid-base balance.

Medical Management

Inotropic and vasopressor agents

Predominant vasoconstrictor with inotrophic property:

Dopamine:

- Low dose: 1 to 3 microgram/kg/min.
- Maintenance dose: 5 to 10 microgram/kg/min.
- High dose: > 10 microgram /kg/min.

Norepinephrine—to maintain cardiac output.

Dose—2 to 20 microgram/min.

Inotropic catecholamine without predominant vasoconstrictor properties: Dobutamine: 2.5 to 5 micro/kg/min and increase to 20 microgram/kg/min depending on hemodynamic and heart rate.

Phosphodiesterase inhibitors, amrinone, nutrinone can increase the contractility without adrenergic stimulation:

- Milrinone: It is given at a 50 mg/kg bolus over 10 minutes followed by an infusion of 3.75 to 0.75 kg/minute infusion

Vasodilators

IV nitroglycerine or a sodium nitroprusside can be used, nitroglycerine is less potent as an arteriolar vasodilator. The starting dose is to 10 to 20 mg/min and is increased to 10 mg/min every few minutes.

Nitroprusside—5 to 10 mg/kg/minute and is titrated to a mean arterial pressure of approximately 70 mm Hg.

Diuretics

Patients with mild pulmonary edema MI can be treated with diuretics such as furosemide. Furosemide is administrated initially 20mg for patients' normal creatinine levels.

Percutaneous therapy

- Circulatory assist device such as an IABP (intraaortic balloon pump) or ventricular assist device (VAD) are used. An IABP should be inserted as soon as possible in patient with cardiogenic shock. It reduces after load, improves cardiac output and decreases the myocardial oxygen requirement by means of reduction in wall stress. The VAD may also be used as a temporary measure for the patient in cardiogenic shock and/or waiting for cardiac transplantation.
- PTCA: Percutaneous transluminal coronary angioplasty—Percutaneous intervention of the infarction related artery has been associated with good prognosis and patients with cardiogenic shock. It reduces afterload, improves cardiac output, and decreases the myocardial oxygen requirement by means of reduction in wall stress.

Surgical therapy

Emergency surgical revascularization is indicated in the care of patients with severe multivessel disease or substantial left main coronary artery stenosis.

NURSING MANAGEMENT

Nursing Assessment

Subjective data

Feeling of anxiety, restlessness, chest pain, breathing difficulty, fear of death.

Objective data

Chest pain, tachypnea, cyanosis, increased capillary refill time.

On lung auscultation: Presence of crackles or rhonchi. The patient's skin will become cooler and mottled, decrease urine output; diminished peripheral pulses and deterioration of neurologic status continue to deteriorate, as the shock progresses.

Nursing Diagnosis

- Decreased cardiac output related to increase after load, increase preload or right-sided heart failure (increase CVP and jugular venous distension), left-sided heart failure (pulmonary edema, crackles in lungs, increase pulmonary capillary wedge pressure).

- Fear related to severity of condition as evidenced by verbalization of anxiety about condition and fear of death, or withdrawal with no communication: restlessness, sleeplessness, increase in heart and respiratory rate.

Planning outcome/Goals

- Maintains normal cardiac function.
- Reports decreased fear and increased psychologic comfort.

Nursing Interventions

Maintains normal cardiac function

- Monitor vital signs, orthostatic blood pressure, mental status, peripheral pulse, capillary refill time and urinary output to assess the baseline data.
- Continuously monitor ECG changes through cardiac monitor.
- Monitor hemodynamic parameters (CVP, PAP, and PAWP) to assess patient's status and detect fluid deficits or excess and to evaluate patient's response to treatment.
- Administer fluids as ordered and maintain intake and output chart.
- Administer inotropes and vasodialators as ordered.
- Provide oxygenation and mechanical ventilation to maximize oxygenation and maintain saturation.
- Administer diuretics as ordered.

Reports decreased fear and increased psychologic comfort

- Assess the level of anxiety and fear.
- Use a calm reassuring approach.
- Listen attentively.
- Administer medications if appropriate to reduce anxiety.
- Stay with patient to promote safety and reduce fear.
- Provide the correct factual information concerning diagnosis, treatment and prognosis.

CARDIOMYOPATHY

Definition

Cardiomyopathy means 'disease of the heart muscle' It damages the muscle tone of the heart and reduces its ability to pump blood to the rest of the body.

Incidence

Cardiomyopathy is a leading cause of heart failure and the most common reason for needing a heart transplant.

Types

There are four main types of cardiomyopathy and they are:

- Dilated cardiomyopathy
- Hypertrophic cardiomyopathy
- Restrictive cardiomyopathy
- Ischemic cardiomyopathy.

Dilated cardiomyopathy

- Dilated cardiomyopathy is the most common form of heart muscle disease.
- Although it is found most often in middle-aged people and more often in men than in women, this condition has been diagnosed in people of all ages, including children.
- Dilated cardiomyopathy also called as 'congestive cardiomyopathy.' It damages the muscle tissue that makes up the heart's pumping chambers.
- If the chamber walls become weak enough, the heart can no longer perform its normal pumping action.

Causes of Cardiomyopathy

Most cases of dilated cardiomyopathy are called idiopathic. According to the research studies some viral infections may be responsible for the cause.

Other causes

- Alcohol and other toxic substances.
- Poor nutrition.
- Inflammation.
- Pregnancy and childbirth.
- Heredity.
- Acquired immunodeficiency syndrome (AIDS).

Pathophysiology

- Dilated cardiomyopathy is characterized by a diffuse inflammation and rapid degeneration of myocardial fibers that results in ventricular dilation, impairment of systolic function, trial enlargement and stasis of blood in the left ventricles.
- Cardiomegaly (enlargement of the heart) results from ventricular dilation. The long-term effect of cardiomegaly is not good.
- The heart tries to increase its rate to pump more blood through the body but when the heart is not able to do so it will affect the circulation and cause excess body fluid to build up in the lungs, abdomen and the legs causing breathing difficulty and edema which are the two common symptoms of heart failure.
- Cardiomegaly sometimes leads to abnormal heart rhythms called as arrhythmias.
- Blood flows more slowly through the enlarged heart, so blood clots may easily form.
- These clots can break free and enter the circulation, ending up in the lungs (called a pulmonary emboli) or blocking a vessel in the brain or heart.

Clinical manifestations

In dilated cardiomyopathy the symptoms most often associated with the common cold or flu—Chills, fever, overall aches, and fatigue.

Other symptoms include
- Chest pain
- Excessive tiredness
- Shortness of breath
- Swelling of the leg and ankles
- Decreased exercise capacity
- Dyspnea at rest
- Paroxysmal nocturnal dyspnea and orthopnea.

As the disease progresses the patient may experience dry cough, palpitations, abdominal bloating, nausea, vomiting, and anorexia.

Signs
- An irregular heart rate with an abnormal S3 or S4.
- Tachycardia or bradycardia.
- Pulmonary crackles.
- Edema.
- Weak peripheral pulses.
- Pallor.
- Hepatomegaly and jugular venous distension.
- Heart murmurs and dysrhythmias are common.
- Decreased blood through an enlarged heart promotes stasis and blood clot formation and may lead to systemic embolization.

Diagnostic Tests

- Chest X-ray: Cardiomegaly,pleural effusion is seen in the X-ray films.
- ECG: It shows areas of the heart that are damaged—Tachycardia,bradycardia and dysrhythmias with conduction abnormalities.
- Echocardiography: It shows the size of the heart and how much damage there is.

- Angiography: Cardiac catheterization procedure gives a detailed view of the arteries, chambers and valves. It gives the percentage of ejection fraction (EF). If the EF< 20% are associated with 50% mortality within 1 year.
- Biopsy: A study of tissue from the wall of the heart can give the idea about the process causing damage.

Treatment

It focuses on relieving the symptoms, as well as on relieving the extra load on the heart. It is divided as follows:

- Life style changes: Includes weight loss, smoking cessation, enough sleep, restrict extra salt intake, moderate exercise program.
- Medicines can help manage symptoms and improve heart action.
  - Diuretics, e.g. lasix reduce excess fluid in the body, decrease preload of the body.
  - Vasodilators such as angiotensin converting enzyme (ACE) inhibitors (captopril), relaxes blood vessels, decrease afterload and help to lower blood pressure.
  - Inotropic agents such digitalis, help to improve the heart's pumping action and keep a regular heart beat and used in the treatment of atrial fibrillation.
  - Calcium channel blockers or beta blockers (metoprolol and Aldosterone antagonist (spironolactone [Aldactone] help to keep a regular heart beat and the lessen the work of heart muscle.

In some cases, patients may need to have oxygen available at all times.

Surgical treatment

1. Latissimus dorsi muscle wrap also known as dynamic cardiomyoplasty.
   The left latissimus dorsi muscle is dissected from the lateral side and back of the chest leaving the medial end of the muscle and the blood supply intact, and the lateral end of the muscle is pulled through the pleural space into the pericardium.
   - The latissimus dorsi muscle flap is then wrapped around the ventricles and sutured in place.
   - Pacemaker leads are implanted into the muscle flap and a pacemaker generator is implanted in the chest wall. For at least 2 weeks following surgery the pacemaker remains turned off to facilitate the development of adhesions between the muscle wrap the ventricles.
   - Eventually the pacemaker is turned on and used to stimulate latissimus dorsi muscle contraction.
   - The ultimate goal is for the latissimus dorsi muscle wrap to augment ventricular contraction and increase cardiac output.
- Heart transplant.

2. Hypertrophic cardiomyopathy/Idiopathic hypertrophic subaortic stenosis: It is a asymmetric left ventricular hypertrophy without ventricle dilation.
   - In one form of the disease, the septum between the two ventricles become enlarged and obstructs the blood flow from the left ventricles.
   - It is termed hypertrophic obstructive cardiomyopathy (HCOM) or asymmetric septal hypertrophy (ASH). HCM is the secondmost common form of cardiomyopathy.

Causes

- HCM can be idiopathic, though about one-half of all cases have a genetic basis.

Pathophysiology

- The four main characteristics of HCM are:
  - Massive ventricular hypertrophy.
  - Rapid, forceful contraction of the left

ventricle, impaired relaxation (diastole) and obstruction to aortic outflow.
- Ventricular hypertrophy is associated with a thickened intraventricular septum and ventricular wall. The end result is impaired ventricular filling as the ventricular becomes noncomplaint and unstable to relax.
- The primary defect of HCM is diastolic dysfunction from the left ventricular stiffness. Demand ventricular filling and obstruction to outflow can result in decreased cardiac output, especially during exertion.

Clinical manifestations

- May be symptomatic.
- Exertional dyspnea, fatigue, angina and syncope. Dyspnea occurs due to increase left ventricular end diastolic pressure (LVEDP).
- Syncope can also be caused by dysrhthymias. Common dysrhythmias include—SVT, Af, VT, Vf, any of these dysrhythmias may lead to loss of consciousness or sudden cardiac death.
- On auscultating—presence of S_4 heart sound.

Diagnostic Tests

- Chest X-ray shows cardiomegaly.
- ECG: It can indicate the hypertrophic changes in the chambers and cardiomegaly, ST wave abnormalities, prominent Q waves in the inferior or precordial leads,left axis deviation , ventricular and atrial dysrhythmias.
- ECHO: It shows the size of the heart and the muscle damage that occurs.

Treatment

Medical treatment

- Betablockers (tab lopressor) are used to reduce the heart rate and blood pressure.
- Ca-channel blockers (tab verapamil) are used for the heart muscle stiffness.
- Antiarrhythmias (amiodarone) regulate the heart rate.

Surgical treatment

1. Left ventricular outflow tract surgery
   - Myectomy (myotomy-myectomy): Some portions of heart tissue is excised.
   - Septal tissue approximately 1cm wide and deep is cut from the enlarged septum below the aortic valve.
   - The length of septum removed depends on the degree of obstruction caused by the hypertrophied muscle.
2. Another procedure is done instead of a septal myectomy, the surgeon may open the left ventricular outflow tract to the aortic valve by mitral valvuloplasty involving the leaflets, chordeii or papillary muscles or the mitral valve is replaced with a disk valve.

Nonsurgical treatment

- Treatment that reduces symptoms and the left ventricular outflow obstruction is alcohol-induced percutaneous transluminal septal myocardial ablation (PTSMA).
- The procedure is performed in the cathlab.
- A special dye is injected through a catheter to locate the exact area of thickened muscle.
- When the area is located tiny amounts of pure alcohol (ethanol) is injected through the catheter.
- The alcohol destroys the area of extra heart muscle causing a 'controlled heart attack', over few minutes , the thickened muscle shrinks to a more normal size allowing more blood to flow through the heart.

Mechanical assist devices and total artificial heart

- Ventricular assist devices circulates blood per minute as the heart. Each

VAD is used to support one ventricle. Some VADs can be combined with an oxygenator; the combination is called extracorporeal membrane oxygenation. (ECHO).

- Total artificial heart designed to replace both ventricles. These are temporary treatments while the patient's own heart recovers or until a donor heart becomes available for transplantation (bridge to transplantation).

Complications

- Bleeding disorders
- Hemorrahge
- Thrombus
- Emboli
- Hemolysis
- Infection
- Renal failure
- Right-sided heart failure
- Multisystem failure
- Mechanical failure.

Restrictive Cardiomyopathy (infiltrative cardiomyopathy)

It is characterized by diastolic dysfunction caused by rigid ventricular walls that impair diastolic filling and ventricular stretch. Systolic function is usually normal.

Causes

- Cardiac amyloidosis (amyloid is a protein substance that is deposited within cells).
- Hemochromatosis—Iron builds up in the body.
- Sarcoidosis—Tiny grain like lump called granulomas most often appear in the lung or lymph node. It effects skin, eyes, liver or heart.

Clinical manifestations

- Weakness
- Tiredness
- Shortness of breath
- Peripheral edema
- Angina
- Dyspnea
- Orthopnea
- Syncope
- Ascites
- Hepatomegaly
- Jugular venous distention
- Palpitation
- Fatigue
- Exercise intolerance
- Dysrhythmias
- Heart block.

Diagnostic tests

- Echocardiography: It shows left ventricular wall thickened but the size of the heart is normal. Dilated right ventricles, dilated atria.
- ECG: Mild tachycardia at rest, supraventricular tachycardia, atrial fibrillation (dysrhythmias) or AV block.
- Chest X-ray: It may be normal or cardiac enlargement, may show cardiac enlargement pleural effusion, or pulmonary congestion.

Management

Currently no specific treatment is present for restrictive cardiomyopathy.

Goals

- Improving diastolic filling and treating underlying disease process.
- Medical and surgical management includes conservative treatment for heart failure and dysrhythmias. Heart transplantation may be considered if required.

NURSING MANAGEMENT OF CARDIOMYOPATHY

Nursing Assessment

Subjective data

Feeling of fatigue, weakness, tiredness, exercise intolerance, dyspnea at rest, swelling of legs and ankles, chest pain.

Objective data

An irregular heart rate with an abnormal S3 or S4, tachycardia or bradycardia, pulmonary crackles, edema, weak peripheral pulses, pallor, hepatomegaly and jugular venous distention, heart murmurs, dysrhythmias.

Nursing Diagnosis

- Decreased cardiac output related to inadequate oxygen and blood supply to the heart muscles as evidenced by tachycardia or bradycardia, weak peripheral pulses, murmurs, dysrhythmias, low BP.
- Activity intolerance related to insufficient oxygenation to the heart and rest of the body as evidenced by weakness, fatigue, shortness of breath, BP changes.
- Excess fluid volume related to heart failure as evidenced by peripheral edema, weight gain, jugular venous distention, pulmonary crackles, heart murmurs.

PLANNING OUTCOMES/GOALS

- Maintains adequate tissue and organ perfusion.
- Achieves optimal level of activity.
- Achieves fluid and electrolyte balance.

Nursing Interventions

Maintains adequate tissue and organ perfusion

- Monitor vital signs,cardiovascular status and respiratory status.
- Monitor for cardiac dysrhythmias including disturbances of both rhythm and conduction.
- Administer inotropic medications as ordered to maintain myocardial contractility.
- Elevate head end of the bed to reduce venous return, reduce oxygen demand and maximize chest expansion.
- Promote bed rest to decrease cardiac workload.

Achieves optimal level of activity

- Monitor cardio respiratory response to activity such as pulse rate, respirations and BP.
- Encourage alternate rest and activity periods to conserve energy and decrease cardiac demands.
- Plan for the activities gradually to increase cardiac tolerance.
- Assist the patient to maintain his activities of daily living.

Achieves fluid and electrolyte balance

- Monitor the serum electrolytes level, intake and output.
- Monitor changes in peripheral edema to detect hypervolemia.
- Monitor respiratory pattern for symptoms of difficulty (dyspnea, tachypnea) to assess for fluid congestion in lung.
- Monitor vital signs, weigh patient daily and record.
- Administer prescribed diuretics to assist with removal of fluid.

ANGINA PECTORIS

Definition

- Angina pectoris derives from Latin word and translates as 'tight chest'. It feels like an oppressive, heavy, crushing pain or a constricting feeling in the center of the chest behind the sternum or on the left side of the front of the chest.
- The pain can radiate out to either one or both arms, more often the left. It can be experienced in the throat, jaw, the stomach and more rarely, between the shoulders.
- Angina is a symptom of a condition called myocardial ischemia. It occurs when the heart muscle (myocardium) doesn't get as much blood (hence as much oxygen) needed. This usually occurs because one or more of the coronary arteries are narrowed or blocked due to the cholesterol deposition. Insufficient blood supply is called ischemia.

Trigger Factors

- Angina is often brought on by:
  - Physical exercise
  - Psychological stress
  - Extreme cold
  - A heavy meal, once these trigger factors stop, the pain generally subsides quickly, usually within 2 to 10 minutes.

Causes

- The most common causes of angina are the following:
  - Coronary atherosclerosis
  - Cardiac arrhythmias
  - Anemia
  - Severe aortic stenosis
  - Hypertrophy of the heart muscle
  - Acute coronary syndrome.

Risk Factors

Numerous risk factors are known to be associated with the development of atherosclerosis:

- A family history of atherosclerosis
- Hypercholesterolemia
- Hypertension
- Smoking
- More in men
- Type I and II diabetes mellitus
- Obesity
- Stress
- Sedentary lifestyle.

Types of Angina

There are various types of angina such as:

Stable angina

Refers to chest pain that occurs intermittently over a long period of time with the same pattern of onset, duration and intensity of symptoms.

They occur on exertion (such as running to catch a bus) or under mental or emotional stress. Normally the chest discomfort is relieved with rest, nitroglycerin or both.

Unstable angina

In people with unstable angina, the chest pain is unexpected and usually occurs while at rest.

The discomfort may be more severe, prolonged than typical angina. In a form of unstable angina called variant or Prinzmetal's angina, the cause is coronary artery spasm.

Variant or Prinzmetal's angina

It occurs spontaneously, and unlike typical angina, it always occurs when a person is at rest, usually in response to spasm of a major coronary artery.

Coronary spasm can be described as a strong contraction of smooth muscle in the coronary artery caused by increase intracellular calcium.

Clinical Manifestations

All symptoms occur in connection with physical exertion or psychological stress. They are:

- A squeezing or heavy pressing sensation on the chest.
- Heaviness or numbness in the arm, shoulder, elbow or hand (usually on the left side).
- A constricting sensation on the throat.
- The discomfort can radiate into arms, jaw, teeth, ears, stomach or between the shoulder blades.
- Increased shortness of breath.

Pathophysiology

- Atherosclerosis in the coronary arteries leading to coronary occlusion.
- Less oxygen and blood supply to the myocardial tissues leading to myocardial ischemia.
- During exercise, oxygen demand increases and work load of the heart increases.
- Hypoxia occurs within 10 seconds of coronary occlusion.
- Anaerobic metabolism begins producing lactic acid and other metabolites as byproduct.
- Irritation of myocardial nerve fibers by the increase lactic acid.
- Transmission of pain message to the cardiac nerves and upper posterior nerve roots.
- Chest pain occurs that may radiate to the left shoulder and arm.

Diagnostic Tests

The diagnosis is based on the presence of typical symptoms, medical history and the immediate effect of tab sorbitrate (glyceryl trinitrate) spray or tablet under the tongue for chest pain.

a. A resting ECG performed during an episode of pain to identify the area of ischemia.
b. Exercise test on a tread mill to determine if the heart muscle is the source of pain.
c. Coronary angiography is done to visualize the blocked arteries due to the plaque deposition by the use of a contrast dye.

Management

Medical management of clients with angina pectoris focuses on two goals:

1. Relief the acute attack
2. Prevention of further attacks to reduce the risk of MI.

The medical management is divided into preventive and therapeutic treatment:

Preventive

Administration of low dose aspirin (e.g. tablet angettes 75) reduces the risk of thrombus formation.

Therapeutic

- Glyceryl trinitrate (GTN sublingual tablets or spray) relax the arteries of the heart and relieve angina attacks.
- Long-acting nitrates reduce the frequency of angina attacks.
- Beta-blockers: block the effect of the hormone adrenaline so that the pulse is slowed and the blood pressure is lowered. This reduces heart's need for oxygen and improves the blood supply to the heart muscle (metoprolol, atenolol).

- Calcium channel blockers: Reduces the muscle tension in the coronary arteries. It relaxes the smooth muscles of the heart thus reducing the oxygen demand an reducing blood pressure(verapamil, nifedipine).

NURSING MANAGEMENT

Nursing Assessment

Subjective data

Chest pain or discomfort, palpitations, a feeling of numbness in the arms, wrists, hands, as well as shortness of breath, dizziness, light-headedness and diaphoresis.

Objective data

Pallor, diaphoresis, nausea, vomiting, cool, clammy peripheries, anxiety, fear, restlessness, tachycardia or bradycardia, pulsus alternans (alternating weak and strong heart beats), dysrhythmias (specially ventricular), presence of S3 and S4, high or low blood pressure, cardiac murmurs.

Nursing Diagnoses

1. Ineffective cardiac tissue perfusion secondary to coronary artery disease as evidenced by chest pain.
2. Anxiety or fear related to perceived or actual threat of death as evidenced by restlessness, agitation and verbalization of feelings.
3. Knowledge deficit about the underlying disease and methods for avoiding complications.
4. Ineffective management of therapeutic regimen related to failure to accept necessary lifestyle changes.

Planning/Goals

- Immediate and appropriate treatment of angina.
- Reduction of anxiety.
- Awareness of the disease process and understanding of the prescribed care, adherence to the self-care program and absence of complications.

Nursing Interventions

Immediate and appropriate treatment of angina

- Monitor and document the clinical manifestations of angina, duration, and the risk factors for CAD and the emotional reaction to chest pain.
- Start cardiac monitoring; Obtain a 12 lead ECG for any significant ST segment and T wave changes.
- Assess the pain—Its intensity, duration, radiation and frequency.
- Give sublingual nitroglycerine or tablets or spray as prescribed.
- Monitor blood pressure as nitroglycerine causes vasodilation and hypotension.
- Administer oxygen 2 L/min by nasal cannula.
- If the pain is not relieved after three nitroglycerine tablets 5 minutes apart or after administer Inj morphine sulfate and to notify the physician.
- Provide complete bed rest and calm and quiet environment.

Reduction of Anxiety

- Provide information about the illness, its treatment and prevention.
- Implement and explain various stress reduction methods such as music therapy.
- Help the patient to meet his spiritual needs.
- Encourage family members to participate in patient care.

Improving Knowledge

- Teach patient about the modifiable risk factors contributing to CAD and angina.

- Explain him to balance activity and rest period.
- Help him to identify the symptoms of MI (myocardial infarction).
- State the action to take when symptoms develop, discuss the methods to prevent chest pain and advancement of CAD.
- Participate in a regular daily program of activities that do not produce chest discomfort, shortness of breath or undue fatigue.
- Avoidusingoverthecountermedications that can increase BP and heart rate.
- Stop smoking and other use of tobacco.
- Eat a diet low in saturated fat, high in fiber.
- Carry NTG at all times state when and how to use it identify its side effects.

MYOCARDIAL INFARCTION

Definition

Myocardial Infarction commonly known as heart attack occurs when blood vessels that supply blood to the heart are blocked, preventing enough oxygenated blood getting into the heart (Fig. 5.1). The heart muscle dies or becomes permanently damaged.

Etiology

Heart attacks are caused by a blood clot that blocks one of the coronary arteries. In atherosclerosis, plaque builds up in the walls of the coronary arteries. This plaque is made up of cholesterol and other cells.

- A heart attack can occur as a result of the following:
  - The slow buildup of plaque may almost blocks one of the coronary arteries. A heart attack may occur if not enough oxygen-containing blood can flow through this blockage. This is more likely to happen during exercise.
  - The plaque itself develops cracks (fissures) or tears. Blood platelets stick to these tears and form a blood clot (thrombus). A heart attack can occur if this blood clot completely blocks the passage of oxygen-rich blood to the heart. This is the most common cause. Occasionally,

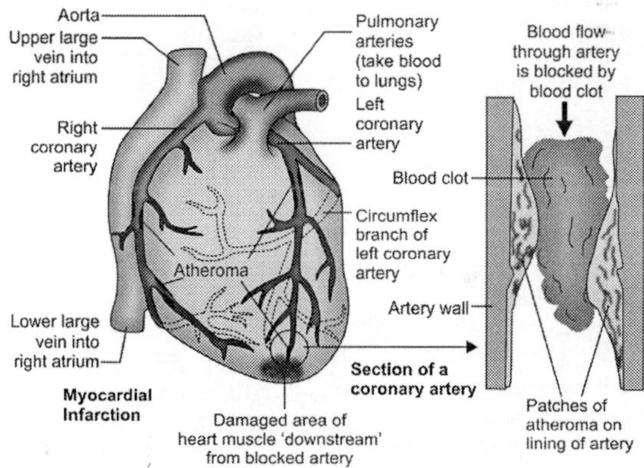

Fig. 5.1: Anterior view of the heart showing myocardial ischemia

sudden, significant emotional or physical stress, including an illness, can trigger a heart attack.

Risk Factors

- Increasing age (over age 65).
- Male gender.
- Diabetes.
- Family history of coronary artery disease (genetic or hereditary factors).
- High blood pressure.
- Smoking.
- Too much fat in diet.
- Unhealthy cholesterol levels, especially high LDL ('bad') cholesterol and low HDL ('good') cholesterol.
- Chronic kidney disease.

Clinical Manifestations

- Chest pain is a major symptom of heart attack. The pain may radiate from the chest to the arms, shoulder, neck, teeth, jaw, belly area, or back. The pain can be severe or mild. Usually lasts longer than 20 minutes. Rest and a medicine called nitroglycerin may not completely relieve the pain of a heart attack. Symptoms may also go away and come back.
- Anxiety.
- Cough.
- Fainting.
- Light-headedness, dizziness.
- Nausea or vomiting.
- Palpitations.
- Shortness of breath.
- Sweating, which may be extreme.
- Some people (the elderly, people with diabetes, and women) may have little or no chest pain. Or, they may experience unusual symptoms (shortness of breath, fatigue, weakness). A 'silent heart attack' is a heart attack with no symptoms.

Diagnostic Tests

A heart attack is always a medical emergency. A detailed physical examination is important.

1. Electrocardiogram (ECG)—It is done once or repeated over several hours: Patterns that occur with an MI include things called pathological Q waves and ST segment elevation.
2. Coronary angiography—It is done to evaluate the extent of coronary occlusion and to determine most appropriate treatment modalities.
3. Echocardiography—It is done to evaluate the ventricular function. Detect hypokinetic and akinetic wall motion and ejection fraction.
4. Blood tests can show the heart tissue damage or a high risk for heart attack. These tests include:

- Troponin I and troponin T—This enzyme is present in heart muscle cells. Damage to heart muscle cells releases troponin into the bloodstream.With an MI, the blood level of troponin increases within 3 to 12 hours from the onset of chest pain, peaks at 24 to 48 hours, and returns to a normal level over 5 to 14 days.
- Creatine kinase (CK) and creatinine phosphokinase (CPK) is released from heart muscle cells during an MI.
- Myoglobin and lactase dehydrogenase (LDH): Myoglobin level starts to increase within 1 to 3 hours and peaks within 12 hours after the onset of symptoms.

Management

Goals

- Successful treatment of the acute attack and prompt alleviation of manifestations.
- Prevention of complications and further attacks.

- Rehabilitation and education of the client and significant others.

Medical management

- Hospital admission possibly in the intensive care unit (ICU).
- Connect an ECG monitor.
- Start oxygen through nasal cannula at the rate of 5 L/min.
- Absolute bed rest to the patient.
- Life-threatening irregular heartbeats (arrhythmias) are the leading cause of death in the first few hours of a heart attack. These arrythmias may be treated with medications or electrical cardioversion/defibrillation.
- Start an intravenous line (IV).

THROMBOLYTIC THERAPY

Purposes of Thrombolytic Therapy

- Dissolve and lyse the thrombus in a coronary artery.
- Allowing blood to flow through coronary artery again (reperfusion).
- Minimize the size of infarction.
- Preserving ventricular function.
- Inj streptokinase (STK) 1.5 million units in 100 mL of normal saline given as IV infusion over 1 hour. Alteplase is a tissue plasminogen activator (tPA) that activates the plasminogen present on the blood clots.
- Analgesics Inj morphine sulfate is administered intravenously to reduce pain and anxiety.
- Nitroglycerin (NTG) helps to reduce chest pain.
- Antiplatelet medicines help prevent clots from forming. Aspirin, clopidogrel (Plavix) and low molecular weight heparin (LMWH) may be used with tPA to prevent another clot from forming at the same lesion site.
- Beta-blockers (such as metoprolol, atenolol, and propranolol) help reduce the strain on the heart and lower blood pressure.
- ACE inhibitors (such as ramipril, lisinopril, enalapril, or captopril) are used to prevent heart failure and lower blood pressure.
- Lipid lowering medications, specially statins (such as lovastatin, pravastatin, simvastatin, atorvastatin, and rosuvastatin) reduce blood cholesterol levels to prevent plaque from increasing. They may reduce the risk of another heart attack or death.

PERCUTANEOUS CORONARY INTERVENTIONS

Angioplasty and Stent Placement

- Angioplasty, a percutaneous coronary intervention (PCI), is the preferred emergency procedure for opening the arteries for some types of heart attacks. It should preferably be performed within 90 minutes of arriving at the hospital and no later than 12 hours after a heart attack.
- Angioplasty is a procedure to open narrowed or blocked blood vessels that supply blood to the heart.
- A coronary artery stent is a small, metal mesh tube that opens up (expands) inside a coronary artery. A stent is often placed after angioplasty. It helps to prevent the artery from closing up again. A drug eluting stent has medicine in it that helps prevent the artery from closing.

Surgical management

Coronary artery bypass graft (CABG): CABG is a surgical procedure in which a blood vessel is grafted to the occluded

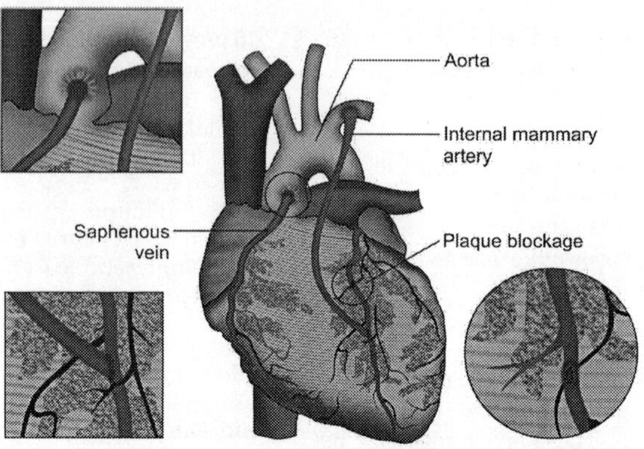

Fig. 5.2: Coronary artery bypass surgery

coronary artery so that blood can flow beyond the occlusion. A vessel commonly used for CABG is the greater saphenous vein, cephalic or basilic veins. The vein is removed from the leg or arm and grafted to the ascending aorta and to the coronary artery distal to the lesion (Fig. 5.2).

Complications

- Cardiogenic shock.
- Congestive heart failure.
- Damage extending past heart tissue (infarct extension), possibly leading to rupture of the heart.
- Damage to heart valves or the wall between the two sides of the heart.
- Inflammation around the lining of the heart (pericarditis).
- Irregular heartbeats, including ventricular tachycardia and ventricular fibrillation.
- Blood clot in the lungs (pulmonary embolism).
- Blood clot to the brain (stroke).
- Side effects of drug treatment.

NURSING MANAGEMENT

Nursing Assessment

Subjective data

Previous history of CAD, angina, MI, heart failure, hypertension, diabetes, anemia, and lung disease. Use of medications such as aspirin, nitrates, betablockers, etc.

Objective data

- Assess and document characteristics of chest pain, including location, duration quality, and intensity, presence of radiation, precipitating factors and alleviating symptoms.
- Assess dyspnea, nocturnal dyspnea, orthopnea, hypertension or hypotension and tachycardia or bradycardia with episode of chest pain.
- Auscultate chest for heart and lung sounds for S3, S4 snaps, clicks, murmers and friction rub.
- Assess for cool, clammy peripheries, jugular venous distension, peripheral pulses present or feeble, peripheral edema and pale skin.

- Check the lab values results of serum cardiac markers, increase serum lipids, increase WBC count, ST segment and T wave abnormalities in ECG, cardiac enlargement in chest X-ray, abnormal wall motion with stress echocardiogram and positive angiography.

Nursing Diagnoses

- Pain related to myocardial ischemia resulting from coronary artery occlusion with loss or restriction of blood flow to an area of the myocardium and necrosis of the myocardium.
- Dysrhythmias related to electrical instability or irritability secondary to ischemia or infarcted tissue as evidenced by increase or decrease in heart rate, change in rhythm, dysrhythmias.
- Decreased cardiac output related to inotropic changes in the heart secondary to myocardial ischemia, injury, or infarction as evidenced by change in level of consciousness, weakness, dizziness, loss of peripheral pulses, abnormal heart sounds, hemodynamic compromise, cardiopulmonary arrest.
- Impaired gas exchange related to decreased cardiac output as evidenced by increased or decreased heart rate, decreased blood pressure, impaired capillary refill, reduced arterial oxygen tension (PaO_2), dyspnea.
- Anxiety and fear related to hospital admission and fear of death as evidenced by client and family appear restlessness, hostile or withdrawn.
- Risk for activity intolerance related to an imbalance between oxygen supply and demand as evidenced by weakness, fatigue, change in vital signs, dysrhythmias, dyspnea, diaphoresis.

PLANNING OUTCOMES/GOALS

- Improved comfort in the chest as evidenced by a decrease in the rating of the chest pain, the ability to rest and sleep comfortably.
- No dysrhythmias, as evidenced by normal sinus rhythm.
- Improved cardiac output as evidenced by cardiac rate, rhythm, and hemodynamic parameters within normal limits.
- Improved gas exchange as evidenced by vital signs within normal limits, absence of cyanosis, absence of dyspnea, arterial blood gas within normal limits.
- Reduced feelings of anxiety and fear as evidenced by demonstrate appropriate range of feeling and effective coping.
- Improved activity tolerance as evidenced by participating in desired activities, meeting his or her own activities of daily living.

Nursing Interventions

Improved comfort in the chest as evidenced by a decrease in the rating of the chest pain, the ability to rest and sleep comfortably

- Assess and document characteristics of chest pain, including location, duration quality, and intensity, presence of radiation, precipitating factors and alleviating symptoms.
- Assess respirations, blood pressure and heart rate with episode of chest pain.
- Obtain a 12 lead ECG on admission then each time when chest pain recur.
- Document the rhythm strip every shift and when required.
- Give antidysrhythmic as ordered.
- Monitor serum potassium levels.
- Administer IV analgesic or vasodilators as ordered.

- Monitor response to drug therapy.
- Provide bed rest, calm and quiet environment. Restrict visitors.

No dysrhythmias, as evidenced by normal sinus rhythm

- Obtain a 12 lead ECG on admission then each time when chest pain recur.
- Document the rhythm strip every shift and when required.
- Check the lab values for negative or positive serum cardiac markers; increase serum lipids, increase WBC count, ST segment and T wave abnormalities in ECG, cardiac enlargement in chest X-ray, abnormal wall motion with stress echocardiogram and positive angiography.

Improved cardiac output as evidenced by cardiac rate, rhythm, and hemodynamic parameters within normal limits

- Auscultate chest for heart and lung sounds.
- Monitor vital signs. Do continuous cardiac monitoring.
- Assess for cool, clammy peripheries, peripheral pulse and pale skin.
- Administer oxygen as ordered, maintain continuous oximetry.
- Administer drugs as ordered.

Improved gas exchange as evidenced by vital signs within normal limits, absence of cyanosis, absence of dyspnea, arterial blood gas within normal limits

- Auscultate chest for heart and lung sounds.
- Assess the respiratory rhythm and rate.
- Monitor arterial blood gases and oxygen saturation.
- Give semi Flowler's position for reducing dyspnea.
- Administer supplemental oxygen as ordered.
- Prepare for intubation and mechanical ventilation if hypoxia occurs.

Reduced feelings of anxiety and fear as evidenced by demonstrate appropriate range of feeling and effective coping

- Allow the patient and family to verbalize fears.
- Allow and encourage the client and family to ask questions.
- Repeat information as necessary because of the reduced attention span of the patient and family.

Improved activity tolerance as evidenced by participating in desired activities, meeting his or her own activities of daily living

- Monitor vital signs before and immediately after activity.
- Monitor for tachycardia, dysrhythmias, dyspnea, diaphoresis or pallor after activity.
- Provide assistance with self care activities and provide frequent rest periods, specially after meals.

CONGESTIVE CARDIAC FAILURE

Definition

Congestive heart failure (CHF) is a condition in which the heart's function as a pump is inadequate to deliver oxygen-rich blood to the body.

Etiology

- Coronary artery disease.
- High blood pressure (hypertension).
- Longstanding alcohol abuse.
- Disorders of the heart valves.

- Viral infections resulting in stiffening of the heart muscle.
- Thyroid disorders.
- Disorders of the heart rhythm.

Pathophysiology

As the heart fails, the body activates neuro-hormonal compensatory mechanisms.

- Systolic heart failure results in decreased blood volume being ejected from the ventricles.
- Decreased ventricular stretch is sensed by baroreceptors in the aortic and carotid bodies.
- Stimulation of sympathetic nervous system (SNS) to release epinephrine and norephinephrine causing increase heart rate and contractility.
- Sympathetic stimulation causes vaso-constriction of the skin, gastrointestinal tract and kidneys.
- Decrease in renal perfusion due to low cardiac output and vasoconstriction then causes the release of renin by the kidney.
- Renin promotes the formation of angiotensin I to angiotensin II a potent vasoconstrictor which then increases the blood pressure and after load.
- Angiotensin II stimulates the release of aldosterone from the adrenal cortex, resulting in sodium and fluid retention by the renal tubules and stimulating the thirst center. Leading to fluid volume overload.
- Angiotensin, aldosterone and other neurohormones lead to an increases stress on the ventricular wall, causing increase workload of heart.
- Contractility of myocardial muscle fibers decrease resulting in increase of end diastolic blood volume in the ventricular, stretching the myocardial muscle fibers and ventricular dilation.
- Resulting in stress of the ventricular wall, increase workload of heart.
- Heart compensates for the increased workload, developing ventricular hypertrophy.
- Hypertrophy results in abnormal proliferation of myocardial cells called ventricular remodeling.
- Diastolic heart failure because of continued increased workload on the heart, ventricular hypertrophy and altered cellular functioning.
- Causing resistance to ventricular filling increase ventricular filling pressure.
- Less blood in the ventricles causing cardiac output.

Clinical Manifestations

- An early symptom of congestive heart failure is fatigue.
- Swelling (edema) of the ankles and legs or abdomen, this can be referred to as 'right-sided heart failure' as failure of the right-sided heart chambers to pump venous blood to the lungs to acquire oxygen results in buildup of this fluid in gravity-dependent areas such as in the legs.
- Right-sided heart failure can also be caused by severe lung disease (referred to as 'cor pulmonale').
- In addition, fluid may accumulate in the lungs, thereby causing shortness of breath, particularly during exercise and when lying flat. In some instances, patients are awakened at night, gasping for air.
- Some may be unable to sleep unless sitting upright.
- Nocturia.
- Accumulation of fluid in the liver and intestines may cause nausea, abdominal pain, and decreased appetite.

Diagnostic Tests

- A thorough patient history may disclose the presence of one or more of the symptoms of congestive heart failure described above. In addition, a history of significant coronary artery disease, prior heart attack, hypertension, diabetes, or significant alcohol.
- The physical examination is focused on detecting the presence of extra fluid in the body (breath sounds, leg swelling, or neck veins) as well as carefully characterizing the condition of the heart (pulse, heart size, heart sounds, and murmurs).
- Electrocardiogram (ECG) and chest X-ray to detect previous heart attacks, arrhythmia, heart enlargement, and fluid in and around the lungs.
- Echocardiogram(ECHO) is very helpful in diagnosing heart muscle weakness.
- Nuclear medicine studies assess the overall pumping capability of the heart and examine the possibility of inadequate blood flow to the heart muscle.
- Cardiac catheterization allows the arteries to the heart to be visualized with angiography (using dye inside of the blood vessels that can be seen using X-ray methods).
- A biopsy of the heart tissue may be recommended to diagnose specific diseases.
- A blood test called a BNP or brain natriuretic peptide level. This level can vary with age and gender but is typically elevated from heart failure and can aid in the diagnosis, and can be useful in following the response to treatment of congestive heart failure.

Management

The main goal in the management of chronic heart failure is:

- To treat the underlying cause and contributing factors.
- maximize cardiac output.
- provide treatment to alleviate symptoms.
- Improve ventricular function.
- Improve quality of life.
- Preserve target organ function.
- Reduce mortality and morbidity.

Lifestyle modification

- Measurement of body weight. An early sign of fluid accumulation is an increase in body weight.
- Aerobic exercise, once discouraged for congestive heart failure patients, has been shown to be beneficial in maintaining overall functional capacity, quality of life and perhaps even improving survival.

Medical Management

Goals

Medications improve symptoms and prolong survival.

- **Diuretics**: Diuretics are used to prevent or alleviate the symptoms of fluid retention. Examples of various classes of diuretics include:
  - Furosemide (lasix)
  - Hydrochlorothiazide (hydrodiuril)
  - Bumetanide (bumex)
  - Torsemide (demadex)
  - Spironolactone (aldactone)
  - Metolazone (zaroxolyn).
- **Vasodilators**: Vasodilators shown to improve survival in heart failure.The goals of vasodilators therapy include: Increasing venous capacity
  - Improving ejection fraction through ventricular contraction.
  - Decreasing heart size.
  - Slowing the process of ventricular dysfunction.

Angiotensin Converting Enzyme (ACE) Inhibitors

- ACE inhibitors have been used for the treatment of hypertension for more than 20 years. Examples of ACE inhibitors include:
  - Captopril (capoten)
  - Enalapril (vasotec)
  - Lisinopril (zestril, Prinivil)
  - Benazepril (lotensin)
  - Ramipril (altace).

For those individuals who are unable to tolerate the ACE inhibitors, an alternative group of drugs, called the angiotensin receptor blockers (ARBs), may be used. These drugs act on the same hormonal pathway as the ACE inhibitors, but instead block the action of angiotensin II at its receptor site directly.

Examples of this class of medications include:

- Losartan (cozaar)
- Candesartan (atacand)
- Telmisartan (micardis)
- Balsartan (diovan)
- Irbesartan (avapro)
- Olmesartan (benicar).

Beta-blockers

Hormones, such as epinephrine (adrenaline), norepinephrine, and other similar hormones, act on the beta receptors of various body tissues and produce a stimulative effect. The effect of these hormones on the beta receptors of the heart is a more forceful contraction of the heart muscle. Carvedilol (coreg) is the most effective drug in the setting of congestive heart failure. Long acting metoprolol (toprol XL) is also very effective in individuals with congestive heart failure.

Digitalis Glycosides (Digoxin)

Digoxin stimulates the heart muscle to contract more forcefully, improves congestive heart failure symptoms and can prevent further heart failure.

Surgical Treatment

Heart transplant

In selected patients, heart transplantation is a viable treatment option. Patients for heart transplantation are generally under age 70 and do not have severe or irreversible diseases affecting the other organs.

Other mechanical therapies

Left ventricular assist devices (LVAD) that are approved for use as a temporary mode of circulatory support in very ill patients until a transplant can be performed.

A less invasive modality, which can be placed without surgery, is the biventricular pacemaker. This device has proved valuable in appropriate types of patients with heart failure and impaired ventricles by improving the synchrony of contraction.

NURSING MANAGEMENT

Nursing Assessment

Subjective data

Past history of disease condition such as—CAD, hypertension, cardiomyopathy, diabetes mellitus, thyroid or lung disease, rapid or irregular heart rate, and use of medication as diuretics, corticosteroids, nonsteroid antiinflammatory drugs, etc.

Objective data

Integumentary system: Cool, diaphoretic skin, cyanosis or pallor, peripheral edema, (right-sided heart failure).

- *Respiratory*: Tachypnea, crackles, rhonchi, wheezes.
- *Cardiovascular*: Tachycardia, S3, S4, murmers, jugular vein distention.
- *Gastrointestinal*: Abdominal distention, hepatomegaly,ascites.
- *Neurologic*: Restlessness, confusion, decreased attention or memory.

Nursing Diagnosis

1. Activity intolerance related to fatigue secondary to CCF as evidenced by dyspnea, SOB, weakness, increase in heart rate on exertion.
2. Excess fluid volume related to cardiac failure as evidenced by edema, dyspnea on exertion, increased weight gain.
3. Impaired gas exchange related to increased preload, mechanical failure, or immobility as evidenced by increased respiratory rate, SOB, dyspnea on exertion.
4. Anxiety related to dyspnea or perceived threat of death as evidenced by restlessness, irritability, expression of life threat.

PLANNING OUTCOMES/GOALS

- Achieve a realistic programme of activity that balances physical activity with energy conserving activities.
- Experiences reduced edema or absence of edema.
- Maintains adequate respiratory rate and rhythm for activities of daily living.
- Verbalizes less anxiety about condition and prognosis.

Nursing Interventions

Achieve a realistic program of activity that balances physical activity with energy conserving activities

- Encourage alternate rest and activity period to reduce cardiac workload.
- Provide diversional activities to promote relaxation to reduce oxygen consumption.
- Monitor patient's oxygen response (pulse rate, cardiac rhythm, and respiratory rate).

Experiences reduced edema or absence of edema

- Weigh patient daily and monitor trends to evaluate fluid retention.
- Monitor abnormal serum electrolytes to assess response to treatment.
- Monitor hemodynamic parameters including CVP, MAP.
- Monitor renal function and intake and output to monitor fluid balance.
- Administer diuretics according to physician's order.

Maintains adequate respiratory rate and rhythm for activities of daily living

- Auscultate breath sounds to assess congestion.
- Monitor rate, rhythm depth and effort of respirations to evaluate changes in respiratory status.
- Administer supplemental oxygen as ordered and monitor effectiveness of oxygen therapy to identify hypoxemia and establish range of oxygen saturation.
- Position the patient to alleviate dyspnea (e.g. semi-Fowler's position).

Verbalizes less anxiety about condition and prognosis

- Assess the level of anxiey.
- Encourage the patient to verbalize his feelings.
- Use calm, reassuring approach to increase confidence in caregiver and relieve anxiety.
- Create an atmosphere to facilitate trust and explain all procedures to promote sense of security.

6

Nursing Management of Patients with Disorders of Hematological System

NURSING ASSESSMENT OF PATIENT WITH HEMATOLOGICAL DISORDERS

Subjective Data

- History of symptoms and chemical/drug exposure: Many prescribed and over the counter drugs are known to produce hematologic effects and bone marrow suppression. Persons when asked about the medications that they are taking overlook periodic use of analgesics, tranquillizers, laxatives and sedatives.
- History of fever as it is a very common manifestation of many hematologic disorders; identification of a pattern of occurrence is helpful, e.g. nighttime sweating may be associated with a fever which is characterized pattern of Hodgkin's disease.

Objective Data

General appearance

- In many hematological disorders there is decrease in RBC's there is progressive fatigue and malaise.
- Due to decreased or altered function of WBC's, there is a progressive lowered resistance to infections and increased time for healing. Relatively minor infections such as a common cold or urinary tract infections, linger and/or recur.
- Due to decreased or altered function of platelets, there is an increase in bruising from relatively minor injuries. Spontaneous nose bleeds or prolonged menses may occur.

Changes in the skin

- Petechiae, ecchymoses and purpura are associated with decreased platelet counts (thrombocytopenia).
- Jaundice may be observed in the sclera, conjunctiva and oral mucosa. It is suggestive of rapid destruction of RBC's and pernicious anemia.
- With iron deficiency anemia, the individual will notice dry skin, dry hair, and brittle nails.
- Severe itching (pruritus) is associated with Hodgkin's disease and polycythemia vera.

Head and neck

- When jaundice of the sclera or pallor of the conjunctiva is observed, the

individual often will have visual disturbances.
- A smooth or sensitive surface of the tongue is associated with pernicious anemia and nutritional deficiencies.
- The neck should be assessed closely for the presence of lymph node enlargement and tenderness. Lymph node enlargement often is the reason for seeking medical attention.

Chest

- Lung fields and heart sounds are within normal limit.
- Tenderness of the sternum may be identified with individuals with the leukemic processes.

Abdomen

- Enlarged liver and/or spleen may be noted.

Extremities

- Bone and joint pain may be noted.

Diagnostic Studies

Laboratory studies

Complete blood count Studies: Hb, Hct, total RBC, red cell indices, RBC morphology, WBC count, WBC differential, platelet count, prothrombin time, INR, aPTT, ACT, TGT, bleeding time, thrombin time, fibrinogen and bilirubin.

ESR, blood typing and Rh factor, iron metabolism (serum iron, total iron-binding capacity (TIBC), serum ferritin, and transferin saturation.

Urine studies: Routine examination of urine for protein, albumin, RBC, specific gravity.

Radioisotope studies: Liver/spleen scan, bone scan.

Radiologic Studies

- CT scan or MRI for evaluating the spleen, liver and lymph nodes. Spiral CT scans are used to evaluate deep lymph nodes.
- Biopsies procedures specific to hematologic assessment are bone marrow examination and lymph node biopsy.
- Skeletal X-ray to rule out any structural abnormalities.

AGRANULOCYTOSIS

Definition

Agranulocytosis or agranulosis is a condition marked by a significant decrease in the number of granulocyte, a type of white blood cells.

- It is usually referred as a severe form of leukopenia.
- It occurs due to a failure of the bone marrow to produce enough granulocytes or an increased destruction of these white blood cells.
- There are three types of granulocytes: Neutrophils, eosinophils and basophils.
- They contain microscopic granules filled with enzymes, which they use to digest foreign invaders or harmful microorganisms.
- When the number of neutrophil granulocytes in the body drops to a significantly low level, it is termed as neutropenia.
- Eosinopenia refers to inadequate numbers of eosinophils.
- Basopenia refers to a low level of basophil.

Causes

- It can be acquired or can be genetic or inherited.
- It develops as side effects of certain drugs such as anticancer drugs, cytotoxic drugs, immunosuppressant drugs,

antibiotics, antithyroid drugs and non-steroid antiinflammatory drugs.
- Aplastic anemia, autoimmune diseases, infections, tumor, and fibrosis of the bone marrow, exposure to radiation and certain toxins, leukemia.

Risk Factors

- A family history of certain genetic diseases.
- Spleen enlargement.
- Folate or vitamin B_{12} deficiency.
- Chemotherapy treatment.

Clinical Manifestations

Agranulocytosis may not produce any symptoms at times. Usually the condition reduces the ability of the immune system to fight infectious agents. The most common symptoms are:
- Sudden, unexplained fever with or without chill.
- Frequent infections.
- Bleeding gums.
- Mouth and anal ulcers.
- Diarrhea.
- Excessive fatigue or tiredness.
- Sore throat.
- Jaundice.
- Septicemia.

Diagnostic Tests

The following tests are done to detect agranulocytosis:
- Complete blood count.
- Bone marrow test.
- Genetic test.
- Test for identifying antineutrophil antibodies are carried out.

Treatment

Treatment of agranulocytosis depends on the underlying causes:
- If infection is present in individual with low white blood cell count then it is treated immediately with the appropriate antibiotics.
- If it is caused by any underlying diseases or disorders then treatment is directed towards curing and managing primary disorders.

HODGKIN'S LYMPHOMA

Definition

It is a malignant condition characterized by proliferation of abnormal, giant, multinucleated cells called Reed-Sternberg cells, which are located in the lymph nodes

Incidence

Lymphomas account for 3% of all cases of cancer.
- Lymphoma is a general term for cancers that develop in the lymphatic system.
- The most common type of lymphoma is called Hodgkin's disease.
- In adults, it is twice as prevalent in men as in women, and its prevalence is increased among patients with HIV infection.
- All other lymphomas are grouped together and are called nonHodgkin's lymphomas.

Pathophysiology

- Lymphomas are diseases of the body's cells. Healthy cells grow, divide and replace themselves in an orderly manner. This process keeps the body in good repair.
- In the non-Hodgkin's lymphomas, cells in the lymphatic system grow abnormally. They divide too rapidly and grow without any order. Too much tissue is formed, and tumors begin to grow. The cancer cells also spread to other organs.

- Malignant lymphocytes may be small and round or cleaved. Others may be large. Combinations of small and large may also be seen.
- Intermediate-sized lymphocytes with rapidly dividing cells are characteristic of aggressive (high grade) lymphomas.
- The main interacting factors include infection with the Epstein-Barr virus, genetic predisposition and exposure to occupational toxins.

Clinical Manifestations

The initial sign is most often an enlargement of the cervical,axillary, or inguinal lymph nodes. The enlarged nodes are not painful unless pressure is exerted on adjacent nerves.

The patient may note:

- Weight loss, fatigue, weakness, fever, chills, tachycardia, or night sweats.
- Generalized pruritis without skin lesions may develop.
- Cough, dyspnea, stridor, and dysphagia may all reflect mediastinal involvement.
- In more advanced disease there is hepatomegaly and splenomegaly. Anemia results from increased destruction as well as decreased production of erythrocytes.
- Jaundice may result from liver involvement.
- Spinal cord compression leading to paraplegia may occur with extra dural involvement.

Diagnostic Test

The following tests are done to confirm the diagnosis of Hodgkin's lymphoma.

- Peripheral blood analysis: Often reveals microcytic hypochromic anemia.
- Excisional lymph node biopsy offers definitive diagnosis. If removed, the node is examined histologically for the presence of Reed-Sternberg cells.
- Bone marrow biopsy is performed as a important aspect of staging.
- CT scan and MRI scans are initial staging tools. PET scans may show increased uptake of carbohydrate by cancer cells.

Management

Medical management

The treatment decisions are made based on the clinical stage of the disease.

- The standard of chemotherapy is the ABVD regimen: Doxorubicin (adriamycin), bleomycin, vinblastine, and dacarbazine given for 2 to 8 cycles of treatment depending on disease stage and prognosis.
- The role of radiation as a supplement to chemotherapy varies depending on site of disease and the presence of resistant disease after chemotherapy.
- Intensive chemoptherapy with or without the use of autologous or allogeneic hematopoietic stem cell transplantation (HSCT) and hematopoietic growth factors is the treatment of choice for advanced, refractory, or relapsed Hodgkin's lymphoma.

ANEMIA

- Anemia describes the condition in which the number of red blood cells in the blood is low.
- Anemia is actually a sign of a disease process rather than a disease itself.

Types

- It is usually classified as either chronic or acute.
- Chronic anemia occurs over a long period of time. In chronic anemia, symptoms typically begin slowly and progress gradually; whereas in acute

anemia symptoms can be abrupt and more distressing.

- Acute anemia occurs quickly.

In general, there are three major types of anemia, classified according to the size of the red blood cells:

a. If the red blood cells are smaller than normal, this is called **microcytic anemia**. The major causes of this type are iron deficiency (low level iron) anemia and thalassemia (inherited disorders of hemoglobin).
b. If the red blood cells size are normal in size (but low in number), this is called **normocytic anemia**, such as anemia that accompanies chronic disease or anemia related to kidney disease.
c. If red blood cells are larger than normal, then it is called **macrocytic anemia**. Major causes of this type are pernicious anemia and anemia related to alcoholism.

Causes

Anemia from active bleeding

Loss of blood through heavy menstrual bleeding or, wounds can cause anemia. Gastrointestinal ulcers or cancers such as cancer of the colon may slowly ooze blood and can also cause anemia.

Iron deficiency anemia

The bone marrow needs iron to make red blood cells. Iron plays an important role in the proper structure of the hemoglobin molecule. If iron intake is limited or inadequate due to poor dietary intake, anemia may occur as a result. This is called iron deficiency anemia. Iron deficiency anemia can also occur when there are stomach ulcers or other sources of slow, chronic bleeding (colon cancer, uterine cancer, intestinal polyps, hemorrhoids, etc).

Anemia of chronic disease

Any long-term medical condition can lead to anemia. The exact mechanism of this process in unknown, but any long-standing and ongoing medical condition such as a chronic infection or a cancer may cause this type of anemia.

Anemia related to kidney disease

The kidneys release a hormone called the erythropoietin that helps the bone marrow make red blood cells. In people with chronic (long-standing) kidney disease, the production of this hormone is diminished, and this in turn diminishes the production of red blood cells, causing anemia. This is called anemia related to chronic kidney disease.

Anemia related to pregnancy

Water weight gain during pregnancy dilutes the blood, which may be reflected as anemia.

Anemia related to poor nutrition

Vitamins and minerals are required to make red blood cells. In addition to iron, vitamin B_{12} and folate are required for the proper production of hemoglobin. Deficiency in any of these may cause anemia because of inadequate production of red blood cells. Poor dietary intake is an important cause of low folate and low vitamin B_{12} levels. Strict vegetarians who do not take sufficient vitamins are at risk to develop vitamin B_{12} deficiency.

Pernicious anemia

There also may be a problem in the stomach or the intestines leading to poor absorption of vitamin B_{12}. This may lead to anemia because of vitamin B_{12} deficiency known as pernicious anemia.

Sickle cell anemia

In some individuals, the problem may be related to production of abnormal hemoglobin molecules. In this condition the hemoglobin problem is qualitative, or functional. Abnormal hemoglobin molecules may cause problems in the integrity of the red blood cell structure and they may become crescent-shaped (sickle cells). There are different types of sickle cell anemia with different severity levels.

Thalassemia

This is another group of hemoglobin-related causes of anemia. There are many types of thalassemia, which vary in severity from mild (thalassemia minor) to severe (thalassemia major). These are also hereditary, but they cause quantitative hemoglobin abnormalities, meaning an insufficient amount of the correct hemoglobin type molecules is made.

Alcoholism

Poor nutrition and deficiencies of vitamins and minerals are associated with alcoholism. Alcohol itself may also be toxic to the bone marrow and may slow down the red blood cell production.

Bone marrow-related anemia

Anemia may be related to diseases involving the bone marrow. Some blood cancers such as leukemia or lymphomas can alter the production of red blood cells and result in anemia. Other processes may be related to a cancer from another organ spreading to the bone marrow.

Aplastic anemia

Occasionally some viral infections may severely affect the bone marrow and significantly diminish production of all blood cells. Chemotherapy and some other medications may pose the same problems.

Hemolytic anemia

The normal red blood cell shape is important for its function. Hemolytic anemia is a type of anemia in which the red blood cells rupture (known as hemolysis) and become dysfunctional. This could happen due to a variety of reasons. Some forms of hemolytic anemia can be hereditary with constant destruction and rapid reproduction of red blood cells (for example, as in hereditary spherocytosis, hereditary elliptocytosis, and glucose-6-phosphate dehydrogenase or G6GD deficiency). This type of destruction may also happen to normal red blood cells in certain conditions, for example, with abnormal heart valves damaging the blood cells or certain medications that disrupt the red blood cell structure.

Anemia related to medications

Many common medications can occasionally cause anemia as a side effect in some individuals. The mechanisms by which medications can cause anemia are numerous (hemolysis, bone marrow toxicity) and are specific to the medication. Medications that most frequently cause anemia are chemotherapy drugs used to treat cancers. Other common medications that can cause anemia include some seizure medications, transplant medications, HIV medications, some malaria medications, some antibiotics (penicillin, chloramphenicol), antifungal medications, and antihistamines.

Other less common causes

Other less common causes of anemia include thyroid problems, cancers, liver disease, autoimmune diseases (lupus), paroxysmal nocturnal hemoglobinuria (PNH), lead poisoning, AIDS, malaria, viral hepatitis, mononucleosis, parasitic infections (hookworm), bleeding disorders and insecticide exposure.

Clinical Manifestations

- Symptoms of anemia may include the following:
  - Fatigue.
  - Decreased energy.
  - Weakness.
  - Shortness of breath .
  - Lightheadedness.
  - Palpitations (feeling of the heart racing or beating irregularly).
  - Looking pale.
- Symptoms of severe anemia may include:
  - Chest pain, angina, or heart attack.
  - Dizziness.
  - Fainting or passing out.
  - Rapid heart rate.
- Some of the signs that may indicate anemia in an individual may include:
  - Change in stool color, including black and tarry stools (sticky and foul smelling), maroon-colored, or visibly bloody stools if the anemia is due to blood loss through the gastrointestinal tract.
  - Rapid heart rate.
  - Low blood pressure.
  - Rapid breathing.
  - Pale or cold skin.
  - Yellow skin called jaundice if anemia is due to red blood cell breakdown.
  - Heart murmur.
  - Enlargement of the spleen with certain causes of anemia.

Diagnosis Studies

- Physical examination and medical history: Some of the important features in medical history are—family history, previous personal history of anemia or other chronic conditions, medications, color of stool and urine, bleeding problems, and occupation and social habits (such as alcohol intake).
- While performing a complete physical examination, the physician may particularly focus on general appearance (signs of fatigue, paleness), jaundice (yellow skin and eyes), paleness of the nail beds, enlarged spleen (splenomegaly) or liver (hepatomegaly), heart sounds, and lymph nodes.

Lab Tests for Anemia

Complete blood count (CBC)

Determines the severity and type of anemia (microcytic anemia or small-sized red blood cells, normocytic anemia or normal-sized red blood cells, or macrocytic anemia or large-sized red blood cells) and is typically the first test ordered. Information about other blood cells (white cells and platelets) are also included in the CBC report.

Stool hemoglobin test

Tests for blood in stool which may detect bleeding from the stomach or the intestines (stool Guaiac test or stool occult blood test).

Peripheral blood smear

Looks at the red blood cells under a microscope to determine the size, shape, number, and color as well as evaluate other cells in the blood.

Iron level

This test is usually accompanied by other tests that measure the body's iron storage capacity, such as transferrin level and ferritin level.

Transferrin level

Evaluates a protein that carries iron around the body.

Ferritin

Evaluates at the total iron available in the body.

Folate

A vitamin needed to produce red blood cells, which is low in people with poor eating habits.

Vitamin B_{12}

A vitamin needed to produce red blood cells, low in people with poor eating habits or in pernicious anemia.

Bilirubin

Useful to determine if the red blood cells are being destroyed within the body which may be a sign of hemolytic anemia.

Lead level

Lead toxicity used to be one of the more common causes of anemia in children.

Hemoglobin electrophoresis

Sometimes used when a person has a family history of anemia; this test provides information on sickle cell anemia or thalassemia.

Reticulocyte count

A measure of new red blood cells produced by the bone marrow.

Bone marrow biopsy

Evaluates production of red blood cells and may be done when a bone marrow problem is suspected.

Management

- If anemia is mild and is found to be related to low iron levels, then iron supplements may be given while further investigation to determine the cause of the iron deficiency is carried out.
- If anemia is related to sudden blood loss from an injury or a rapidly bleeding stomach ulcer, then hospitalization and transfusion of red blood cells may be required to relieve the symptoms and replace the lost blood. Blood transfusion may be required in other less critical circumstances as well.

Medications

- Iron may be taken during pregnancy and when iron levels are low. It is important to determine the cause of iron deficiency and treat it properly.
- Vitamin supplements may replace folate and vitamin B_{12} in people with poor eating habits. In people with pernicious anemia who are unable to absorb sufficient amounts of vitamin B_{12}, monthly injections of vitamin B_{12} are commonly used to replete the vitamin B_{12} levels and correct the anemia.
- Epoetin alfa (Procrit or Epogen) injection can be used to increase red blood cell production in people with kidney problems. The production of erythropoietin is reduced in people with advanced kidney disease, as described earlier.
- If alcohol is the cause of anemia, then in addition to taking vitamins and

maintaining adequate nutrition, alcohol consumption needs to be stopped.

Surgery

There are no specific surgical interventions for the treatment of anemia. However, depending on the causes of the anemia, surgery may be a treatment option. For example, if colon cancer or uterine cancer that slowly bleeds is the cause of anemia, then surgical removal of the cancer could potentially treat the anemia.

NURSING MANAGEMENT

Nursing Assessment

Subjective data

Fatigue, weakness, general malaise, tachycardia, tachypnea, dyspnea during work or rest. Lethargy, withdrawn, apathetic, lethargic and less interested in its surroundings. Muscle weakness and decreased strength. A history of chronic blood loss, such as chronic gastrointestinal bleeding, heavy menstruation, angina, CHF (due to excessive cardiac work). History of chronic infective endocarditis. Palpitations (tachycardia compensation) A history of pyelonephritis, kidney failure. Flatulence, malabsorption syndrome. Hematemesis,melena, diarrheaorconstipation. Decrease in urine output. Abdominal distension.

Objective data

Blood pressure: systolic to diastolic steady improvement and widening pulse pressure, postural hypotension. Dysrhythmias: ECG abnormality, ST segment depression and T wave leveling or depression; tachycardia, systolic murmur. Extremity (color)—pale skin and mucous membranes (conjunctiva, mouth, pharynx, lips) and the base of the nail. Decreased dietary input. Painful mouth or tongue, difficulty swallowing (pharyngeal ulcers). Nausea/vomiting, dyspepsia, anorexia, weight loss.

Nursing Diagnoses

- Ineffective tissue perfusion related to the decrease in the cellular components required for the delivery of oxygen/nutrients to the cells.
- Imbalanced nutrition, less than body requirements related to failure to ingest or inability to digest food/absorb nutrients necessary for formation of normal RBCs possibly evidenced by weight loss, decreased triceps skin-fold measurement; changes in gums, oral mucous membranes; and decreased tolerance for activity, weakness, and loss of muscle tone.

PLANNING OUTCOMES/GOALS

- Maintain adequate tissue perfusion.
- Demonstrate progressive weight gain or stable weight, with normalization of laboratory values.
- Experience no signs of malnutrition.
- Demonstrate behaviors, lifestyle changes to regain and/or maintain appropriate weight.

Nursing Interventions

Maintain adequate tissue perfusion

- Monitor vital signs assess capillary refill, color of skin/mucous membranes, nail beds.
- Elevate head of bed as tolerated.
- Monitor respiratory effort; auscultation of breath sounds adventitious note sounds.
- Investigate complaints of chest pain/palpitations.
- Avoid using a bottle warmer or hot

water bottle. Measure the temperature of bath water with a thermometer.
- Keep an eye on the results of laboratory examination. Give a complete red blood cell/blood product packed as indicated.
- Provide supplemental oxygen as indicated.

Demonstrate progressive weight gain or stable weight, with normalization of laboratory values

- Review nutritional history, including food preferences.
- Observe and record patient's food intake.
- Weigh periodically as appropriate (e.g. weekly)
- Recommend small, frequent meals and/or between-meal nourishment.
- Suggest bland diet, low in roughage, avoiding hot, spicy or very acidic foods as indicated.
- Have patient record and report occurrence of nausea/vomiting, flatus, and other related symptoms such as irritability or impaired memory.
- Encourage/assist with good oral hygiene; before and after meals, use soft-bristled toothbrush for gentle brushing. Provide dilute, alcohol-free mouthwash if oral mucosa is ulcerated.
- Consult with dietitian.
- Monitor laboratory studies, e.g. Hb/Hct, blood urea nitrogen (BUN), pre-albumin/albumin, protein, transferrin, serum iron, vitamin B_{12}, folic acid, TIBC, serum electrolytes.
- Administer medications as indicated, e.g. vitamin and mineral supplements, e.g. cyanocobalamin (vitamin B_{12}), folic acid (folvite), ascorbic acid (vitamin C).

POLYCYTHEMIA VERA

Definition

Polycythemia vera (also known as erythremia, primary polycythemia and polycythemia rubra vera) is a myeloproliferative blood disorder in which the bone marrow makes too many red blood cells. It may also result in the overproduction of white blood cells and platelets.

Incidence

More common in the elderly and may be symptomatic or asymptomatic. Polycythemia vera occurs in all age groups, although the incidence increases with age.

Pathophysiology

- Polycythemia vera (PCV), being a primary polycythemia, is caused by neoplastic proliferation and maturation of erythroid, megakaryocytic and granulocytic elements to produce what is referred to as panmyelosis.
- In contrast to secondary polycythemias, PCV is associated with a low serum level of the hormone erythropoietin (EPO).

Clinical Manifestations

- Patients with polycythemia vera can be asymptomatic.
- A classic symptom of polycythemia vera is pruritus or itching, particularly after exposure to warm water (such as when taking a bath), which may be due to abnormal histamine release or prostaglandin production. Such itching is present in approximately 40% of patients with polycythemia vera.
- Gouty arthritis may be present in upto 20% of patients.
- Peptic ulcer disease is also common in patients with polycythemia vera; the reasons for this are unclear, but may be related to an increased susceptibility to infection with the ulcer-causing bacterium *H. pylori.* Another possible mechanism for the development for

peptic ulcer is increased histamine release and gastric hyperacidity related with polycythemia vera.

- A rare but classic symptom of polycythemia vera (and the related myeloproliferative disease essential thrombocythemia) is erythromelalgia.
- Erythromelalgia: A sudden, severe burning pain in the hands or feet, usually accompanied by a reddish or bluish coloration of the skin. Erythromelalgia is caused by an increased platelet count or increased platelet stickiness (aggregation), resulting in the formation of tiny blood clots in the vessels of the extremity; it responds rapidly to treatment with aspirin (Fig. 6.1).
- Patients with polycythemia vera are prone to the development of blood clots (thrombosis). A major thrombotic complication, e.g. heart attack, stroke, deep venous thrombosis, may sometimes be the first symptom or indication that a person has polycythemia vera.

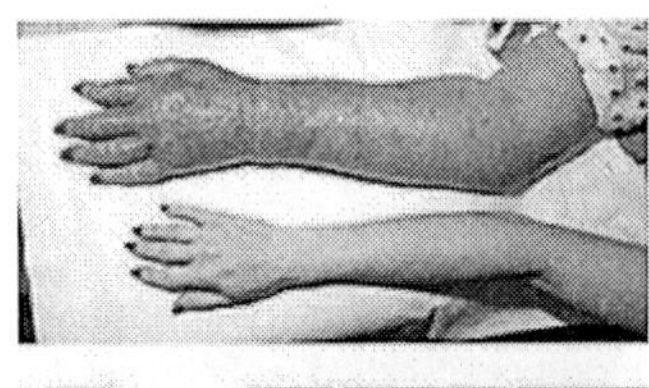
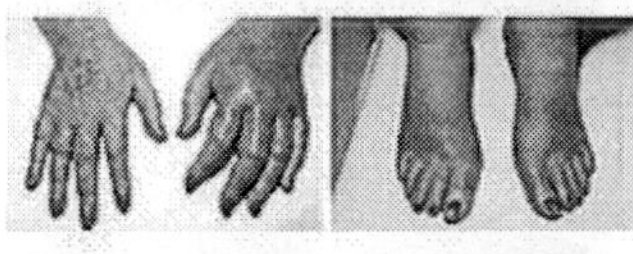
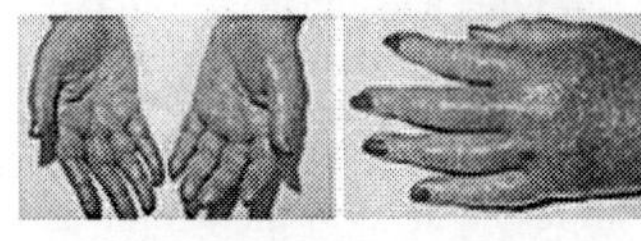

Fig. 6.1: Erythromelalgia in a patient with longstanding polycythemia vera

- Headaches, lack of concentration and fatigue are common symptoms that occur in patients with polycythemia vera as well.

Diagnostic Tests

- Physical exam findings are nonspecific, but may include enlarged liver or spleen, plethora, or gouty nodules.
- Laboratory tests: Common findings include an elevated hemoglobin level or hematocrit, reflecting the increased number of red blood cells; the platelet count or white blood cell count may also be increased. The erythrocyte sedimentation rate (ESR) is decreased due to an increase in zeta potential. Because polycythemia vera results from an essential increase in erythrocyte production, patients have a low erythropoietin (EPO) level.

Management

- Untreated, polycythemia vera can be fatal.
- Venesection or phlebotomy: The removal of blood from the body reduces the blood volume and brings down the hematocrit levels; in patients with polycythemia vera, this reduces the risk of blood clots. Venesection is typically performed in people with polycythemia vera to bring their hematocrit (red blood cell percentage) down below 45 for men or 42 for women. It has been observed that phlebotomy also improves cognitive impairment.
- Low dose aspirin (75–81 mg daily) is often prescribed. Aspirin reduces the risk for various thrombotic complications.
- Chemotherapy may be used for maintenance, or when the rate of phlebotomy required maintaining normal hematocrit is not acceptable, or when

there is significant thrombocytosis or intractable pruritus. This is usually with a cytoreductive agent (hydroxyurea, also known as hydroxycarbamide).

- Bone marrow transplants are rarely undertaken in polycythemia patients; since this condition is nonfatal if treated and monitored, the benefits rarely outweigh the risks involved in such a procedure.
- Use of certain genetic markers, Erlotinib may be an additional treatment option for this condition.

NURSING MANAGEMENT

Nursing Assessment

Subjective data

Ask the patient about the history of any peptic ulcer disease, itching all over the body, burning sensation in the hands and feet, fatigue, headache.

Objective data

Development of blood clots (thrombosis) e.g. heart attack, stroke, deep venous thrombosis, lack of concentration, gouty arthritis, pruritus or itching, particularly after exposure to warm water (such as when taking a bath).

Nursing Diagnosis

- Altered tissue perfusion related to increased blood volume as evidenced by increase serum level of RBC, WBC and platelets.
- Impaired skin integrity related to abnormal histamine release in blood as evidenced by pruritus all over the body.

Planning Outcomes/Goals

- Maintain a normal blood volume
- Maintain normal skin integrity.

Nursing interventions

Maintain a normal blood volume

- Assess the serum RBC, WBC and platelets.
- Assess the signs of abnormal blood volume such as headache, fatigue, burning sensation in hands and feets, lack of concentration.
- Administer low dose of aspirin to prevent thrombosis.
- Explain the patient about phlebotomy.
- Assist the patient in the procedure.

Maintain normal skin intergrity

- Assess the condition of skin.
- Encourage the patient to take bath intepid or cool water.
- Apply cocoa butter lotions and bath products to moisture the skin.
- Report for any kind of allergic reaction over the body.

LEUKEMIA

Definition

Leukemia is cancer of the blood cells. It starts in the bone marrow, the soft tissue inside most bones.

- In case of leukemia, the bone marrow starts to make many abnormal white blood cells, called leukemia cells. They don't do the work of normal white blood cells, they grow faster than normal cells, and they don't stop growing when they should.
- Over time, leukemia cells can crowd out the normal blood cells. This can lead to serious problems such as anemia, bleeding, and infections. Leukemia cells can also spread to the lymph nodes or other organs and cause swelling or pain.

Types

There are two major types of leukemia.

Acute or chronic and acute leukemia

It refers to a disorder of rapid onset. In the acute myelocytic leukemias, the abnormal cells grow rapidly and do not mature.In acute lymphocytic leukemias, cell growth is not so rapid as that of the myelocytic cells. Rather the cell tends to accumulate.

Chronic leukemia

The onset tends to be slow, and the cells generally mature abnormally and often accumulate in various organs. Their ability to fight infections and assist in repairing injured tissue is impaired.

- It may be lymphocytic or myelogenous. Lymphocytic (or lymphoblastic) leukemia affects white blood cells called lymphocytes. Myelogenous leukemia affects white blood cells called myelocytes.

The four main types of leukemia

- Acute lymphoblastic leukemia or ALL.
- Acute myelogenous leukemia or AML.
- Chronic lymphocytic leukemia or CLL.
- Chronic myelogenous leukemia or CML.

In adults, chronic lymphocytic leukemia (CLL) and acute myelogenous leukemia (AML) are the most common leukemias. In children, the most common leukemia is acute lymphoblastic leukemia (ALL). Childhood leukemias also include acute myelogenous leukemia (AML) and other myeloid leukemias, such as chronic myelogenous leukemia (CML) and juvenile myelomonocytic leukemia (JMML).

Other types

- Hairy cell leukemia: Accounts for only 2%. Male over 40 years of age are mostly affected. It is a chronic disease of lymphoproliferation predominantly involving B-lymphocytes that infiltrate the bone marrow and spleen. Cells have hairy appearance under the microscope.
- There are also subtypes of leukemia—such as acute promyelocytic leukemia (a subtype of AML).
- Unclassified leukamia occasionally the subtype cannot be classified. The malignant leukemia cells may have lymphoid, myeloid, or mixed. They have a poor prognosis and does not respond to treatment.

Causes

The exact cause of leukemia is unknown. The following are some of the risk factors for leukemia:

- Smoking.
- Long-term exposure to chemicals such as benzene or formaldehyde.
- Prolonged exposure to radiation.
- Previous chemotherapy.
- Infection with Human T cell leukemia virus1 (HTLV-1).
- Myelodysplastic syndromes.
- Down syndrome and other genetic disease.
- Family history.

Clinical Manifestations

- Fever and night sweats.
- Frequent infections.
- Fatigue.
- Headache.
- Confusion.
- Blurred vision.
- Seizures.
- Bruising or bleeding easily.
- Bone or joint pain.
- A swollen or painful abdomen from an enlarged spleen.

- Swollen lymph nodes in the armpit, neck or groin.
- Losing weight and not feeling hungry.

Diagnosis Tests

History

The health care provider should collect a detailed history regarding symptoms, current medical situations, medications, medical and surgical history, family history, work history, habits and lifestyle.

- The physical examination includes a thorough evaluation of all symptoms, not merely lymph nodes and/or possible enlargements of the liver and spleen.

Blood tests

Complete blood count.

Biopsy

Biopsy means to take a small sample of the relevant tissue to check for abnormal cells. In leukemia, a biopsy of the bone marrow must be taken and examined. Samples of both liquid (aspirate) and solid bone marrow (biopsy) are taken, usually from a hip bone. The bone marrow is examined under a microscope, where the presence of leukemic cells confirms the suspected diagnosis.

Genetic studies

The chromosomes of the abnormal cells are examined to look for irregularities. This helps in classifying the various types of leukemia.

Lumbar puncture

Because the collection of leukemia cells in the central nervous system can affect mental processes, it is extremely important to know whether the fluid surrounding the brain and spinal cord (cerebrospinal fluid) is affected. The fluid is examined for the presence of leukemia cells.

Lymph node excision

If the lymph nodes are enlarged, a node may require a biopsy if the bone marrow is difficult to interpret for some obscure reason. This is exceedingly uncommon.

Chest X-ray

A chest X-ray is frequently taken to look for signs of infection or lymph node involvement by leukemia.

Staging

- Staging is the way cancers are classified. Staging indicates the size or extent of spread of the cancer, the degree to which other parts of the body are affected. In general, leukemias are classified rather than staged in order to determine the most appropriate therapy.
- All leukemias are classified according to their genotypes, or their unique chromosomal arrangements.
- Chronic myelogenous leukemia is classified by phase. The three phases are chronic phase, accelerated phase, and blast phase (or blast crisis) and are defined by the number of blasts (immature leukemia cells) in the blood and bone marrow.
- Chronic lymphocytic leukemia is classified by two different staging systems, both based on the parts of the body affected by the leukemia.

Management

Medical management

- Leukemia treatment falls into two categories—treatment to fight the cancer and treatment to relieve the symptoms of the disease and the side effects of the treatment (supportive care).

- The most appropriate treatment is chemotherapy, that is, the use of powerful drugs to kill leukemia cells.
- Treatment usually involves combinations of chemotherapy.
- The chemotherapeutic drugs are administered intravenously (IV).
- Patients who have leukemia in their cerebrospinal fluid, or who are at high risk of having leukemic cells migrate to the spinal fluid, receive chemotherapy directly into the cerebrospinal canal. This is known as intrathecal chemotherapy.

Intrathecal chemotherapy: It is necessary because drugs given via IV do not sufficiently penetrate into the cerebrospinal fluid or brain and, thus, cannot kill leukemia cells there. Insufficient penetration of drugs into the cerebrospinal fluid results in uncontrolled growth of leukemic cells in the cerebrospinal fluid. Sometimes the therapy is inserted into a sac placed in one of the larger fluid-filled areas of the brain, a ventricle. The sac is known as an Ommaya reservoir, so named after its developer.

- The reservoir stays in place for the duration of the treatment.
- Newer agents are being developed that target leukemia cells and only minimally affecting healthy cells. These agents are known as targeted therapy.
- These agents greatly reduce the severity of side effects.
- Imatinib (Gleevec), an agent used in the treatment of CML, is an example of such a targeted therapy drug.

Chemotherapy is usually given in cycles

- Each cycle consists of intensive treatment over several days followed by a few weeks without treatment for rest and recovery from side effects caused by the chemotherapy, particularly anemia and low white blood cells. The sequence is then repeated.
- Chemotherapy regimens may be administered for 2 to 8 cycles, depending on the subtype of leukemia and risk factors involved.
- In accordance with particular treatment regimens, bone marrow exams may be carried out prior to each cycle of chemotherapy. After completion of treatment, the patient is evaluated again to see the effect of the chemotherapy on the leukemia.

Phases of chemotherapy

Induction: The purpose of this first phase is to kill as many leukemia cells as possible and bring about a remission.

Consolidation: In this phase, the goal is to seek out and kill the residual leukemia cells not killed by induction. Often, these cells are not detectable, but they are assumed to be still present.

Maintenance: The third phase is used to keep numbers of leukemia cells low, that is, to keep the disease in remission. The doses of chemotherapy are not as high as in the first two phases. This phase can last as long as 2 years.

- The fundamental goal of chemotherapy is to cure the patient. Cure means that blood tests and bone marrow biopsy show no evidence of leukemia and the leukemia does not come back (relapse) over time. Only time can determine whether a remission (with no evidence of disease) will lead to disease-free survival (cure).
- In effect, remission may be short-lived, thereby requiring administration of new, previously unseen therapy. Results

of this approach, often referred to as second-line therapy, are rarely curative. Stem cell transplant, if available, has the best chance of a second-line therapy cure.

Biological drug therapy

- This type of therapy uses biological drugs that act similarly to the body's natural immune system, such as monoclonal antibodies, interferon, or interleukins.
- Biological therapy consists of proteins like those produced naturally by the body's immune system to promote the body's innate ability to fight cancer.
- Patients with chronic lymphocytic leukemia or acute myelogenous leukemia receive a monoclonal antibody. This is an antibody specifically designed to fight their type of leukemia cells.
- People with chronic myelogenous leukemia receive injections of interferon, a protein produced by some of the body's lymphocytes, which on occasion may slow the growth of leukemia cells but which has many unpleasant side effects.

Radiation therapy

Radiotherapy is another treatment occasionally used in some types of leukemia.

- A high-energy beam is targeted at an organ, such as the brain, bones, or spleen, where large numbers of leukemia cells have collected. The radiation kills these cells.

Stem cell transplantation

It is a treatment that allows use of very high doses of chemotherapy along with total body irradiation in order to kill the leukemic cells.

- At the completion of high-dose (lethal) therapy, the patient's immune system is essentially depleted, and the patient is at high risk of developing serious life-threatening infections. Accordingly, these patients are treated in specially designed, sterile, air-filtered marrow transplant rooms.
- Immediately upon completion of the high-dose therapy, stem cells from a healthy, complete blood cell matched donor, usually a sibling or less commonly a parent, are transplanted into a vein whereupon they migrate to the marrow where they grow and multiply before entering the circulation, a process that may take 2 to 3 weeks to be completed.
- On rare occasions, when a donor is not available, one's own marrow cells, usually pretreated in order to remove residual, but otherwise unseen, leukemic cells, are infused. This approach is far less successful than the use of matched donor cells.
- If a patient receives stem cells from a matched donor, the type of stem cell transplant is called allogeneic. If the patient's own stem cells are reintroduced back into the patient following high dose therapy, the infusion is called autologous. Marrow or stem cells from an identical twin are referred to as syngeneic.

NURSING MANAGEMENT

Nursing Assessment

Subjective data

Patients complain about weakness, fatigue resulting in complications of anemia and infection.

Objective data

Dry cough, mild dyspnea, diminished breath sounds, fever suggesting pulmonary infection. Decreased WBC and platelets, increase in creatinine levels, a swollen or painful abdomen from an enlarged spleen. Swollen lymph nodes in the armpit, neck, or groin, loosing and not feeling hungry.

Nursing Diagnoses

- Risk for infection related to neutropenia or leukocytosis secondary to leukemia or treatment.
- Decreased cardiac output related to thrombocytopenia secondary to either leukemia or treatment.
- Imbalanced nutrition: Less than body requirement RT anorexia, pain or fatigue.
- Disturbed body image resulting from alopecia, weight loss and fatigue.

Planning Outcomes/ Goals

- Prevent or manage infection
- Improve cardiac output
- Maintain adequate nutrition
- Positive body image.

Nursing Interventions

Prevent or manage infection

- Assess the cause of fever.
- Send the specimens of blood, sputum, central lines sites for culture.
- Administer antibiotic as ordered.
- Hand washing and maintain other infection control policies.
- Monitor the client closely for manifestations of fungal or viral infections (R/R, rales, dyspnea, changed oral mucosa).

Improve cardiac output

- Assess the vital signs, oxygen saturation, ABG parameters, etc.
- Check the platelet count, Hb% level, and Hct daily.
- Provide a soft toothbrush for oral hygiene.
- Do not give any IM or SC inj.
- Remove all potential hazards and sharp objects from the environment.
- Administer packed RBCs and platelets as ordered.

Maintain adequate nutrition

- Assess the nutritional status of the patient.
- Monitor weight daily.
- Administer local and IV analgesics as ordered.
- Provide high CHO diet and encourage small and frequent meals.
- If the client cannot tolerate food, begin total parenteral nutrition.

Positive body image

- Assess the psychological state of the patient.
- Encourage the patient to ventilate his/ her feelings.
- Encourage the patient to use hats, wigs, as desired.
- Alopecia may be permanent with whole brain radiation therapy (WBXRT).
- Encourage the client to balance rest with exercise and activities to maintain muscle tone.
- Provide high CHO diet.

DISSEMINATED INTRAVASCULAR COAGULOPATHY (DIC)

Definition

DIC is a serious bleeding and thrombotic disorder. It involves abnormal, excessive generation of thrombin and fibrin in the circulating blood. The condition is characterized by the profuse bleeding that result from the depletion of platelets and clotting factors.

Predisposing Conditions

Acute DIC

- **Shock**
  - Hemorrhage
  - Cardiogenic
  - Anaphylactic.
- **Septicemia**
  - Hemolytic processes
  - Transfusion of mismatched blood
  - Acute hemolysis from infection or immunologic disorders.
- **Obstetric conditions**
  - Abruptio placenta
  - Amniotic fluid embolism
  - Septic abortion.
- **Malignancies**
  - Acute leukemia
  - Lymphoma
  - Tumor lysis syndrome.
- **Tissue damage**
  - Extensive burns and trauma.
  - Heatstroke.
  - Severe head injury.
  - Transplant rejection.
  - Postoperative damage, specially ECMO.
  - Fat and pulmonary emboli.
  - Snakebites.
  - Glomerulonephritis.
  - Acute anoxia.
  - Fulminant hepatitis.

Subacute DIC

- **Malignant disease**
  - Myeloproliferative malignancies
  - Metastasic cancer.
- **Obstetric**
  - Retained dead fetus

Chronic DIC

- Liver disease
- Systemic lupus erythematosus(SLE)
- Localized malignancy.

Pathophysiology (Fig. 6.2)

- DIC can occur as an acute, catastrophic condition, or it may exist at a subacute or chronic level. Each condition may have one or multiple triggering mechanism to start the clotting cascade.
- For example, tumors and traumatized or necrotic tissue release tissue factors into circulation. Endotoxin from gram-negative bacteria activates several steps in the coagulation cascade.

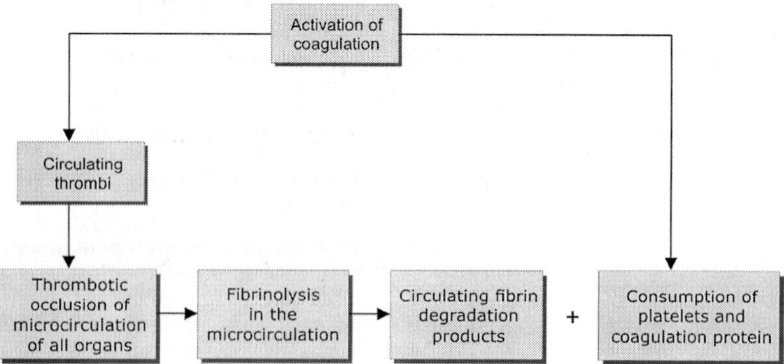

Fig. 6.2: The sequence of events that occur during DIC

- Tissue factor is released at the site of tissue injury and by some malignancies such as leukemia causes normal coagulation mechanisms to be enhanced.
- Abundant intravascular thrombin, the most powerful coagulant, is produced. It catalyzes the conversion of fibrinogen to fibrin and platelet aggregation.
- There is widespread fibrin and platelet deposition in capillaries and arterioles resulting in thrombosis; this can lead to multi organ failure.
- In addition, clotting inhibitory mechanism, such as antithrombin III (AT III) and protein C are depressed.
- This excessive clotting activates the fibrinolytic system, which in turn breaks down the newly formed clot creating fibrin split products.
- These products have anticoagulant properties and inhibit normal blood clotting.
- Ultimately with fibrin split products accumulating and clotting factors being depleted, the blood loses its ability to clot.
- Therefore a stable clot cannot be formed at injury sites. This situation predisposes the patient to hemorrhage.

Clinical Manifestations

See Table 6.1 for clinical mainifestion.

Diagnosis tests

DIC is suspected in patients with unexplained bleeding or venous thromboembolism especially if a predisposing condition exists. The following laboratory test is conducted if DIC is suspected.

- Blood for: Platelet count, plasma fibrinogen level, prothombin time, partial thromboplastin time and activated partial thromboplastin time.
- Special test: Plasma D–dimer, antithrombin III(AT III).

Management

Prehospital care

- Monitor vital signs, assess and document extent of hemorrhage and thrombosis, correct hypovolemia and administer basic hemostatic procedures when indicated.

Emergency department care

- The management of acute and chronic forms of DIC should primarily be directed at treatment of the underlying disorder. Typically, DIC results in

Table 6.1: Clinical manifestations of DIC

Signs of microvascular thrombosis	Signs of hemorrhage
• Neurologic: Multifocal, delirium,coma • Integumentary: Focal ischemia,superficial • Renal: Oliguria,azotemia, cortical necrosis • Pulmonary: Acute respiratory distress syndrome • Gastrointestinal: Paralytic ileus.	• Neurologic: Intracerebral bleeding • Integumentary: Petechiae, ecchymoses, gangrene, venipuncture, oozing • Renal: Hematuria • Pulmonary: Respiratory congestion, dyspnea hemoptysis • Mucous membrane: Epistaxis, gingival oozing • Gastrointestinal: Massive bleeding

significant reductions in platelet count and increases in coagulation times (PT and APTT).
- If a patient is bleeding therapy is directed toward providing support with necessary blood products while treating the primary disorder.

Blood components

- Blood components are used to correct abnormal hemostatic parameters. These products should be considered only after initial supportive and anticoagulant therapy.
- Washed PRBCs and platelet concentrates are considered safe in uncontrolled DIC. Specialized blood components (cryoprecipitate, FFP) may interfere with or improve DIC.

Packed red blood cells

- Preferred to whole blood since they limit volume, immune, and storage complications.
- Obtain PRBCs after centrifugation of whole blood.
- Use washed or frozen PRBCs in individuals with hypersensitivity transfusion reactions.

Adult

- 1 unit of PRBCs should raise hemoglobin by 1 gm/dL or raise hematocrit by 3%.

Fresh frozen plasma

- This treatment entails removing blood from body, spinning it to separate cells from plasma, and replacing cells suspended in fresh frozen plasma, albumin, or saline. Contains coagulation factors as well as protein C and protein S. Recommended with active bleeding and fibrinogen <100 mg/dL.

Adult

- 15 to 20 mL/kg IV or based on clinical situation

Cryoprecipitate or Fibrinogen Concentrates

Not commonly recommended except when fibrinogen is needed.

Adult

- Each bag contains 80 to 100 U of factor VIII; base administration on fibrinogen levels, antithrombin III levels, and coagulation parameters.

Medications

- Therapy should be based on etiology and aimed at eliminating the underlying disease. Therapy should be appropriately aggressive for the patient's age, disease, and severity and location of hemorrhage/thrombosis.
- Treatment for acute DIC includes anticoagulants, blood components, and antifibrinolytics.
- Hemostatic and coagulation parameters should be monitored continuously during treatment.

Anticoagulants: Heparin or low molecular weight heparin

- Use and dose of heparin is based on severity of DIC, underlying cause, and extent of thrombosis.

Dosage in adult

- 80 to 100 U/kg SC 4 to 6h or 20,000 to 30,000 IU for IV continuous infusion.
- Heparin augments antithrombin III activity and prevents conversion of fibrinogen to fibrin.
- Does not actively lyse but inhibits further thrombogenesis.

- Prevents reaccumulation of a clot after spontaneous fibrinolysis.

Antithrombin III (AT native)

- Used for moderately severe to severe DIC or when levels are depressed markedly. Alfa-2-globulin that inactivates thrombin, plasmin, and other serine proteases of coagulation, including factors IXa, Xa, XIa, XIIa, and VIIa. These effects inhibit coagulation.
- Dosage: Total Units = (Desired Level - Initial Level) (0.6 × Total Body Weight kg) IV 8 hourly with a desired level >125% or loading dose of 100 U/kg IV over 3 hours; followed by continuous infusion of 100 U/kg.

Recombinant human activated protein C (Drotrecogin alfa [Xigris])

- These agents inhibit factors Va and VIIIa of the coagulation cascade. They may also inhibit plasminogen activator inhibitor-1 (PAI-1).
- Indicated for reduction of mortality in patients with severe sepsis associated with acute organ dysfunction and at high risk of death. Recombinant form of human activated protein C that exerts antithrombotic effect by inhibiting factors Va and VIIIa. Has indirect profibrinolytic activity by inhibiting PAI-1 and limiting formation of activated thrombin-activatable-fibrinolysis-inhibitor. May exert anti-inflammatory effect by inhibiting human tumor necrosis factor (TNF) production by monocytes, blocking leukocyte adhesion to selectins and limiting thrombin-induced inflammatory responses within micro vascular endothelium.

NURSING MANAGEMENT

Nursing Assessment

Subjective data

Ask the patient about any history of gum bleeding, oozing from wounds, previous injection sites, respiratory distress, hematuria, tarry stool, anxiety ,headache, visual disturbances, decreased urine output.

Objective data

Decreased temperature, increase pain sensation, cyanosis in extremities,nose, earlobes, bradycardia, hypoxia, heartburn, decreased urine output,decreased alertness and orientation, petechia, tachycardia, hemoptysis.

Nursing Diagnosis

- Potential for fluid volume deficit related to bleeding.
- Potential for impaired skin integrity secondary to ischemia or bleeding.
- Potential for diminished tissue perfusion secondary to microthrombi.

Planning Outcomes/Goals

- Maintain hemodynamic status
- Intact skin integrity
- Maintain normal tissue perfusion.

Nursing interventions

Maintain hemodynamic status

- Monitor vital signs closely including neurological status.
- Avoid procedures/activities that can increase intracranial pressure.
- Avoid medication that can interfere with platelet function such as NSAIDs, beta lactum antibiotics.
- Avoid IM injection.

- Monitor amount of external bleeding carefully.
- Give mouth care carefully avoid hydrogen peroxide, or commercial mouthwashes. Use normal saline.

Intact skin integrity

- Assess skin, particularly bony prominences and skin folds.
- Position carefully, provide water or air mattress.
- Perform skin care every 4 hourly interval.
- Provide comfort devices such as extra pillows, air cushion, air rings, etc.

Maintain normal tissue perfusion

- Assess neurologic, pulmonary, circulatory and integumentary system.
- Monitor response to heparin therapy.
- Assess extent of bleeding.
- Monitor fibrinogen level.
- Administer IV fluids and give blood transfusion as ordered.
- Monitor and record intake and output.

7

Nursing Management of Patients with Disorders of Gastrointestinal System

ASSESSMENT OF PATIENTS WITH DISORDERS OF GASTROINTESTINAL SYSTEM

Subjective Data

Chief complaints of abdominal pain, nausea, vomiting, diarrhea, constipation, abdominal distention, heart burn, dyspepsia, changes in appetite, indigestion, excessive gas, bloating, food intolerance or allergies, hematemesis, melena, hemorrhoids, rectal bleeding, jaundice, anemia.

Presence or past history of diseases such as gastritis, peptic ulcer, colitis, hepatitis, gallstone, cancer, hernias.

Unexplained weight loss or gain, dieting, changes in taste or smell, sensitivity to hot or cold.

Past and current use of medications, prescription drugs, over the counter medications, herbal medications, supplements, appetite suppressants, hepatotoxic medications, e.g. acetaminophen, NSAIDs (potential to gastrointestinal bleeding); antibiotics (potential to change bacterial composition of gastrointestinal tract leading to diarrhea); antacids and laxatives.

Treatments and surgery for major diseases, blood transfusion.

Maintenance of proper body weight, oral care and hygiene, elimination pattern, nutritional practices such as strict vegetarian (may lead to anemia).

Recent travel, immunization of hepatitis A and hepatitis B.

Consumption of alcohol and smoking.

Activity and exercises, immobility, sleep disturbances due to gastrointestinal problems, stress and anxiety.

Self-perception about being very thin or obese, body image disturbances due to presence of jaundice, ascites, colostomy, etc.

Objective Data

Height, weight, skin fold thickness.

Color of lips, sore in lips, ulcer or growth in lips, lesion in mouth, condition of teeth, swelling, bleeding from gums, pigmentation on buccal mucosa or tongue, mouth odor. Scar on abdomen, striae, dilated veins, rashes, umbilicus for location, contour of the abdomen, observable masses, movement (peristalsis) and pulsation on inspection.

Bowel sounds normal (high-pitched gurgling sound, 5 to 35 per minute); absent or less than 5 in 1 minute; loud gurgles or borborygmi due to hyperperistalsis on auscultation.

Tympany (higher pitched hollow sound) or dullness (short high pitched sound with no resonance) on percussion.

Location, size, shape of abdominal organs, tenderness, rebound tenderness on palpation.

Color, texture, lumps, scars, rashes, erythema, fissures, external hemorrhoids on inspection of perianal and anal areas. Nodules, tenderness, or any other abnormality on palpation of the rectum.

Findings of the Diagnostic Studies

1. Fecal analysis for presence of undigested material, mucus, blood, pus, parasites, fat content and occult blood.
2. Stool culture for presence of bacteria.
3. Blood test for hemoglobin percentage. Serum amylase and serum lipase for pancreatic functioning.
4. Gastric analysis to determine hyperchlorohydria (excessive gastric acid secretion) and achlorhydria (absence of gastric acid secretion).
5. Abdominal ultrasound to detect tumor, cysts enlargement of organs and fluid in abdomen, gallstones, etc.
6. X-ray (plain) in upright position detects level of fluid and gas pockets in intestinal obstruction.
7. X-ray using contrast medium (Barium solution):
   a. Upper gastrointestinal series (Barium meal and Barium swallow) taken to identify conditions of esophagus, stomach and small intestine such as esophageal varices, strictures, tumors, polyp, foreign bodies, ulcers, gastric ulcer and duodenal ulcer.
   b. Lower gastrointestinal series (Barium enema) reveals polyps, tumor and other lesions in the colon.
8. CT scan and MRI detect status of biliary tract, liver and pancreas.
9. Nuclear imaging scan is the intravenous injection of radioactive isotope followed by scanning, done to show size shape and position of organs.
10. Gastric emptying study. In this procedure radioactive isotope is ingested by the patient with food or drink and then scanning is done to assess ability of stomach to empty its content.
11. Cholangiography (Percutaneous transhepatic cholangiogram, Surgical cholangiogram, Magnetic resonance cholangiopancreatography) obtains images of hepatic duct, biliary duct and pancreatic ducts.
12. Endoscopy is the visualization of the mucosal lining of the gastrointestinal tract. Esophagogastroduodenoscopy visualizes mucosal lining of esophagus, stomach and duodenum with flexible fiberoptic endoscope. Varices may be treated and biopsies are obtained also through endoscope.
13. Sigmoidoscopy visualizes rectum and sigmoid colon, Colonoscopy visualizes entire colon with lighted flexible endoscope and detects tumors, polyps, fissures, fistulas, hemorrhoids, inflammatory and infectious diseases.
14. Endoscopic retrograde cholangiopancreatography visualizes common bile duct and pancreatic ducts. The procedure may also treat gallstone in common bile duct, obtain biopsy of tumors.
15. Laparoscopy visualizes peritoneal cavity and its contents with the help of a laparoscope.

ORAL CANCER

Incidence

Cancers of the oral cavity is most common in the developing countries.

Highest incidence is recorded in India. 4 in 10 of all cancers are oral cancers.

It is the most common cancers in male (rank 1) and third common cancers in women (rank 3).

Site

Oral cancer is a type of head and neck cancer.

It may form on the lips or in any part within the mouth, e.g. tongue, floor of the mouth, hard palate, soft palate, buccal mucosa, pharyngeal walls and tonsils.

Etiology

Definite cause of oral cancer is unknown.

Predisposing factors

- Use of tobacco in any form, e.g. cigar, cigarette, pipe, snuff and chewing tobacco.
- Excessive alcohol intake.
- Intake of very hot beverages and food.
- Chronic irritation from ill fitting dentures or bad teeth or pipe resting on the lips.
- Constant overexposure to ultraviolet rays from the sun especially in fair complexion persons.
- Elderly persons.
- Poor oral hygiene.
- Deficient diet, ingestion of smoked meat.
- Recurrent herpetic lesion, syphilis.
- Immune suppression.

Pathophysiology

- The most common types of oral cancers are squamous cell carcinoma and basal cell carcinoma.
- Squamous cell carcinoma arises from the squamous cells of the mucous membrane that lines the oral cavity. Common sites are tongue, lower lip, floor of the mouth, buccal mucosa and tonsils.
- It is usually well-differentiated.
- Disease advances by direct invasion to buccal fat and even to the mandible.
- Rate of metastasis is less common. Metastasis takes place by direct infiltration of local lymph nodes.
- Basal cell carcinoma primarily occurs on the lips due to excessive exposure to sunlight particularly in fair-skinned persons.

Clinical Manifestations

1. White patches (leukoplakia) or red patches (erythroplakia) or a combination of red and white patches inside the mouth or lips (considered as precancerous).
2. A sore or lesion in the mouth or on the lips which bleeds easily and does not heal.
3. A mild irritation of the tongue, sore throat, difficulty in wearing dentures or loose teeth.
4. Difficulty in swallowing, chewing, moving the jaw.
5. Earache, toothache, pain in tongue, difficulty in moving the tongue and speaking, slurred speech, increased salivation, drooling.
6. Coughing of blood-tinged sputum or enlarged cervical lymph nodes.

Diagnostic Tests

1. Biopsy of the suspicious lesion with cytological examination is the definitive diagnostic study for oral cancer.
2. Oral exfoliative cytology (scraping the suspicious lesion and forming a smear on a slide for examination) and toluidine blue test (when toluidine blue is applied to the suspicious area, cancer cells if present take up the dye) may be used for initial screening as negative results do not always rule out malignancy.
3. CT scan and MRI may be done if metastasis is suspected.

Medical Management

Depending on the site and stage of cancer, management consists of surgery, radiation therapy, chemotherapy or a combination of these therapies.

Surgical therapy

Surgical therapy is the most effective treatment of oral cancers.

Various surgical procedures are carried out depending on the site and stage of cancer:

1. Hemiglossectomy is the removal of half of the tongue.
2. Glossectomy is removal of the tongue.
3. Mandibulectomy is removal of the mandible.
4. Resection of the buccal mucosa or floor of the mouth, or lips along with modified neck dissection (removal of superficial and deep cervical lymph nodes along with their channels).
5. Wide excision of the involved structures along with radical neck dissection (removal of superficial and deep cervical lymph nodes along with their channels, removal of all tissues under the skin from the jaw to clavicle, the sternocleidomastoid muscle, the spinal accessory nerve, internal jugular vein, mandible, submaxillary glands, part of the thyroid and parathyroid) is commonly performed along with a tracheostomy when disease is advanced.
6. Gastrostomy as a palliative surgery may be conducted in advanced inoperable cases to provide nutrition.

Radiation therapy

1. Teletherapy (external beam therapy) may be used when the disease is more advanced or involves several structures in the oral cavity.
2. Brachytherapy (interstitial radiation therapy) which involves implantation of radioactive seeds or needles in the tissue may be carried out for small localized lesion.

Chemotherapy

Chemotherapy may be used along with radiotherapy in case of advanced cancer or when surgery and radiation therapy has failed or as the initial stage therapy for a smaller tumor.

The drugs include 5-fluorouracil, bleomycin, adriamycin, methotrexate, cyclophosphamide, cisplatin, carboplatin, hydroxyurea, vincristine, paclitaxel, docetaxel, etc.

NURSING MANAGEMENT

Assessment

Subjective data

History of present illness—Sore in mouth or tongue or lip, painful ulcer, difficulty in chewing food and speaking, increased salivation, intolerance to certain foods or temperatures of foods, toothache, earache, white or red patches on the oral mucosa, bleeding in the mouth, foul odor, difficulty in wearing dentures, loss of body weight.

Past history of illness—Recurrent oral herpetic lesion, syphilis, removal of previous tumor or lesion, use of immunosuppressants.

Personal habits—Use of alcohol, tobacco in any form, poor oral hygiene, sun exposure for prolonged period.

Objective data

Ulcer on lip, mouth or tongue, areas of thickening or roughness, leukoplakia or erythroplakia on the tongue or oral mucosa, limited movement of the tongue, increased salivation or drooling, foul odor, slurred speech, painless neck mass or lump, anxious look, not mixing with others.

Diagnostic test findings—Positive exfoliative smear cytology and positive biopsy.

Nursing Diagnoses

1. Impaired oral mucous membrane related to the tumor or due to surgery or radiation therapy or chemotherapy as evidenced by sore, ulceration, increased salivation, xerostomia (dryness of mouth due to radiation or chemotherapy), halitosis, bleeding from mouth.
2. Deficient nutrition related to painful ulceration, difficulty in chewing and swallowing, surgical excision and radiation therapy as evidenced by loss of body weight.
3. Pain related to oral lesion, surgery or radiation therapy as evidenced by patient's complain of pain.
4. Social isolation related to change in body image secondary to oral lesion, impaired verbal communication or disfiguring surgery as evidenced by patient not mixing with others, covering mouth.
5. Risk for infection related to the disease or it's treatment regimen, i.e. surgery, radiotherapy or chemotherapy.
6. Anxiety related to the diagnosis of cancer, prognosis, possible disfiguring surgery or potential for recurrence as evidenced by anxious look, frequent questioning to the health team members or expression of sadness.
7. Deficient knowledge about disease process, treatment and self-care as evidenced by frequent questioning, expression of feelings of inadequacy.

Planning and Goals

- **Major goals for the patient will be**:

1. Improvement of oral mucous membrane.
2. Adequate nutritional intake.
3. Relief of pain and discomfort.
4. Attainment of a positive body image and establishing an alternate communication system.
5. Prevention of infection.
6. Relief of anxiety.
7. Understanding of the disease process, treatment regimen and self-care.

Nursing Interventions

Improvement of oral mucous membrane

- Teach patient to perform careful oral hygiene by avoiding physical, chemical or thermal trauma at least four times a day with a soft brush soaked in warm water. If unable to brush, gently irrigate mouth with normal saline or baking soda solution.
- If patient is unable to perform on his own then the nurse should provide such care to the patient.
- Instruct patient to take a lot of fluid if he experiences xerostomia (a complication of radiation therapy).
- Avoid dry, bulky, and irritating foods and fluids, alcohol and tobacco in any form.
- Encourage chewing of sugarless gums if dryness of mouth (xerostomia).
- Encourage patient to visit dental department before radiotherapy.

Maintaining adequate nutritional intake

- Monitor patient's body weight, level of activity and amount of foods and fluids ingested to find out the adequacy of daily calorie intake.
- Encourage small frequent feeds, non-irritating, soft in consistency and at room temperature.
- Teach patient how to obtain nutritious foods according to his means. Refer patient to a dietician if needed.

- Provide or encourage oral care before each feed to stimulate appetite.
- Administer analgesic as ordered one hour before meal.
- If unable to take food orally provide nutrition by nasogastric, gastrostomy or parenteral route.

Relief of pain and discomfort

- Assess patient's pain and discomfort with the help of a pain scale.
- Administer analgesic as ordered and monitor it's effectiveness.
- Encourage patient to avoid foods that are hot, hard in consistency and spicy.
- Teach patient frequent mouth care to get relief from discomfort.

Developing a positive body image

- Encourage verbalization of patient's feelings regarding his disfigurement or potential disfigurement secondary to surgery. Listen attentively, provide acceptance and support.
- Explain to patient the actual loss or gain.
- Explain patient that person's worth is not determined by his appearance only.
- Reinforce patient's achievements and positive attributes and strengths.
- Refer patient to a counselor or spiritual counselor or support group if needed.

Maintaining a meaningful communication system

- Assess patient's ability to communicate in writing.
- Provide magic slate or paper and pencil.
- If unable to write provide communication board with commonly used pictures or words so that he is able to point to the needed item.
- Refer the patient to the speech therapist if communication impairment is permanent.

Preventing infection

- Assess patient's oral lesion or incision site and dressing for presence of infection.
- Check patient's temperature (fever) regularly to find out early evidence of infection.
- Obtain periodical WBC count if patient on radiotherapy or chemotherapy since leukopenia indicates risk for infection.
- Provide nutritious diet to build resistance.
- Restrict visitors with any infection.
- Avoid trauma during mouth care and dressing. Use aseptic technique during dressing.

Understanding of the disease process, treatment regimen and self-care

- Teach patient the predisposing factors of oral cancer, i.e. tobacco, alcohol and other irritants and to abstain from all of these irritants.
- Explain the patient the treatment regimen planned for him by the physician.
- Discuss with the patient the preoperative preparation and postoperative feeding and communication problem and ways to overcome them beforehand.
- The need for radiotherapy and chemotherapy if any and their consequences should be explained to the patient.
- Demonstrate the technique of gentle mouth care, enteral feeding and gastrostomy feeding if any to the patient or a significant family member.
- Importance of proper nutrition to be explained to the patient. Demonstrate to relative how to make suitable meals for this patient according to his preference and means.
- When the patient is recovering from the disease teach him to regularly examine his mouth for signs of recurrence.

ACHALASIA

Definition

Achalasia is a rare disease of the muscles of the esophagus (swallowing tube). The term achalasia means "failure to relax" and refers to the inability of the lower esophageal sphincter to open and let food pass into the stomach.

Incidence

Achalasia is a rare disorder.

It may occur at any age, but is most common in middle-aged or older adults of both sexes.

Etiology and Risk Factors

- The cause of achalasia is unknown.
- Theories on causation suggest infection, heredity or autoimmune disease.
- No identifiable risk factors are known.

Pathophysiology

- Lower esophageal sphincter, which normally relaxes during swallowing, fails to relax and open to let food pass into the stomach. The reason for this problem is damage to the nerves of the esophagus.
- In addition to abnormal function of the lower esophageal sphincter, the peristalsis of the lower-half to two-thirds of the esophagus is absent.
- Food and fluids are not passed down and accumulate in the lower esophagus resulting in its dilation and increased lower esophageal sphincter pressure.

Clinical Manifestations

- Dysphagia occurring with both solids and liquids.
- Globus sensation (feeling of food sticking in the chest after it is swallowed).
- Feeling of heaviness in chest or substernal chest pain (like angina pain) occurring during or soon after meal.
- Halitosis.
- Inability to belch.
- Regurgitation of sour tasting food and fluids while lying down.
- Weight loss.

Complications

1. Esophagitis or esophageal ulcer due to the irritating effect of collected food and fluid in the esophagus.
2. Aspiration pneumonia from aspiration of regurgitated gastric contents in the lung.

Diagnostic Studies

1. X-ray studies after barium swallow (video esophagram) detects nonpropulsive waves and esophageal dilation. Barium retains in the esophagus for a longer time.
2. Endoscopy determines the status of the lower esophageal sphincter, esophageal dilation and presence of food in the esophagus.
3. Manometry reveals elevated lower esophageal sphincter pressure or slow or absent peristalsis.

Medical Management

Drug therapy

1. Nitrates, e.g. isosorbide dinitrate (Isordil) and calcium channel blockers, e.g. nifedipine (procardia) and verapamil (calan) taken immediately before meals improves dysphagia by relaxing the lower esophageal sphincter. Effectiveness of the drugs is short-term and side effects are common.
2. Antacids, H_2 receptor antagonists and proton pump inhibitor minimize pain.

3. Modification of diet, e.g. small and frequent feedings with semisoft warm foods, drinking fluids with meals, improves symptoms. Patient should avoid hot, spicy, iced foods, tobacco and alcohol.
4. Alternate positions, e.g. arching the back while swallowing or sitting or standing after eating may reduce pressure in lower esophageal sphincter (LES). Sleeping with head of the bed elevated on 4 to 6 inch blocks prevents nocturnal reflux of food.
5. Injection of botulinum toxin endoscopically into LES improves esophageal emptying and provides short-term relief of symptoms for 1 to 2 years. Botulinum toxin promotes smooth muscle relaxation by inhibiting the release of acetylcholine from nerve endings.

Conservative management

Pneumatic dilation: Endoscopic pneumatic dilation is done as an outpatient procedure. Under sedation and radiologic guidance a balloon tipped tube is placed endoscopically to the narrowed part of the esophagus and the LES. Sudden inflation of the balloon stretches and tears the muscle fibers in the esophagus and the LES.

Surgical management

Esophagomyotomy or Heller myotomy is done to enlarge the opening by surgical incision of the circular muscle fibers of the LES laparoscopically. GERD being a common complication of this procedure, antireflux surgery is often combined at the same time.

NURSING MANAGEMENT

Assessment

Subjective data

Dysphagia with solid and liquid foods, globus sensation, heaviness in chest, substernal chest pain occurring during or soon after meal, regurgitation of sour tasting food and fluids while lying down, unintentional weight loss.

Objective data

Evidence of malnourishment, anemia.

Possible diagnostic test findings

Absence of peristalsis and esophageal dilation in video esophagram, esophageal dilation and presence of food in the lower esophagus seen by endoscopy, elevated lower esophageal sphincter pressure by manometry.

Nursing Diagnoses

1. Imbalanced nutrition less than body requirement related to dysphagia as evidenced by the complain of weight loss, manifestation of malnutrition and anemia.
2. Acute pain related to episodes of gastric reflux as evidenced by patient's verbal complaints.
3. Deficient knowledge related to preoperative preparation and postoperative care.

GOALS

1. Maintenance of adequate nutritional intake.
2. Relief of pain.
3. Understanding of the surgical procedure (if planned), preoperative preparation and postoperative care.

Nursing Interventions

Maintenance of adequate nutritional intake

- Observe patient during meal time and assess the amount of food the patient is able to consume.
- Discuss with patient regarding his di-

etary habits and amount of nutrient consumed daily.

- Obtain body weight of patient on admission and monitor body weight daily.
- Teach the patient to:
  - Eat slowly in small amounts and frequent intervals.
  - Chew food thoroughly to ease swallowing.
  - Eat semisoft, warm foods.
  - Avoid cold, hard, spicy, iced foods as well as tobacco and alcohol.
  - Adopt certain positions, e.g. arching the back while swallowing.
  - Administer medications, e.g. nitrates or calcium channel blockers as ordered before meal.
  - Remain upright by standing or sitting after eating.
- Administer feeding through gastrostomy tube if patient is unable to consume adequate amount of food orally.

Relief of pain

- Assess pain by a pain scale.
- Explain patient the reason for pain.
- Administer medications as ordered, e.g. H_2 blockers, proton pump inhibitors.
- Teach patient modification of diet, alternate positions during eating and sleeping with head elevated.
- Reassess pain every shift to find out the effectiveness of medications, dietary modifications and alternate positions.

Understanding of the surgical procedure, preoperative preparation and postoperative care

- Explain patient that:
  - Pneumatic dilation, if planned will be carried out as an OPD procedure.
  - He/she has to be on liquid diet 12 hours to 2 days before the procedure depending on the severity of the condition.
  - He/she will not feel pain, as physician will spray anesthetic agent to the throat.
  - He/she has to cooperate by swallowing the tube and by taking slow long breaths during tube insertion.
  - Slight discomfort may be felt during tube insertion.
  - Severe pain should be reported to the physician.
  - He/she may consume oral feeding after 6 hours of the procedure.

GASTROESOPHAGEAL REFLUX DISEASE

Introduction

Occasional back flow of stomach content into the esophagus or gastroesophageal reflux (GER) is normal both in adults and children but persistent GER (more than twice a week for a prolonged period) in some individuals giving rise to a more serious health problem is considered as gastroesophageal reflux disease (GERD).

Definition

Gastroesophageal reflux disease (GERD) refers to a syndrome resulting from excessive reflux of gastric contents into the esophagus giving rise to significant clinical manifestations or histopathologic changes. This condition is also known as reflux esophagitis.

Incidence

GERD may occur at any age group but increased incidence is found in aged population.

10% of populations in the United States have daily manifestations of GERD.

Etiology and Predisposing Factors

- Exact cause of GERD is still unknown. It is believed to be due to:
  - Inappropriate relaxation of the lower esophageal sphincter (LES).

- Anatomic alteration of gastroesophageal region, e.g. hiatal hernia, incompetent LES.
- Impaired esophageal motility resulting into ineffective emptying of food and fluids from the esophagus into the stomach.
- Decreased emptying of stomach.

Other contributing factors

- Obesity, pregnancy.
- Smoking, chewing tobacco.
- High levels of estrogen and progesterone.

Common foods that increase symptoms of GERD

- High fat, spicy and fried foods.
- Citrus fruits.
- Carbonated beverages, alcohol, caffeinated drinks.
- Foods containing peppermint flavorings.

Pathophysiology

- The region of gastroesophageal sphincter normally is a high pressure area.
- Due to high pressure, food and fluids that enter in the stomach cannot get back into esophagus.
- Reflux occurs when there is an alteration of pressure in this area.
- The reflux commonly contains gastric and duodenal contents consisting of hydrochloric acid, pepsin, bile salts, bile acids, intestinal enzymes which are corrosive to the esophageal mucosa.
- Reflux of these corrosives for a prolonged period cause inflammation of esophagus or esophagitis.
- The degree of esophagitis depends on frequency and content of reflux; buffering ability of the saliva and mucus; rate of gastric emptying.

Clinical Manifestations

1. Pyrosis (Heart burn). Intermittent burning pain behind the sternum which spreads upward to the throat, jaw or back. Pain occurs after meals and is relieved by drinking milk or fluids, antacids, standing or walking. Activities that increase intraabdominal pressure, e.g. straining, lifting increases discomfort.
2. Dyspepsia.
3. Dysphagia/odynophagia.
4. Acid regurgitation (hot bitter or sour liquid).
5. Hyper salivation (water brash).
6. Respiratory symptoms, e.g. wheezing, coughing, dyspnea, disturbed sleep pattern due to nocturnal coughing.
7. Otolaryngologic symptoms, e.g. hoarseness, sore throat, sense of lump in the throat and choking.
8. Gastric symptoms, e.g. early satiety, post meal bloating, nausea, vomiting due to delayed gastric emptying.

Complications

- Esophagitis.
- Esophageal strictures.
- Barret's esophagus—It is a precancerous condition. Normal squamous epithelium of the esophagus is replaced by columnar epithelium. A potential risk for adenocarcinoma.
- Cough, laryngospasm, cricopharyngeal spasm.
- Asthma, chronic bronchitis.
- Dental erosion.

Diagnostic Tests

1. Endoscopy with biopsy and cytological studies—It detects LES competence,

scarring, strictures in esophagus and Barret's esophagus or malignancy.
2. Barium swallow—It detects hiatal hernia and other anatomical problems of esophagus and stomach.
3. Esophageal manometry—It determines pressure in esophagus and LES.
4. Gastric pH study and acid perfusion test detect hyperchlorohydria.
5. Radio nuclide studies—It detect reflux of gastric content and rate of esophageal clearance.

Management

Management consists of:
- Lifestyle changes
- Nutritional therapy
- Drug therapy
- Surgical therapy
- Endoscopic therapy.

Lifestyle changes

The patient is taught to avoid factors that increase symptoms by affecting LES, increasing acid secretion and delays gastric emptying, e.g.
- Lose weight, if overweight, to decrease LES pressure gradient.
- Avoid tobacco, salicylates, etc. as they may aggravate gastritis.
- Wear loose-fitting clothes.
- Avoid lying down for 3 hours after a meal.
- Elevate the head of the bed to 6 to 8 inches by securing wood blocks under the bedposts to prevent nocturnal reflux.

Nutritional therapy

- To take small frequent feeds comprising of 4 – 6 feeds per day.
- Chew food thoroughly and eat slowly to add saliva to the food.
- Avoid extremely hot or cold foods, spices, fats, coffee, alcohol, chocolate and citrous juices to decrease acid production. Avoid milk products especially at bed time.
- Avoid drinking fluids with meals. Drink adequate fluids in between meals.

Drug therapy

1. Antacids 1 to 3 hours after meals and at bed time are effective to relieve mild to moderate symptoms of heart burn.
2. H_2 R blockers, e.g. cimetidine, ranitidine, famotidine decrease HCl acid secretion by the stomach, reduce symptoms and promote esophageal healing in 50% patients.
3. Proton pump inhibitors, e.g. omeprazole, pantoprazole, lansoprazole, etc.- decrease HCl acid secretion and heal the esophageal lining in 90% of patients.
4. Cytoprotective, e.g. sucralfate and alginic acid antacid (Gaviscon) are effective in protecting esophagus against acid.
5. Cholinergic, e.g. bethanechol increases LES pressure, improves esophageal and gastric emptying.
6. Prokinetic (motility increasing) e.g. metoclopramide (reglan) increases muscle action in the digestive tract promoting gastric emptying and prevents reflux.

Surgical therapy

- **Indications**:
1. Lifestyle changes, nutrition therapy and medicine do not help to manage GERD symptoms.
2. Hiatal hernia is present.
3. Presence of complications, e.g. chronic esophagitis, esophageal strictures, bleeding.
- **Operative procedures**:
1. Fundoplication (Nissen/Belsey/Toupet)—The upper part of the stomach is wrapped around the LES to strengthen

the sphincter, prevent acid reflux, and repair a hiatal hernia. The procedure may be performed laparoscopically.

2. Hill gastropexy—The procedure involves attachment of the stomach subdiaphragmatically to prevent reherniation.

Endoscopic therapy

1. Endoscopic intraluminal valvuloplasty—It increases integrity of LES with the help of gastric tissue.
2. Endoscopic radiofrequency therapy—It delivers radiofrequency energy to the smooth muscle of the LES, resulting in contraction of collagen thus forms a barrier against reflux.
3. Endoscopic injection or implantation of foreign material in LES as gate keeper to prevent reflux.

NURSING MANAGEMENT

Assessment

Subjective data

Heart burn, burning pain behind sternum radiating to throat and jaw, dysphagia, odynophagia, dyspepsia, acid eructation in mouth, water brash, early satiety, post meal bloating, nausea, vomiting, intolerance to certain foods or beverages, wheezing, coughing, dyspnea, hoarseness, sense of lump in throat, choking, presence of hiatal hernia.

Habit of smoking, chewing tobacco, drinking alcohol.

Objective data

Obesity, hiatal hernia, dental erosion.

Possible diagnostic findings

Hiatal hernia or anatomical abnormality in Barium swallow; esophagitis, strictures and incompetent LES in endoscopy; low LES pressure in esophageal manometry; presence of reflux by radionuclide study.

Nursing Diagnoses

1. Heart burn or burning pain under sternum radiating to throat and jaw related to esophagitis secondary to reflux of acid gastric content into the esophagus as evidenced by complaints of burning and pain.
2. Ineffective therapeutic regimen management related to lack of knowledge regarding disease process, aggravating factors, lifestyle modification and medication as evidenced by recurrence of pain, frequent questioning.

GOALS

1. Relief of heart burn and burning pain.
2. Understanding of the disease process, aggravating factors, lifestyle modifications and therapeutic regimen.

Nursing Intervention

Relief of heart burn and burning pain

- Assess pain and burning with the help of pain scale.
- Reassure patient that every possible measure will be taken to relieve his pain and discomfort and obtain his cooperation.
- Administer drugs as prescribed by the physician and record their effectiveness.
- Raise head end of the bed on 6 inch blocks to elevate head at 30 degree angle.
- Provide small and frequent feeds containing high protein and low fat.
- Instruct the patient not to lie down within 2 to 3 hours after meals.

Understanding of the disease process, aggravating factors, lifestyle modifications and therapeutic regimen

- Discuss with patient the cause, manifestations, treatment regimen and complications of GERD.
- Assist patient to identify risk factors of GERD, e.g. obesity, hiatal hernia, etc.
- Teach him necessary lifestyle changes to reduce risk factors, e.g. – small frequent high protein low fat diet, to chew food thoroughly to add saliva to the diet, to take adequate fluids in between meals, not to lie down within 2 to 3 hours of meal, raise head end of beds over 4 to 6 inch blocks, avoid bending, straining, wearing tight clothes, smoking, chewing tobacco, drinking alcohol, citrus juices, caffeinated and carbonated beverages.
- Assist patient to identify factors which aggravate his symptoms, e.g. high fat meal, straining, bending or tight clothing.
- Teach patient to continue drugs even if symptoms are relieved since the underlying problems remain.
- Teach patient the action, side effects of the drug and when to report to the physician.
- Explain patient the reason for surgical intervention or endoscopic therapy if any planned for him.
- Explain preoperative care if surgery is planned.

HIATAL HERNIA

Definition

A hiatal hernia is a condition in which the portion of the upper part of the stomach is herniated or displaced in the lower part of the thorax through an opening or hiatus in the diaphragm.

It is also known as esophageal or diaphragmatic hernia.

Incidence

It is most common abnormality of upper gastrointestinal tract found on X-ray examination.

It is found more often in women than men.

High incidence is found in elderly people over 60 years of age.

Types

Sliding or type I: The upper stomach and gastroesophageal junction are displaced upward through the esophageal opening of the diaphragm into the thorax. 90% of all hiatal hernias are sliding hernias.

Rolling or paraesophageal or type II: The gastroesophageal junction remains below the diaphragm but all or part of the stomach pushes upward in the thorax beside esophagus through the diaphragm.

Etiology and risk factors

- **Cause of hiatal hernia is related to**:
  - Weakness of the muscles of the diaphragm around the esophageal opening.
  - Increased intraabdominal pressure.
- **Factors predisposing to muscle weakness are**:
  - Congenital weakness, trauma, surgery, increased age, poor nutrition, prolonged illness.
- **Factors which increase intraabdominal pressure are**:
  - Obesity, pregnancy, tumors, ascites, heavy lifting, severe physical strain, tight belt around waist.

Clinical Manifestations

Majority are asymptomatic. Symptoms vary with types.

Sliding hiatal hernia

Heart burn after ½ to 1 hour of meal which is worse during bending or lying down, and relieved by sitting or standing. Alcohol and smoking also precipitate pain. Pain is common at night specially when the person has eaten before lying down.

- Dysphagia.
- Regurgitation.
- Substernal pain similar to that of angina.

Rolling hiatal hernia

- Feeling of fullness after meal or difficulty in breathing.
- Angina like chest pain in some patients, specially when lying down.
- Symptoms of reflux is absent.

Complications

1. GERD.
2. Esophagitis.
3. Hemorrhage from erosion.
4. Esophageal stenosis.
5. Regurgitation with tracheal aspiration.
6. Ulceration of the herniated portion of the stomach.
7. Strangulation, obstruction of hernia.

Diagnostic Studies

1. Barium swallow may reveal protrusion of gastric mucosa through esophageal opening.
2. Endoscopic study may reveal degree of mucosal inflammation or other abnormalities.

Management

Medical management

Medical management and nursing management of a patient with hiatal hernia is same as that described in gastroesophageal reflux disease (GERD).

Surgical management

The patients who do not respond to medical treatment may undergo the following surgical procedures:

1. Reduction of the herniated stomach into the abdomen.
2. Herniotomy.
3. Herniorrhaphy
4. Antireflux procedures, e.g. fundoplications (see GERD).
5. Gastropexy.

These procedures may be performed by open surgical approach or by laparoscopic approach.

Nursing Management

Assessment

- Same as described for medical patient in addition routine preoperative and postoperative assessment.
- Evidence of respiratory distress (if chest tube is in situ), wound infection, patency of nasogastric tube, abdominal distention, venous thrombosis.

Nursing Diagnoses

1. Deficit knowledge related to impending surgery, preoperative care and expected post operative outcome as evidenced by frequent questioning.
2. Fear and anxiety related to pain, unfamiliar surroundings, and prognosis as evidenced by anxious look, sleeplessness.
3. Pain related to surgical incision as evidenced by patient's complain of pain.
4. Risk for respiratory complications related to high abdominal incision.
5. Risk for gas-bloat syndrome related to the fundoplication surgery (if any).
6. Risk for infection, related to the surgery, invasive lines, presence of chest tube if any.

Goals

1. Acquisition of knowledge
2. Relief from fear and anxiety
3. Relief of pain
4. Prevention of respiratory complications
5. Prevention of gas-bloat syndrome
6. Prevention of infection.

Nursing Interventions

Acquisition of knowledge

- Explain to the patient the surgery planned for him
- Explain preoperative care, e.g. shaving from nipple line to midthigh including axilla, nil orally from 10 pm onwards, nasogastric tube, enema, etc.
- Teach preoperative deep breathing and coughing to be practiced post-operatively. Demonstrate use of incentive spirometer.
- Explain patient the need for continuing medical regimen (medications, diet changes, lifestyle changes) after surgery to prevent recurrence.

Relief from fear and anxiety

- Assess extent of anxiety and fear in patient.
- Allow to verbalize his concerns.
- Provide explanations as much as the patient wants.
- Reassure patient that a nurse will be present with him throughout the total surgical experience.

Relief of pain

- Assess pain after surgery with the help of pain scale.
- Administer pain medication as ordered by the physician at the onset of pain and before pain becomes severe.
- Document date and time of medication and effectiveness of pain medication.
- Schedule timing of pain medication in such a way so that patient cooperates during postoperative exercises and ambulation.
- Institute comfort measures, e.g. change of position, back massage as and when required.

Prevention of respiratory complications

- Encourage patient to take deep breath and cough to remove secretions. Provide incentive spirometer and steam inhalation to loosen secretions.
- Auscultate chest for air entry in both the lungs.
- Encourage patient to turn side to side every 2 hours and maintain semi-Fowler's position to facilitate breathing.
- Assess chest tube for proper functioning and explain patient the purpose of chest tube.

Prevention of gas-bloat syndrome

- Maintain nasogastric suction every 1or 2 hourly to decompress the stomach.
- Assess tube patency, amount and color of gastric drainage, bowel sounds.
- Withheld food and fluid till peristalsis returns.
- Administer small and frequent meals to prevent overloading of stomach.
- Teach patient to report if he experiences dysphagia, epigastric fullness, bloating or excessive borborygmi.
- Reassure patient that these symptoms are temporary and help him to ambulate for the easy passage of gas from the gastrointestinal tract.
- Teach patient to avoid carbonated beverages and gas producing foods.

Prevention of infection

- Assess patient's body temperature, wound drainage for color and odor for the presence of infection.

- Institute hand washing and other infection control measures strictly as per hospital protocol.

CANCER OF THE ESOPHAGUS

Definition

The esophagus is one of the common sites of malignancy in the gastrointestinal tract and cancer of the esophagus is malignancy arising in tissues lining the esophagus.

Types

Esophageal cancers are primarily two types:

Squamous cell carcinoma

It arises from the cells that line the upper part of the esophagus.

Adenocarcinoma

It arises from glandular cells that are present at the junction of the esophagus and stomach.

Incidence

The incidence of cancer of the esophagus in the United States was rare.

In the last decade the incidence has increased fivefold, particularly adenocarcinoma.

In India the problem is seen very frequently.

At the Tata Memorial Hospital, between 800 and 1000 patients of cancer esophagus are registered every year. Unlike in the west, the majority of these are squamous carcinoma.

The reported five year survival worldwide ranges from 5% to 30%.

Etiology and Risk Factors

The cause of esophageal cancer is unknown.

There are a number of risk factors for esophageal cancer:

- Age: Most patients are over 60.
- Sex: It is more common in men.
- Heredity: It is more likely in people who have close relatives with cancer.
- Tobacco smoking and heavy alcohol use increase the risk, and together appear to increase the risk more than either individually.
- Gastroesophageal reflux disease (GERD) and its resultant Barrett's esophagus increase esophageal cancer risk due to the chronic irritation of the mucosal lining.
- Corrosive injury to esophagus by swallowing strong alkali or acids.
- Radiation therapy for other conditions in the mediastinum.
- Celiac disease predisposes towards squamous cell carcinoma.
- Obesity increases the risk of adenocarcinoma fourfold. It is suspected that increased risk of reflux may be behind this association.
- Thermal injury as a result of drinking hot beverages.

Pathophysiology

- Cancer of the esophagus begins as slow-growing tissue changes but extends locally and rapidly.
- The cancers are typically intraluminal, ulcerating lesions that encircle the esophageal wall and extend upward and downward. The tumor may penetrate the muscular layer and even extend outside the wall of the esophagus.
- Due to rich lymphatic supply in this area the disease spreads quickly to the lymph nodes and metastasizes widely.
- Many patients develop pulmonary complications, e.g. aspiration due to

formation of tracheoesophageal fistula.
- Infiltration into blood vessels may predispose the patient to hemorrhage.
- Obstruction of esophagus occurs in the later stages.

Signs and Symptoms

Appearance of symptoms is usually late. When symptoms appear the disease is usually far advanced:
- Dysphagia, initially with solid foods and later with soft and liquids.
- Sensation of mass in the throat (globus sensation).
- Pain in substernal, epigastric or back areas which increases with swallowing (odynophagia). Pain often of a burning nature is severe and may be spasmodic in character. Pain may radiate to the neck, jaw, ears and shoulders.
- Sore-throat, choking, and hoarseness if the tumor is in the upper-third of the esophagus.
- Weight loss due to poor nutrition and active cancer.
- Nausea, vomiting, regurgitation of food due to impairment in normal peristalsis of esophagus.
- Hematemesis due to bleeding from tumor surface.
- Cough, fever due to pneumonia occurring from aspiration or tracheoesophageal fistula.

Diagnostic Studies

1. Endoscopy of esophagus with biopsy to identify malignant cells.
2. Barium swallow with fluoroscopy detects narrowing of the esophagus at the tumor site.
3. Endoscopic ultrasonography to determine the stage of cancer.
4. Bronchoscopy to detect malignant involvement of the trachea.
5. Computed tomography scans of the chest and abdomen to determine the extent of the disease.

Medical Management

Treatment of the cancer of the esophagus depends on tumor's location and size, metastasis and condition of the patient. A combination of surgery, radiation and chemotherapy is used to obtain best results.

Endoscopy

Photodynamic or laser therapy by endoscopic approaches is used to ablate mucosal adenocarcinoma or Barret's esophagus. Photodynamic therapy involves intravenous injection of a light sensitive drug, photofrin. The photofrin is absorbed by all tissues but in a greater degree by malignant tissue. After 2 days a fiberoptic probe with a light bearing tip is placed in the esophagus through endoscope. The light activates the photofrin and kills only cancer cells.

Surgery

1. Esophagectomy —In this procedure part of the esophagus is resected and replaced by Dacron graft.
2. Esophagogastrostomy—It is the resection of a portion of the esophagus and anastomosis of the remaining part to the stomach.
3. Esophagoenterostomy—It involves resection of a portion of the esophagus and anastomosis of a segment of colon to the remaining portion.

Surgery may be performed by thoracic or abdominal incision or by laparoscopy.

Radiation

Radiation therapy may be used alone or before or after surgery to slow the progression of the cancer.

Chemotherapy

Chemotherapy, by combining several agents is used for symptomatic relief and increased survival. Cisplatin and 5-FU are very commonly used before surgery to decrease the tumor size and its invasiveness.

Palliative therapy

Palliative therapy carried out to keep the esophagus open, to assist with nutrition and to control saliva. Procedures are:

1. Dilation of the esophagus.
2. Placement of an endoprosthesis to allow passage of food and fluid through the stenosed esophagus.
3. Gastrostomy or esophagostomy with tube placement.

NURSING MANAGEMENT

Assessment

Subjective data

History of GERD, hiatal hernia, achalasia, Barrett's esophagus.

Dysphagia, odynophagia, type of food causing dysphagia or odynophagia, pain behind sternum, epigastric region or back areas, choking, heartburn, hoarseness, cough, anorexia, weight loss and regurgitation.

Objective data

Cough, hoarseness, choking, increased secretions, poor nutritional status, e.g. low body weight, dehydration, anemia, etc.

Possible diagnostic findings

Obstruction of esophagus in barium swallow with fluoroscopy, endoscopy with biopsy detects malignant cells.

Nursing Diagnoses

1. Imbalanced nutrition, less than body requirements related to dysphagia, odynophagia, radiotherapy or chemotherapy.
2. Pain due to the tumor compressing surrounding areas, dysphagia from esophageal stenosis.
3. Risk for aspiration related to impaired esophageal function or presence of tracheoesophageal fistula.
4. Risk for ineffective coping related to changes in body image and potentially terminal prognosis.
5. Ineffective health maintenance related to lack of knowledge of disease process and therapeutic regimen.

Goals

1. Attainment of optimum nutritional intake.
2. Relief of symptoms, e.g. pain and dysphagia.
3. Avoidance of respiratory compromise from aspiration.
4. Achieving a quality of life appropriate to the stage of the disease.
5. Effective coping from alteration in body image and potentially terminal prognosis.

Nursing Interventions

Attainment of optimum nutritional intake

- Monitor patient's nutritional status throughout treatment by measuring intake and output, calories consumed and daily weight.
- Teach patient change of diet, e.g. from solid to soft and liquid that will be easier to eat.
- Encourage patient to chew thoroughly and eat slowly.

- Provide small, frequent, nonirritating but appealing diet.
- Provide tube feeding as the disease advances and patient is unable to eat orally.
- Assess skin around tube for erosion from gastric leakage.
- Wash skin with soap and water around the opening of the tube twice a day, dry thoroughly and apply protective ointment for protection of the skin.

Relief of symptoms

- Assess pain with a pain scale.
- Provide analgesic if ordered before pain becomes severe.

Avoidance of respiratory compromise from aspiration

- Provide or assist with frequent oral care.
- Suction excessive secretion if patient is unable to spit out.
- Teach patient to carry a receptacle to receive saliva if drooling.
- Keep patient in semi-Fowler's position to decrease the risk of aspiration.

Achieving a quality of life appropriate to the stage of the disease

- Explain patient and relatives about the disease, treatment options planned for him, and expected outcome.
- Provide preoperative teaching if surgery is planned.
- Explain the side effects of radiotherapy or chemotherapy if planned for him and the measures to minimize those side effects.
- Teach patient and relatives the technique of tube feeding and the skin care around the tube.

Effective coping from potentially terminal illness and body image changes

- Assess patient's mental status.
- Explain information given by physician regarding the patient's condition.
- Provide emotional support.
- Refer patient to psychological therapist if needed to prepare for the patient's death.

NURSING MANAGEMENT OF THE PATIENT SCHEDULED FOR SURGERY

Assessment

Routine preoperative and postoperative assessment, nutritional status, ability to swallow, respiratory status, and ability to cope with the diagnosis.

Nursing Diagnoses

1. Risk for injury related to the surgical procedure.
2. Ineffective health maintenance due to knowledge deficit regarding self-care.

GOALS

1. Prevention of injury, e.g. atelectasis, infection, problems arising with chest tubes.
2. Experience quality life and independence by managing self-care.

Nursing Interventions

Prevention of injury

- Improve nutritional status of the patient by providing nutritional support with tube feeding or TPN and monitoring of nutritional status for 2 to 3 weeks before surgery.
- Provide preoperative teaching regarding:
  - Postoperative deep breathing, turning, coughing and chest physiotherapy.
  - Incision, wound drainage tubes, feeding tubes, chest tubes that will be present after surgery.

- Preoperative bowel care in case of esophagoenterostomy and 4 hourly mouth care after surgery.
- Maintain patent airway postoperatively by:
  - Placing the patient on ventilator or by frequent turning, coughing and deep breathing.
  - Monitoring respiratory status of patient frequently.
  - Providing supplemental oxygen.
  - Scheduling analgesic before deep breathing and coughing.
  - Placing patient in semi-Fowler's position to prevent reflux.
  - Monitoring chest tube drainage for amount color and patency.
- Maintain fluid and electrolyte balance by:
  - Assessing fluid and electrolyte status every shift.
  - Monitoring drainage from the nasogastric, gastric and all drainage tubes every shift.
  - Reporting to the physician, if the drainage from nasogastric or gastric tube remains bloody after 24 hours.
  - Checking dressings for bleeding.
  - Keeping patient NPO and providing fluid and nutrition parenterally for 4 to 5 days until peristalsis returns.
- Advance diet as tolerated by:
  - Allow sips of water when peristalsis returns, increase quantity if tolerated.
  - Keep patient in upright position while feeding and 1 hour after meals to prevent over distention and reflux.
  - Assess patient for manifestations of leakage at the anastomosis site, e.g. shock, fever, fluid accumulation at the wound site and inflammation.
  - Provide patient pureed and semisolid food in small amount and frequent intervals when water is tolerated.

Managing self-care

- During discharge provide written instructions regarding wound healing, nutritional support, medications and respiratory care.
- Teach patient manifestations of respiratory and wound complications that should be reported immediately.
- Refer patient to a community health nurse for continued care and teaching at home.

GASTRITIS

Definition

Inflammation of the gastric or stomach mucosa is known as gastritis.

Types

1. Acute
2. Chronic
3. Localized
4. Diffuse.

Etiology and Risk factors

Acute

- Consumption of contaminated or irritating or highly seasoned foods.
- Overuse of drugs, e.g. aspirin, digitalis, steroids, NSAIDs, chemotherapeutic drugs, etc.
- Excessive alcohol intake.
- Bile reflux.
- Radiation therapy.
- Ingestion of acids or alkalis.
- Excessive amounts of tea, coffee, mustard, cloves, pepper, foods with rough texture.
- Very hot food.
- Diseases, e.g. uremia, shock, hepatic cirrhosis, portal hypertension, central nervous system lesion, and prolonged emotional tension.

Chronic

- Benign or malignant ulcers of the stomach.
- Infection with *Helicobacter pylori.*
- Autoimmune disease.
- Pernicious anemia.
- Use of caffeine.
- Use of medications, e.g. NSAIDs, alcohol, smoking.
- Reflux of intestinal contents into the remaining stomach after gastric surgery.
- Intense emotional tension.
- Bacterial, viral or fungal infections such as Mycobacterium tuberculosis, syphilis, cytomegalovirus, etc.

Pathophysiology

- Injury to the protective mucous membrane of stomach occurs due to any noxious substance.
- Hydrochloric acid comes into contact with gastric mucosa and injury to small blood vessels occurs leading to edema and hyperemia.
- Gastric mucosa secretes scanty amount of gastric juice containing little hydrochloric acid but much mucus.
- Gastric mucosa undergoes superficial erosion leading to ulceration or hemorrhage.

Clinical Manifestations

Many people with gastritis remain asymptomatic.

Most common symptoms are:

- Abdominal pain — Located in the epigastric region.
  - Patient describes pain as dull, aching or burning, gnawing or sharp or cramping.
- Epigastric tenderness.
- Feeling of fullness.
- Headache, lassitude.
- Nausea, anorexia.
- Vomiting—Vomitus may be clear, green or yellow, blood-streaked or bloody.
- Reflux.
- Hiccuping.
- Belching.
- Weight loss and manifestations of cobalamine (vitamin B_{12}) deficiency may occur in chronic cases.

Diagnostic Studies

1. Endoscopic study—Visualizes inflamed gastric mucosa.
2. Biopsy of gastric tissue specimen obtained during endoscopy detects *H. pylori* infection.
3. Breath test, urine, stool and serum test—Detect presence of *H. pylori.*
4. Complete blood count to detect anemia.
5. Gastric analysis detects presence of achlorhydria
6. Stool for occult blood detects evidence of melena.

Medical Management

Acute

Medical management in patients with acute gastritis is supportive in nature and includes:

- Rest and sedative.
- Keep patient in nothing per mouth status.
- IV fluids to maintain hydration.
- Antiemetics to control vomiting.
- Nasogastric tube may be inserted to give lavage, observe for bleeding and to keep stomach empty and free of offending stimuli.
- Drug therapy, e.g. antacid, H_2R blockers (cimetidine, ranitidine), proton pump inhibitors (omeprazole, lansoprazole), cytoprotective agents (sucralfate, bismuth subsalicylates), etc.

Chronic

- Elimination of causative factors, e.g. alcohol abuse, over use of drugs, smoking.
- Adherence to nonirritating food, taking small and frequent meals and antacids after food.
- Promoting rest and reducing stress.
- Following a strict drug regimen to eradicate *H. pylori. H. pylori* infection is treated by several combined drug therapy, e.g.
  - Two drug therapy—Clarithromycin, ranitidine bismuth citrate
  - Three drug therapy—Proton pump inhibitor, amoxicillin, clarithromycin
  - Four drug therapy—Proton pump inhibitor, bismuth, tetracycline, metronidazole.

NURSING MANAGEMENT

Assessment

Subjective data

Abdominal discomfort, feeling of fullness, anorexia, nausea, vomiting, cramping, belching, reflux, history of ingestion of spicy/ irritating foods, drugs, alcohol, loss of weight, headache, lassitude, anxiety, stress, fatigue, history of food poisoning (similar symptoms in others).

Objective data

Epigastric tenderness, dehydration, evidence of any systemic disorder, previous scar of gastric surgery.

Possible diagnostic findings

Evidence of inflammation and erosion by endoscopy, presence of *Helicobacter pylori* in histopathological examination, gastric analysis reveals achlorhydria, occult blood in stool examination and anemia in complete blood count.

Nursing Diagnoses

1. Pain related to irritated gastric mucosa as evidenced by paient's complain of abdominal pain, cramping or abdominal discomfort.
2. Ineffective health maintenance due to lack of knowledge about disease process, medical and dietary management.

GOALS

1. Relief of pain
2. Promotion of health by acquiring knowledge about the disease, its medical management and dietary modifications.

Nursing Interventions

Relief of pain

- Explain patient about causes of gastritis and the various factors that aggravate the disease.
- Help patient to identify factors that increases the severity of symptoms, e.g. fatigue, stress, anxiety, taking certain drugs, consuming certain foods or beverages, alcohol and smoking.
- Instruct patient to adhere to a modified diet schedule and to take antacids and other drugs regularly as ordered.
- Assess patient's level of pain and the amount of comfort attained by drug therapy and dietary modifications.

Promotion of health by acquiring knowledge about the disease, it's medical management and dietary modifications

- Assess patient's level of knowledge about the disease and its medical management and dietary modifications.
- Develop an individual teaching plan that will include the disease process, medications, dietary modifications and other lifestyle changes.

- Provide information about prescribed medications, e.g. antibiotics, bismuth salts, antacids, etc.
- Provide information about patient's daily caloric needs, food preferences, and food and fluids to be avoided, e.g. spicy, irritating or highly seasoned foods, caffeine, nicotine, alcohol.
- Teach patient with chronic gastritis the importance of follow-up visits.
- Teach patients with pernicious anemia to take long-term vitamin B_{12} injections.

PEPTIC ULCER DISEASE

Definition

Peptic ulcer disease is a condition characterized by a break in the continuity of the gastrointestinal mucosa that comes into contact with hydrochloric acid and pepsin of gastric juices.

A peptic ulcer refers to an ulcer (excavation or hole formed in the mucosal layer) in the lower esophagus, stomach or duodenum, in the jejunum after surgical anastomosis to the stomach, or rarely in the ileum adjacent to a Meckel's diverticulum.

Incidence

- Occurs in 10% of population.
- Common in men aged 40 to 60 years.
- Less common in women of child bearing age, but after menopause the incidence is almost equal to that of men.

Types

Duodenal ulcers

- Incidence of duodenal ulcers is more than gastric ulcers.
- Occur within 1.5 cm of the pylorus.
- Characterized by increased gastric acid secretion and or rapid gastric emptying.
- Combined effect of increased gastric acid secretion and rapid gastric emptying reduces the buffering effect of food resulting into large acid load or low pH in the duodenum for a longer time.
- Pancreatic secretion, which is alkaline may be insufficient to raise the pH of the duodenum.

Gastric ulcers

- May occur at any part of the stomach but most commonly found in the lesser curvature of stomach near to the antral junction.
- Usually single but more than one may also occur.
- Characterized by normal to low secretion of gastric acid.
- Caused by a break in the mucosal barrier.
- Incidence is high in persons over 50 years of age.
- The mortality rate is greater in persons with gastric ulcer than that from duodenal ulcer.
- Acute ulcers tend to heal within a few weeks.
- Recurrence rate is lower than that of duodenal ulcer.

Acute ulcers

- Acute ulcers are characterized by superficial erosion and minimal inflammation.
- They are of short duration, resolve quickly when cause is known and removed.

Chronic ulcers

- Chronic ulcers are of long duration.
- Thye are present continuously for many months or intermittently throughout the person's life time.
- Ulcer erodes deep in the muscularis layer with formation of fibrous tissue.

- They are more common than acute ulcers.

Stress induced and drug-induced ulcers

- Acute gastric erosion commonly called stress ulcers or stress erosive gastritis can occur after an acute medical crisis.
- Conditions that give rise to gastroduodenal ulcerations include:

Severe burns (Curling's ulcer), Major illness, severe trauma, head injury or intracranial disease (Cushing's ulcer), shock, sepsis, ingestion of alcohol, drugs like NSAIDs, steroids.

Etiology

1. *Helicobacter pylori* infection is found to be the most important causal factor. About 90% of duodenal ulcer patients and 70% of gastric ulcer patients are infected with *Helicobacter pylori.*
2. Nonsteroidal antiinflammatory drugs damage the gastric mucosal barrier. 30% of gastric ulcers and a small proportion of duodenal ulcers are due to use of NSAIDs. In preexisting gastric or duodenal ulcers these drugs increase the risk of bleeding and perforation.
3. Smoking causes increased risk of gastric ulcer and to a lesser extent duodenal ulcer. Smoking delays the healing of ulcers and increases the risk of complications.
4. Acid-pepsin versus mucosal resistance. Ulcer forms when there is an imbalance between the aggressive factors (the digestive power of hydrochloric acid and pepsin) and defensive factors (ability of the gastric and duodenal mucosa to resist the digestive power of gastric juices). Ulcer occurs in the presence of acid and pepsin. Most duodenal ulcer patients have markedly exaggerated acid secretion. Patients with gastric ulcer may have normal acid secretion but have impaired mucosal resistance due to the effect of *Helicobacter pylori* infection, NSAIDs and smoking.

Risk Factors

- Stress and anxiety.
- Ingestion of milk, caffeinated beverages
- Smoking and alcohol.
- Familial tendency.
- Individual with blood group O (increased incidence of duodenal ulcer).
- People living in crowded environment and poor sanitation facilities tend to be infected with *H. pylori.*
- Ingestion of hot, rough or spicy foods.
- Eating hurriedly or irregularly.

Pathology

- Normally the gastric mucosal barrier protects the stomach from auto digestion by hydrochloric acid and pepsin.
- Several factors, e.g. *H. pylori*, NSAIDs, aspirin, steroids and hypersecretion of acids due to various causes lead to disruption of mucosal barrier.
- Disrupted mucosa allows back diffusion of acid into the gastric epithelial wall resulting in cellular destruction and inflammation.
- Disrupted mucosa may increase blood flow as a compensatory mechanism. Increased blood flow dilutes and buffers the excess hydrochloric acid, brings nutrients for cell function and increases the rate of mucosal cell replication resulting in minor or no injury.
- Damaged mucosa releases histamine, which stimulates further secretion of acid and pepsin.
- Further damage of mucosal wall, destruction of blood vessels take place resulting in ulceration and bleeding.

Clinical Manifestations

- Acute pain—It is the principal manifestation of ulcers. Patient describes pain as aching, burning, cramp like and gnawing. It has three notable characteristics:
  1. Localization—Gastric ulcer pain occurs in the upper epigastrium with localization to the left of the midline, Pain in duodenal ulcer localizes in right epigastrium. Patient can point the location of pain—so it is called point sign.
  2. Relationship to food—In gastric ulcer food may cause the pain and vomiting may relieve it. Pain occurs after 1 to 2 hours of eating. Duodenal pain occurs when the stomach is empty. Food or antacid relieves pain.
  3. Episodic occurrence—Pain in duodenal ulcer occurs regularly each day for weeks or months, then disappears only to reappear some months later without any notable cause. The cause may be psychological stress, dietary irregularities or excessive alcohol consumption.

  For some patients pain may be absent. Perforation or hemorrhage or gastric outlet obstruction may be the presenting symptom. Some patients may not complain of pain but may complain of some distention in epigastrium or unease after eating, heart burn or water brash.
- Nausea and vomiting—It may occur in patients with duodenal ulcer complicated with pyloric obstruction. Patients with uncomplicated duodenal ulcer usually have normal appetite. For them vomiting may occur after experiencing severe pain. Patients with gastric ulcer may have anorexia, nausea, frequent vomiting and loss of weight. Vomiting results from gastric stasis or pyloric obstruction. Vomits are of large amounts and contain undigested food.
- Constipation and diarrhea may occur as a result of diet and medications.

Complications

- Three major complications of peptic ulcer are:
  1. Hemorrhage
  2. Perforation
  3. Gastric outlet obstruction.
- Hemorrhage
  - It is the most common complications of Peptic ulcer disease.
  - It occurs when the ulcer erodes through a blood vessel.
  - Hemorrhage may be massive or may be occult with slight oozing.
  - Hemorrhage from duodenal ulcers are more common than that of gastric ulcers.
- Perforation
  - It is the most lethal complication of peptic ulcer disease.
  - Commonly seen in large penetrating duodenal ulcers located on the posterior mucosal wall and gastric ulcers located in the lesser curvature of stomach.
  - Perforation occurs when the ulcer penetrates the serosal surface spilling gastric and duodenal contents into the peritoneum. Within 6 to 12 hours bacterial peritonitis occurs.
  - The patient experiences sudden severe abdominal pain that quickly spreads all over the abdomen. Abdomen appears rigid and board like. Bowel sounds are usually absent. Patient's respiration become shallow and rapid. Nausea and vomiting may occur.
  - Perforation is usually a surgical emergency.
- Gastric outlet obstruction
  - Gastric outlet obstruction or pyloric obstruction occurs when long-standing ulcer distal to the pylorus

becomes scarred and stenosed from spasm or edema or from scar tissue formed due to repeated ulcerations and healing.
- Patient experiences generalized abdominal discomfort, which increases at the end of the day.

Diagnostic Studies

1. **Endoscopy**—It allows direct visualization of gastric and duodenal mucosa, detects degree of healing of ulcer after treatment and obtains tissue specimen to identify *H. pylori* infection and to rule out carcinoma.
2. **Barium X-ray**—It is not useful to detect superficial shallow ulceration. It cannot rule out malignancy but may be helpful to diagnose gastric outlet obstruction.
3. **Gastric analysis**—It detects achlorhydria and Zollinger–Ellison syndrome.
4. **Stool examination**—It reveals occult blood.
5. **Breath test**—It detects *H. pylori.*
6. Serologic Test for antibodies of *H. pylori* detects presence of H. pylori.
7. **Complete blood count**—It detects anemia.

Medical Management

Goals of medical management are to eradicate *H. pylori* and to control gastric acidity, which are achieved by medications and lifestyle changes.

Medications

Antibiotics in combination are given to eradicate *H. pylori* :

- 3 drug therapy— Proton pump inhibitor.
  Amoxicillin 1 gm 12 hourly.
  Clarithromycin 500 mg 12 hourly.
  Or
  Metronidazole 400 mg 12 hourly, given for 7 days.
  Or,
- 4 drug therapy— Proton pump inhibitor.
  Bismuth 120 mg 6 hourly.
  Metronidazole 400 mg 12 hourly.
  Tetracycline 500 mg 6 hourly given for 14 days.
- Other drugs those are available to control gastric acidity as short term measures are:
  1. Histamine (H_2)-receptor blockers, e.g. Cimetidine 400 mg 12 hourly, Ranitidine 150 mg 12 hourly.
  2. Proton pump inhibitors, e.g. Omeprazole 20 to 40 mg once daily, pntoprazole 40 mg once daily, rabeprazole 20 mg once daily.
  3. Cytoprotective, e.g. sucralfate 2 gm 12 hourly, colloidal bismuth 125 mg 6 hourly, misoprostol 200 microgram 6 hourly.
  4. Antacids, e.g. magnesium salts or aluminium hydroxide singly or in combination, e.g. gaviscon, aludrox, gelusil, etc.

Lifestyle changes

- Rest— Physical and mental rest help in healing. A regular rest period during the day in acute period is recommended. Biofeedback, hypnosis or behavior modifications help in reducing stress.
- Cessation of smoking.
- Aspirin and NSAIDs to be avoided.
- Dietary modifications— Eat 3 regular meals (6 meals not needed when on antacids and H_2-receptor blockers). Avoid extremes of temperature,

alcohol, coffee, caffeinated beverages, foods rich in milk and cream. Eat foods that are tolerated and avoid foods that produce pain.

Surgical management

Surgery is done for patients who are unresponsive to medical treatment or who have life-threatening complications. (discussed later).

NURSING MANAGEMENT

Assessment

Subjective data

Acute or chronic pain or burning in midepigastric or back pain occurring 2 to 4 hours after meals and relieved by food, nocturnal pain (duodenal ulcer). High epigastric pain occurring 1 to 2 hours after meals, pain precipitated or aggravated by food and relieved by vomiting (gastric ulcer). Nausea, vomiting, anorexia, loss of weight (gastric ulcer), hematemesis or black tarry stool.

Objective data

Pain and tenderness, abdominal distention, anemia, loss of body weight (gastric ulcer).

Possible findings

Low hemoglobin and hematocrit level, evidence of ulcer in endoscopy, achlorhydria or hyperchlorohydria in gastric analysis, occult blood in stool, presence of *H. pylori* in breath test or serological test.

Nursing Diagnoses

1. Acute or chronic pain related to injury in gastrointestinal mucosa secondary to increased gastric secretion or decreased mucosal resistance as evidenced by patient's complain of pain in epigastrium and abdomen 1 to 2 hours of meal (gastric ulcer) or 2 to 4 hours after meal and at night (duodenal ulcer).
2. Risk for ineffective therapeutic regimen management related to lack of knowledge regarding the cause of disease, long-term treatment regimen, complications as evidenced by frequent questioning about home care, incorrect responses to questions about the disease and noncompliance with treatment regimen.

Potential Complications

1. Hemorrhage secondary to eroded mucosal tissue.
2. Perforation of ulcer secondary to impaired mucosal tissue integrity.

GOALS

1. Relief of pain.
2. Understanding of the disease, treatment regimen, complications and ways to prevent complications and recurrence.
3. Absence of complications.

Nursing Interventions

Relief of pain

- Assess pain and determine its character from patient's verbal description.
- Administer medications (antacids, H_2 receptor blockers, proton pump inhibitors or cytoprotective drugs) as ordered to reduce pain.
- Assess the effectiveness of the drugs the patient is taking and report to the physician.
- Help the patient to take rest both physically and mentally. Provide calm environment to promote rest. Restrict visitors until the patient's condition is improved.

- Encourage patient who is on normal work to schedule some physical rest periods in between daily activities.
- Teach patient different nonpharmacologic techniques, e.g. relaxation, music therapy, distraction, etc. and encourage using those along with medications before after and during pain.
- Provide bland, nonirritating, low fiber diet in acute phase. Encourage patient to eat small amount at regular intervals.
- Discourage use of alcohol, cola, tobacco, tea, coffee, milk or foods that cause discomfort.

Understanding of the disease, treatment regimen, complications and ways to prevent complications and recurrence

- Explain to the patient the pathogenesis of ulcer to help him understand the disease.
- Help patient identify factors that caused the condition and ways to lessen their effects.
- Explain patient that ulcer tends to heal rapidly when irritating factors are removed.
- Explain the importance of continuing the medical regimen till healing is complete even if symptoms subside.
- Provide information on action and side effects of drugs to help the patient regarding safe self-administration of medicine.
- Help patient identify stressors and encourage modification in daily routine.
- Discuss with patient and family members the required modification in diet.
- Discourage use of alcohol, cola, tobacco, tea, coffee, milk or spicy foods.
- Inform patient what to do if symptoms recur or if any complication.

Absence of complications

Hemorrhage

- Assess for hematemesis (coffee ground color vomiting), melena (black tarry stool), abdominal pain or discomfort, weakness, diaphoresis or symptoms of shock.
- If ulcer is actively bleeding, insert a nasogastric tube as ordered and assess amount of bleeding and start gastric lavage with saline to remove blood from the stomach.
- Take vitals every 15 to 30 minutes.
- Maintain intravenous infusion line to replace fluid and blood as ordered.
- Record intake and output.
- Monitor urine output by a Foley catheter. Inform physician if urine output is less than .5 mL/kg/hour.
- Monitor hematocrit and hemoglobin percentage to assess the severity of blood loss and need for blood and fluid replacement.
- Observe for transfusion reaction when the patient is having blood transfusion
- Reassure patient and family to reduce anxiety.
- Remain calm and confident to make the patient and family understand that best possible care is being provided by the health team members.
- Prepare patient for possible endoscopy or surgery.

Absence of complications

Perforation

- Observe for sign and symptoms of perforation, e.g. sudden severe abdominal pain increasing in intensity, radiating pain to shoulder, tender, rigid abdomen, vomiting, increasing distention, decreasing or absent bowel sounds for early detection and treatment.
- Monitor vital signs every 15 to 30 minutes to assess the hemodynamic

status of the patient to detect early signs of shock.

- Maintain nasogastric suction to decompress the stomach to prevent further leak of stomach content into the abdominal cavity.
- Administer intravenous infusion as ordered to maintain hemodynamic status and fluid and electrolyte balance
- Administer analgesics as ordered to reduce pain and anxiety.
- Prepare patient for emergency diagnostic procedure and surgery for timely intervention.

Surgical Therapy for Peptic Ulcer Disease

Commonly performed surgical procedures are:

Billroth I

Partial gastrectomy with removal of the distal two-third of the stomach and anastomosis of the gastric stump to the duodenum is called a gastroduodenostomy or Billroth I operation (Fig. 7.1).

Billroth II

Partial gastrectomy with removal of the distal two-third of the stomach and anastomosis of the gastric stump to the jejunum is called a gastrojejunostomy or Billroth II operation (Fig. 7.2).

Vagotomy

Cutting of the vagus nerve at the point of innervation to the stomach is called vagotomy and is performed to eliminate the acid secreting stimulus to gastric cells. Truncal vagotomy is cutting of the entire vagus nerve innervating the stomach and selective vagotomy is the cutting of a branch of the vagus nerve in order to denervate only a portion of the stomach.

Pyloroplasty

Surgical enlargement of the pyloric sphincter to promote easy passage of gastric contents is called pyloroplasty. The procedure is commonly done after vagotomy. Vagotomy decreases gastric motility and emptying. So pyloroplasty with vagotomy increases gastric emptying (Fig. 7.2).

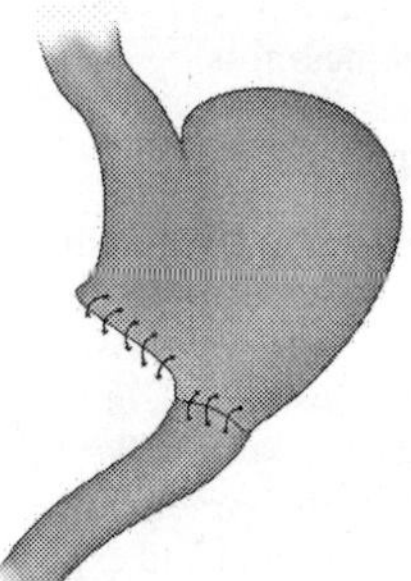

Fig. 7.1: Partial gastrectomy with Billroth I anastomosis

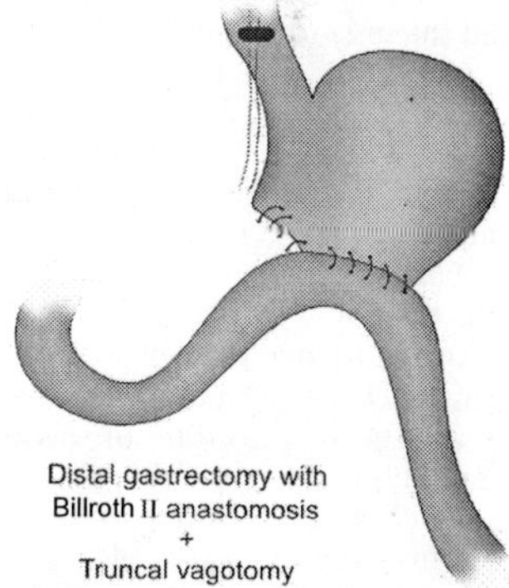

Fig. 7.2: Partial gastrectomy with Billroth II anastomosis + truncal vagotomy

Postoperative Complications

Marginal ulcers

Marginal ulcers develop when gastric acids come in contact with the operative site either at the site of anastomosis or in the jejunum.

Dumping syndrome

- This complication is the result of surgical removal of a large portion of the stomach and the pyloric sphincter.
- Usually occurs when patient consumes meals of hyperosmolar composition.
- As the pyloric sphincter is absent large amounts of hyperosmolar chime enters the intestine at a time. This is followed by drawing of large volume of extracellular fluid into the bowel lumen to dilute the hyperosmolar chime resulting into a decrease in plasma volume. distention of the bowel lumen and rapid passage of intestinal content.
- Symptoms of dumping syndrome appear at the end of the meal or 15 to 30 minutes after eating and usually last for 1 hour. Patient experiences generalized weakness, sweating, palpitations, dizziness, abdominal cramps, borborygmi and the urge to defecate.

Postprandial hypoglycemia

- Occurs due to uncontrolled gastric emptying of a bolus of fluid high in carbohydrate content into small intestine.
- Bolus of concentrated carbohydrate results in hyperglycemia and the release of excessive amounts of insulin in circulation. A secondary hypoglycemia then occurs after 2 hours of meal.
- Patient experiences sweating, weakness, mental confusion, palpitations, tachycardia and anxiety.

Bile reflux gastritis

- Bile reflux gastritis results from surgery that involves removal or reconstruction of pylorus.
- Prolonged contact of bile, bile salts damages gastric mucosa.
- Patient experiences continuous epigastric distress that increases after meals and decreases temporarily with vomiting.
- The condition may be treated with cholestyramine that binds with bile salts and is administered before or during meal.

NURSING MANAGEMENT OF PATIENTS UNDERGOING SURGERY FOR PEPTIC ULCER DISEASE

Preoperative Care

Assessment

Assess knowledge of patient and significant family members regarding purpose of surgery, preoperative and postoperative routine and expectations.

Assess loss of body weight, vomiting, hematemesis, melena, bowel sounds decreased or exaggerated, anxiety, apprehension, sleeplessness.

Nursing Diagnoses

1. Anxiety related to the surgical procedure as evidenced by frequent questioning about the prognosis, anxious and apprehensive look or sleeplessness.
2. Deficient knowledge about surgical procedures, preoperative and postoperative routine and expectations.

GOALS

1. Reducing anxiety
2. Increasing knowledge.

Nursing Interventions

Reducing anxiety

- Observe for verbal and nonverbal signs of anxiety.
- Encourage verbalization of feelings, apprehension, fears and encourage verbalization of concerns.
- Introduce patient to other patients recovering from similar types of surgeries.
- Provide calm, efficient and knowledgeable care and explain what is being done.
- When emergency surgery is required, stay with patient to promote safety and reduce fear.

Increasing knowledge

- Provide teaching regarding the purpose of surgery, the surgery planned, expectation after surgery, pain relief and comfort measures.
- Explain patient the preoperative routines, e.g. skin preparation, bowel preparation, preoperative medications, nasogastric tube insertion, intravenous infusion line, etc.
- Demonstrate and discuss the importance of deep breathing and coughing exercises, use of an incentive spirometer and early ambulation.

Postoperative Care

Assessment

Routine postoperative assessment, abdominal distention, patency of nasogastric tube, gastric aspirate for color (bright red initially, changes to yellow green within 36 to 48 hours) and amount, bowel sounds, incision site for early signs of infection, bleeding and drainage from the wound, etc.

Nursing Diagnoses

1. Acute pain related to surgical incision as evidenced by patient's complain of pain.
2. Risk for postoperative complications, e.g. hemorrhage, distention, atelectasis as evidenced by bloody drainage from the nasogastric tube, abdominal distention and diminished breath sounds.
3. Imbalanced nutrition less than body requirement related to poor nutrition before surgery and altered gastrointestinal system after surgery.

GOALS

1. Relieving pain.
2. Prevention and early detection of postoperative complications.
3. Achieving optimum nutritional status.

Nursing Interventions

Relieving pain

- Assess pain with a pain scale.
- Administer analgesics liberally as ordered to relieve pain and discomfort which will ultimately help in breathing, coughing and ambulation. Avoid sedating the patient.
- Place patient in Fowler's position to promote emptying of the stomach, increase comfort and help in breathing.
- Maintain nasogastric tube functioning to prevent distention that increases pain.

Prevention and early detection of postoperative complications

- Assess drainage from nasogastric tube for color, consistency and amount, record findings.
- Maintain nasogastric tube patency with saline irrigations. Do not try to reposition the nasogastric tube.

- Ensure that the nasogastric tube is attached with suction and maintain low suction as ordered.
- Assess operative site for excessive drainage or bleeding.
- Assess and monitor vital signs, blood pressure frequently (every 15–30 minutes for first 2 hours) for shock or hemorrhage; lung sounds for pulmonary problems; infections; thrombosis; bowel sounds for paralytic ileus; intake and output for fluid balance.

Achieving optimum nutritional status

- Continue parenteral nutrition to meet caloric needs, replace fluid lost through drainage and vomits till bowel sounds return.
- When bowel sounds return, clamp nasogastric tube and allow patient to take orally clear water 30 mL at a time.
- Suction after 1 hour to determine whether fluid has been retained.
- If patient tolerates clear water, remove nasogastric tube and allow patient gradually liquid to soft diet and then normal diet of 5 to 6 small meals a day.
- Teach patient to assume Fowler's position during meal time and to lie down for 20 to 30 minutes after meal to delay stomach emptying.
- Discourage fluid intake during meal. Fluid may be taken 1 hour before and 1 hour after meals.
- Meals should contain less liquid items and more dry items.
- Diets should be low in carbohydrate contents. Concentrated sources of carbohydrate should be avoided.
- Encourage to continue dietary supplementations, e.g. vitamin B_{12}, and iron as ordered by the physician.

GASTRIC CANCER

Definition

Gastric cancer refers to the malignant neoplasm found in the stomach.

Incidence

Worldwide it is the second most common cancer.

Found more in men of urban lower socioeconomic group.

Incidence in male is twice than that of female.

The condition is more common in Hispanics, African, American and Asians than in Whites.

Etiology and Risk Factors

No single causative agent has been identified but several risk factors are believed to be associated with the condition. The risk of gastric cancer increases in people:

- With *Helicobacter pylori* infection, chronic atrophic gastritis, achlorhydria, pernicious anemia.
- Consuming diet high in smoked foods, salted fish and meat, pickled vegetables, foods preserved with nitrite preservatives and low in whole grains, fruits and vegetables.
- With repeated exposure to irritants, e.g. bile, antiinflammatory drugs and smoking.
- With gastric surgery for peptic ulcer disease.
- Who are first degree relative of patients with stomach cancer.
- Working in dusty and smoky environment.

Pathophysiology

- 95% of gastric cancers are adenocarcinomas. Rest of the 5% is sarcomas comprising lymphomas and leiomyomas.
- Gastric cancers may occur in any part of the stomach but most of them occur in the lesser curvature of the stomach in the pyloric and antrum area.

- They spread by direct extension and infiltration of the surrounding mucosa; penetrate the wall of the stomach and adjacent organs and structures, e.g. liver, pancreas, esophagus and duodenum.
- Seeding of tumor cells into the peritoneal cavity and metastasis through lymph to the peritoneal cavity occur late in the disease.

Clinical Manifestations

The disease is asymptomatic in the early stage. Early manifestations are vague and indefinite and may resemble peptic ulcer disease or dyspepsia.

Early symptoms if appear consist of:

- Abdominal pain or epigastric distress relieved by antacids or modification of diet.
- Vague epigastric fullness, feeling of early satiety after meals.

As disease progresses:

- Dysphagia, constipation (if disease is near the cardia).
- Nausea, vomiting and hematemesis (if disease is near the pylorus).
- Anorexia, loss of body weight, anemia.
- Fatigue, weakness, dizziness due to anemia from chronic blood loss.
- On examination patient looks pale and lethargic, cachectic.
- Mass may be felt beneath the abdominal wall.

For some patients the first presenting symptoms may be:

- Presence of palpable mass in abdomen.
- Ascites or bone pain due to metastasis.

Diagnostic Studies

1. Endoscopy with biopsy and cytological study confirms the disease.
2. Endoscopic ultrasound and CT scanning helps in staging of the disease.
3. Upper GI barium studies may demonstrate abnormality in gastric contractility and emptying. Cancer may be seen as excavated central lesion with irregular elevated edges. Small lesion at cardia or pylorus may not be visible.
4. Complete blood count and hemoglobin level detect anemia and its severity.
5. Elevated level of serum amylase and liver enzymes indicate metastasis to pancreas and liver.
6. Stool examination detects occult blood or visible blood.
7. Tumor markers, e.g. carcinoembryonic antigen (CEA) and carbohydrate antigen (CA) predict prognosis.

Medical Management

Surgery

It is the primary treatment of gastric cancer. Surgical procedure depends on location, extent of the lesion and condition of the patient. The purpose is to remove the tumor with a margin of normal tissue. Operative procedures commonly performed are:

1. Total gastrectomy with esophagojejunostomy if the lesion is in fundus (Fig. 7.3).
2. Partial gastrectomy with Bilroth I or II if the lesion is in antrum or in the pylorus region (Fig. 7.1 and 7.2).

Radiotherapy

It is not much effective as primary treatment. It may be used as a palliative measure to decrease the tumor mass and provide temporary relief from obstruction.

Radiotherapy and chemotherapy

Radiotherapy and chemotherapy in combination is used following surgery to prevent disease recurrence. Drugs commonly used

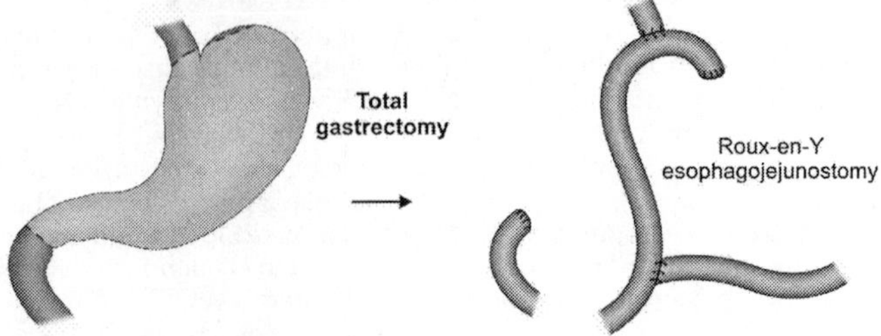

Fig. 7.3: Total gastrectomy with esophagojejunostomy

are 5-FU, cisplatin, mitomycin, etoposide, leucovorin and adriamycin.

Total parenteral nutrition

It is provided in advanced stages to bypass the diseased stomach.

Nursing Management

Assessment

- **Subjective data**: Feelings of early satiety, vague epigastric fullness, dyspepsia, symptoms of gas pain, loss of body weight, abdominal pain, epigastric distress, nausea, vomiting, fatigue, weakness, dizziness, history of chronic gastritis, pernicious anemia, previous gastric surgery, presence of *H. pylori* infection, smoking, frequent ingestion of nitrites, smoked fish, salty fish or pickled vegetables.
- **Objective data**: Pallor, lethargy, cachexia, presence of mass in abdomen.

Nursing Diagnoses

1. Acute pain related to the disease process and postoperative pain related to high surgical incision as manifested by patient's verbal complaints.
2. Imbalanced nutrition less than body requirements related to inability to take food, digest and absorb nutrients as manifested by reduced energy, anemia, cachexia,
3. Activity intolerance related to dizziness, weakness, epigastric discomfort.
4. Anxiety related to lack of knowledge about diagnostic tests, disease process, treatment regimen and outcome of treatment.
5. Grieving related to the diagnosis of cancer and impending death.

GOALS

1. Control of pain and minimum discomfort.
2. Attainment of optimum nutritional status and physical well-being.
3. Reduced anxiety and adjustment to the diagnosis, treatment schedule and anticipated lifestyle changes appropriate to the disease stage.

Nursing Interventions

Control of pain and minimum discomfort

- Assess pain by a pain scale.
- Administer pain medication liberally as ordered but avoid sedating the patient so that the patient participates in postoperative breathing and coughing.

- Assess the effectiveness of pain medication and report to the physician.
- Instruct patient to splint his incision with a pillow while coughing in order to lessen pain and tension on sutures.
- Place the patient in Fowler's position to promote emptying of the stomach after partial gastrectomy, which will reduce distention, lessen pain and increase comfort.
- Maintain nasogastric suction as ordered to reduce distention and pain.
- Help patient to change position frequently and provide backrub to increase comfort.
- Teach patient various nonpharmacologic methods of pain relief, e.g. relaxation, distraction, imagery and music to get relief from chronic pain.

Attainment of optimum nutritional status and physical well-being

- Provide patient high caloric diet with adequate vitamins A and C and iron to improve poor nutritional status and enhance postoperative tissue repair and prevent infection and complications.
- Encourage the patient to eat small amount at frequent intervals. Innovate ideas and take help from family members to encourage the anorexic and depressive patient to eat.
- Administer antiemetic as ordered if nausea and vomiting.
- Provide enteral feedings and parenteral nutrition if the patient is unable to eat.
- Administer blood or packed cells as ordered to correct anemia. Watch closely for transfusion reaction.
- Monitor nutritional status, body weight, hematocrit and hemoglobin level, intake and output to ensure that the patient is gaining weight.
- Postoperatively administer small amounts of clear fluid when intestinal peristalsis starts. Observe for leakage of fluid from anastomosis site by elevation of body temperature and dyspnea.
- Increase fluid intake and small amount of solid foods when clear fluid is well tolerated.
- Advise patient to prevent and manage postoperative dumping syndrome by taking six small dry meals with low carbohydrate contents and drinking fluids in between meals.
- Replace vitamins, e.g. B complex, C, K and cobalamine as ordered, if a total gastrectomy.

Reduced anxiety and adjustment to the diagnosis, treatment schedule and anticipated lifestyle changes appropriate to the disease stage

- Help the patient to express fears, concerns and grief about the diagnosis.
- Answer the patient's questions honestly; provide explanations to all procedures and treatment options.
- Encourage patient to participate in treatment planning.
- Involve family members or any significant person, e.g. religious guru, social worker, psychiatrist, psychiatric nurse or counselor to provide emotional support.
- Refer the patient to a dietician or a community health nurse or a hospice team as appropriate to ensure ongoing assessment, treatment and emotional support after discharge.

GASTROENTERITIS

Gastroenteritis is an inflammation of the gastrointestinal tract that particularly affects the stomach and intestine.

Etiology

Pathogens that cause gastroenteritis include

- Bacteria, e.g. *E. coli, Shigella, Salmonella, Staphylococcus aureus, Clostridium per-*

fringens, Clostridium difficile, Campylobacter, etc.
- Viruses, e.g. Rotavirus, Norwalk.
- Parasites, e.g. *Giardia lamblia. Entamoeba hystolytica, Cryptosporidium.*

Mode of transmission of pathogens is from person to person by fecal oral route through ingestion of contaminated food and water. Common sources of pathogen transmission are:
- Unclean hands after defecation.
- Contaminated eggs, raw or undercooked meat and chicken, focally contaminated shellfish, unpasteurized milk, ice cream, fruit juices.

Risk Factors

- Person with oral antibiotics.
- Person practicing unsafe food preparation and storage.
- Aged and the children.
- Person with immune disorders or on immunosuppressive drugs.

Pathophysiology

- Normal flora of the intestine usually protects the bowel from colonization of pathogens.
- Use of oral or parenteral antibiotics and invasion of certain pathogens that cause tissue damage result into inflammation and disruption of normal flora respectively.
- Invasion of pathogens in the intestine releases endotoxins that stimulate its mucosal lining, resulting in greater secretion of water and electrolytes in the intestinal lumen.
- Greater electrolyte concentration in the intestinal secretion inhibits sodium reabsorption.
- To dilute the extra sodium and electrolyte, load large amount of protein-rich fluid is secreted in the bowel.
- The large bowel is unable to reabsorb this extra fluid load and give rise to diarrhea.
- Inflammation and disruption of mucous membrane of the intestine gives rise to ulceration and bleeding.
- Impaired integrity of the gastrointestinal tract affects its digestive and absorptive functions.

Clinical Manifestations

- Diarrhea of variable intensity
- Nausea, vomiting and anorexia
- Abdominal pain, cramp, borborygmi
- Fever.

Diagnostic Studies

1. Stool test shows presence of white blood cells, mucus, blood and causative organisms.

Management

Medical management

1. Keep patient in nothing per oral status until the vomiting subsides.
2. Replace fluids and electrolytes—
   - IV infusion of dextrose saline or Ringer's lactate, if severe diarrhea or vomiting.
   - Clear liquid containing glucose and electrolytes orally when nausea and vomiting subsides.
3. Soft diet as tolerated after 24 hours.
   If diarrhea continues beyond 2 to 3 days
   - Identify organism.
   - Start metronidazole or other antibiotics to eliminate the offending organism.

NURSING MANAGEMENT

Assessment

Subjective data

Increase in number and looseness of stool, change in character and odor of stool, abdominal tenderness, cramping, bloating, nausea, vomiting, thirst, reduced urinary output, perianal skin irritation, history of eating outside/travel/greasy spicy food, food intolerances.

Objective data

Lethargy, sunken eyeballs, pallor, dry mucous membranes, poor skin turgor, abdominal distention, tachycardia, hypotension, hyperactive bowel sounds, loose watery stools, presence of pus, mucus, blood in stool, decreased urine output, concentrated urine, perianal skin inflammation.

Possible findings

Leukocytosis, abnormal serum electrolytes levels, positive stool cultures, presence of ova, parasites, blood, white blood cells in stools.

Nursing Diagnoses

1. Diarrhea related to acute infectious process of the gastrointestinal tract as evidenced by frequent passage of liquid stools.
2. Risk of transmission of infection to others.
3. Deficient fluid volume related to excessive fluid loss and decreased fluid intake, secondary to diarrhea and vomiting as evidenced by sunken eyes, dry skin and mucous membrane, poor skin turgor, decreased urine output, tachycardia, hypotension, altered serum electrolytes.
4. Impaired skin integrity related to frequent passage of loose stools as evidenced by redness and excoriation of perianal skin.

GOALS

1. Prevention of transmission of infection.
2. Controlling diarrhea and resuming normal bowel pattern.
3. Maintaining fluid electrolyte and acid-base balance.
4. Maintaining perianal skin integrity.

Nursing Interventions

Prevention of transmission of infection

- Admit the patient in a private room and initiate contact isolation procedure, e.g. strict hand washing, wearing gown and gloves, meticulous cleanliness of the environments, use of disposable equipments, disinfection of equipments, etc. as per institution's protocol.
- Teach patient and family members proper hand washing, infection control precaution, proper food handling, cooking and storage.

Controlling diarrhea and resuming normal bowel pattern

- Keep patient in nil orally status till nausea and vomiting subsides.
- Obtain stool for culture if diarrhea continues beyond 2 days.
- Teach patient to report each episode of diarrhea to monitor the effectiveness of treatment.
- Instruct family members to record color, volume, frequency and consistency of stools to monitor effectiveness of treatment.
- Administer antidiarrheal medications as ordered.
- Teach patient proper use of over the counter antidiarrheal medications to prevent self-administration of antiperistaltic agent (e.g. lomotil) that prolongs exposure to infecting organisms.

Maintain fluid, electrolyte and acid-base balance

- Periodically observe for signs of dehydration.

- Encourage oral fluid intake when nausea vomiting subsides and patient tolerates.
- Maintain intravenous fluid infusion and replace fluid and electrolytes as ordered.
- Monitor intake output, body weight to determine fluid balance.
- Monitor vital signs to determine risk for hypovolemia.
- Monitor serum electrolytes, hematocrit, blood urea nitrogen, serum osmolality, urine specific gravity levels to indicate response to treatment.

Maintaining perianal skin integrity

- Carefully assess patient's perianal area for signs of inflammation e.g. redness, excoriation and irritation.
- Clean perianal area after each bowel movement with mild soap and water.
- Pat dry the area and apply some moisturizing cream or lotion according to the preference of the patient.
- Take special care while offering and removing of bed pan.
- Teach and demonstrate care to the patient and significant family member.

INTESTINAL OBSTRUCTION

Definition

Partial or complete impairment of forward flow of intestinal contents is known as an intestinal obstruction.

Both the small and large intestine may get obstructed.

Majority of the obstruction occur in the small intestine specially the ileum.

Obstruction in the large intestine usually occurs in the sigmoid colon.

Classification

- Dynamic obstruction/mechanical. In dynamic obstruction intestinal peristalsis works against a mechanical obstruction.
- Adynamic obstruction/functional. In this type of obstruction intestinal peristalsis is usually absent or it may be present in a nonpropulsive form.

Clinically intestinal obstruction may be classified as

- Small bowel obstruction high or low
- Large bowel obstruction.

According to the period of onset

- Acute—usually occurs in small intestine.
- Chronic—usually occurs in large intestine.
- Acute on chronic.
- Subacute.

Etiology

Dynamic or mechanical obstruction is usually caused by narrowing of the intestinal lumen by

- Intraluminal factors, e.g. impaction, foreign bodies, bezoars (collection of undigested fibers in food), gallstones.
- Intramural factors, e.g. strictures, neoplasms.
- Extramural factors, e.g. adhesions/bands, hernia, volvulus, intussusception.

Adynamic or functional obstruction is caused by cessation of peristaltic activity due to

- Vascular factors, e.g. mesenteric occlusion due to thrombosis or embolism.
- Neurogenic factors, e.g. paralytic ileus after abdominal surgery.

Pathophysiology

- Below the obstruction intestinal activity remains normal with normal peristalsis and absorption until it becomes empty.

- Empty distal intestine contracts and ultimately become immobile.
- Above the obstruction, proximal peristalsis increases to overcome the obstruction.
- If obstruction is not relieved proximal bowel gradually dilates.
- Dilated bowel gradually looses peristaltic strength. Ultimately paralytic ileus occurs.
- The dilated bowel proximal to obstruction fills with accumulation of gas and fluid resulting into abdominal distention.
- Absorption of fluid from the obstructed bowel diminishes.
- Defective absorption in the intestine, reduced oral intake and vomiting result into dehydration and electrolyte imbalance.

Clinical Features

Clinical features depend upon

- The level of obstruction, i.e. high or low, small bowel or large bowel obstruction:
- Acute (usually in small bowel) or chronic (usually in large bowel) onset of obstruction.
- Simple obstruction with no interference of blood supply or obstruction with severe impairment of blood supply in the intestine.

Major clinical features of intestinal obstruction

- Abdominal pain
  - Sudden, severe and colicky pain due to increased peristaltic activity is usually the early manifestation of acute obstruction.
  - Pain is felt around the umbilicus in small bowel obstruction and in lower abdomen in large bowel obstruction.
  - Development of severe pain occurs in strangulation.
  - Pain is absent in intestinal obstruction due to paralytic ileus.
  - Colicky pain changes to a mild diffuse constant pain as distention increases and intestinal peristalsis stops.
- Vomiting
  - Vomiting is accompanied by nausea.
  - Vomiting occurs early in proximal small bowel obstruction and vomiting is delayed in distal small bowel and large bowel obstruction.
  - Vomitus initially contains undigested food later watery and contains bile. Finally dark fecal materials appear due to enteric bacterial overgrowth.
- Distention
  - It is minimal in high small bowel obstruction.
  - It is greater in low small bowel obstruction.
  - It is delayed and pronounced in large bowel obstruction.
  - It is minimal or absent in mesenteric vessel obstruction.
- Constipation
  - Constipation in intestinal obstruction may be absolute (neither flatus nor feces is passed) or relative (only flatus is passed).
  - Absolute constipation or obstipation occurs in complete intestinal obstruction.
  - Relative constipation occurs after the onset of symptoms due to evacuation of distal bowel contents.
  - Constipation may be absent in obstruction due to mesenteric vascular occlusion, gallstone impaction, pelvic infection in which diarrhea may often occur.
- Dehydration
  - It commonly occurs in small bowel obstruction due to repeated vomiting and defective fluid absorption.

- It is manifested as dry skin and mucous membrane, sunken eyes, feeble pulse, oliguria, increased blood urea level and hematocrit concentration.
- Hypokalemia
  - It is not a common feature in simple obstruction but present in strangulation.
- Leukocytosis.
- Pyrexia
  - It ay be present in intestinal perforation, ischemia or inflammation associated with the obstructing disease.
- Hypothermia
  - It is present in septicemic shock.
- Abdominal tenderness
  - Localized tenderness indicates ischemia, perforation or peritonitis.
- Bowel sounds
  - High pitched bowel sounds are heard on the area above the obstruction.
  - It may also be absent.

Diagnostic Studies

1. X-ray
   - X-ray of the abdomen in upright and supine positions reveal bowel distention and presence of multiple (more than six) gas-fluid levels.
   - Presence of intraperitoneal air indicates perforation.
2. Barium X-ray
   - Barium enema or small bowel series is helpful to determine the level of obstruction or the nature or cause of obstruction (barium is not used if perforation is suspected).
3. CT scan may also be used for diagnosis.
4. Sigmoidoscopy or colonoscopy provides direct visualization of an obstruction in the colon.
5. CBC
   - Elevated leukocytosis indicates strangulation or perforation.
   - Elevated hematocrit level indicates dehydration.
   - Decreased hematocrit level and hemoglobin level indicates bleeding from a tumor or strangulation with necrosis.
6. Serum electrolytes
   - Decreased level of serum sodium, potassium and chloride concentration is seen in small bowel obstruction.
7. Stool examination may reveal occult blood if obstruction due to neoplasm.

Management

Conservative management

1. Gastrointestinal drainage
   - Patient is placed on nil per oral status.
   - Nasogastric tube or long intestinal tube is passed and connected with continuous or intermittent suction.
   - Often an intestinal tube both decompresses the bowel and breaks up the obstruction.
   - It helps recover adynamic obstruction by relieving distention and providing bowel rest.
2. Fluid and electrolyte replacement
   - Normal saline and lactated Ringer's solution is administered.
   - Fluid and electrolyte balance is maintained by monitoring of hematocrit and serum electrolytes concentration.
3. Analgesics are given to control pain.
4. Antibiotics are given to control bacterial overgrowth.

Surgical management

- Surgery is done when patient's condition does not improve within 24 to 48 hours.

- Early surgery is done if strangulated or obstructed external hernia or internal intestinal strangulation is suspected or there is acute obstruction.
- Surgical procedures involve resecting the obstructed segment of bowel and anastomosing the remaining healthy bowel back together.
- Partial or total colectomy, colostomy or ileostomy may be required depending upon the extent of obstruction.

NURSING MANAGEMENT

Assessment

Subjective data

Abdominal pain in lower abdomen or around the umbilicus, colicky, severe pain or constant dull pain, nausea, vomiting, abdominal distention, relative or absolute constipation, borborygmi, thirst.

Objective data

Abdominal distention, tenderness and rigidity in abdomen, visible peristalsis, scar of previous operation, visible masses, absent or hyperactive bowel sounds, vomitus containing bile, fecal materials, elevated body temperature, tachycardia, feeble pulse, hypotension, dry skin and mucous membrane, oliguria.

Possible findings

Multiple fluid and gas level in supine and erect abdominal X-rays, positive findings in Barium X-rays of lower and upper gastrointestinal tract, positive findings in colonoscopy or sigmoidoscopy, leukocytosis if strangulation or perforation, elevated hematocrit level, low serum sodium and potassium level, occult blood in stool.

Nursing Diagnoses

1. Abdominal pain related to increased peristalsis and distention as evidenced by patient's verbal complaints.
2. Fluid and electrolyte imbalance related to decreased fluid absorption by the intestine, vomiting and nasogastric suction as evidenced by dry skin and mucous membrane, sunken eyes, tachycardia, feeble pulse, hypotension, oliguria.
3. Fear and anxiety related to the sudden nature of the disease and knowledge deficit regarding the disease, treatment options and prognosis as evidenced by repeated questioning.

GOALS

1. Relief of abdominal pain.
2. Relief of the obstruction and return to normal bowel function.
3. Maintenance of normal fluid and electrolyte balance.
4. Freedom from fear and anxiety by acquisition of knowledge.

Nursing Interventions

Relief of abdominal pain

- Assess the location and character of pain.
- Determine the severity of pain by a pain scale.
- Introduce a nasogastric or intestinal tube and attach it to suction.
- Administer analgesics as per physicians order.
- Assess the effectiveness of analgesics and report to the physician.
- Institute comfort measures like comfortable position, change of position, 4 hourly back rub to promote comfort.
- Provide restful environment by restricting visitors and avoiding distractions.

Relief of the obstruction and return to normal bowel function

- Introduce nasogastric tube or intestinal tube as ordered and attach it to suction.
- Note and document the amount, color, odor, consistency of the drainage.
- Check patency of nasogastric tube every 4 hours.
- Monitor patient's condition whether relief from distention and nausea occurs or not.
- Provide frequent mouth care to remove distaste from patient's mouth due to vomiting.
- Observe patient's nose for signs of irritation due to the presence of nasogastric tube and apply lubricant to this area as needed.

Maintenance of normal fluid and electrolyte balance

- Monitor vital signs, blood pressure, hourly urine output and skin turgor for evidence of dehydration.
- Monitor hematocrit level and serum electrolyte level for signs of dehydration and electrolyte imbalance.
- Administer intravenous fluids as ordered.
- Maintain strict intake output chart by carefully taking into account all vomitus and intestinal tube drainage.

Freedom from fear and anxiety by acquisition of knowledge

- Assess patient's current level of knowledge about the disease, treatment options, routine preoperative preparations if any and future outcome.
- Explain patient in simple language the information given by the physician.
- Provide time for the patient to discuss his questions and concerns.
- Demonstrate calm and confidence and reassure patient that every possible care is being provided to him.

Postoperative nursing management is like any other abdominal surgery explained in previous sections.

HERNIA

Definition

A hernia is the protrusion of an organ, fascia or part of an organ through an abnormal opening or a weakened area in the wall of the cavity that normally contains it.

Hernia can occur in any part of the body but most commonly occurs in abdominal cavity.

Types

Inguinal hernia

- It is the most common type of hernia. Up to 75% of all abdominal hernias are inguinal hernia.
- It occurs at the point of weakness in the abdominal wall where spermatic cord in men and the round ligament in women pass.
- It is subdivided into two types
  - Indirect inguinal hernia in which the inguinal canal is entered via a congenital weakness in the internal inguinal ring.
  - Direct inguinal hernia in which the hernia contents push through a weak spot in the posterior wall of the inguinal canal.

Femoral hernia

- It occurs when abdominal contents pass into the weak area at the posterior wall of the femoral canal.
- It appears as a bulge below the inguinal ligament.

- It is common in women.
- The incidence of strangulation in this hernia is high.

Umbilical hernia

- In this type of hernia abdominal organs protrude through a weakness at the site of passage of the umbilical cord through the abdominal wall.
- It is common in African infants, specially boys.
- In adults umbilical hernias are acquired and are frequent in obese and pregnant women.

Incisional hernia

- It occurs when the defect or weakness is the result of an incompletely healed surgical wound.
- It is common in persons who are obese, had multiple operation in same site or had inadequate wound healing due to poor nutrition or infections.
- Incisional hernia on median incision is also called ventral hernia.

Etiology and Risk Factors

Hernias develop when there is a defect in the integrity of the muscular wall (muscle weakness) along with increased intraabdominal pressure.

- Factors causing muscle weakness may be due to: Congenital or occur with aging or is associated with other conditions, e.g. stretching of muscles during pregnancy, losing weight in obese people or scars from previous surgery.
- Increased intraabdominal pressure may be due to: Pregnancy, ascites, COPD, dyschezia, benign prostatic hypertrophy, improper weight lifting, traumatic injuries from blunt pressure.

Pathophysiology

- When muscular weakness and intraabdominal pressure coexist hernia develops.
- Intraabdominal pressure without weakness is not likely to cause hernia.
- Beside congenital weakness acquired weakness may occur as part of aging.
- With aging muscular tissues become infiltrated and are replaced by adipose and connective tissues.
- When the contents of the hernial sac go back to the abdominal cavity by manipulation or by lying down the hernia is said to be reducible.
- When the contents of the sac can not be returned to the abdominal cavity by manipulation the hernia is said to be irreducible or incarcerated hernia.
- An irreducible hernia often turns into strangulated hernia when pressure from the hernial ring on the hernial contents compromises blood supply (specially the veins because of their low pressure) causing venous congestion. The bowel becomes edematous at first causing it more irreducible and finally becomes necrosed and gangrenous. The result of this condition is often fatal.
- An irreducible hernia often cause intestinal obstruction as the herniated segment of the bowel cannot propel intestinal contents forward. This also gives rise to an emergency situation.

Clinical Manifestations

Uncomplicated hernia

- A visible or palpable lump in the groin or in another abdominal area.
- The bulge becomes more prominent during standing; bulge reduces by simple manipulation or by lying in bed.
- Discomfort or dragging sensation at the site due to tension.

- Pain and swelling at the scrotum in male.

Complicated hernia

- Severe pain followed by tenderness if hernia becomes strangulated.
- Cramping abdominal pain, distention, vomiting, inability to have bowel movement or pass flatus, and fever may occur due to bowel obstruction.
- The hernia bulge may turn red, purple, or dark and pink if strangulation.

Diagnostic Studies

Diagnosis is based on history and physical examination findings.

Management

Conservative management

Wearing a truss, a firm pad placed over the hernia and held in place by a belt. Patient wears the truss to keep the hernia reduced. The pad is placed after the hernia is reduced and is left in place to prevent the hernia from recurring. Patient should be taught to apply the truss daily before arising.

Surgical management

Surgery is the treatment of choice. Timely surgery prevents hernia become strangulated and obstructed.

- **Surgical procedures**

1. Herniorrhaphy: In this operation a small incision over the weakened area is given. The intestine is pushed back to the abdominal cavity, the hernia sac is excised and muscle is closed tightly over the area.
2. Hernioplasty: Hernia repair by using wire, fascia or mesh graft to reinforce the weakened area due to absence of muscle mass is performed in hernioplasty.
3. Laparoscopic extraperitoneal (LEP) herniorrhaphy is a new surgical technique which may be performed as an outpatient procedure.

NURSING MANAGEMENT

Preoperative Nursing Care

Preoperative preparation of the patient is like any other abdominal surgery.

Postoperative Nursing Care

Helping in voiding

- Assess urinary bladder for distention.
- If patient is having difficulty in voiding help him by giving proper position to evacuate the bladder.
- Maintain an intake output chart.

Preventing scrotal edema and pain

- Assess the degree of swelling in the scrotum.
- Apply an ice bag on the scrotum to relieve pain and swelling in the scrotum.
- Position patient so that his scrotum is elevated.
- Teach patient to wear a scrotal support when he is out of bed.

Teaching self-care

- Teach patient to do deep breathing exercises but not coughing.
- Instruct patient to splint incision during coughing.
- Teach the patient that if he has sneezing he must do so with mouth open.
- Teach patient to carry out normal activity gradually and not to do heavy lifting for at least 6 to 8 weeks.
- Reassure patient that hernia will not recur once surgery is done.

INFLAMMATORY BOWEL DISEASE

Definition

Inflammatory bowel disease (IBD) refers to two chronic inflammatory disorders of gastrointestinal tract namely, Crohn's disease or regional enteritis and ulcerative colitis, which are characterized by chronic inflammation of the intestine with alternate periods of remission and exacerbation usually extending over years.

Incidence

- Incidence varies widely between populations.
- Incidence of Crohn's disease is less common than that of ulcerative colitis.
- Both diseases start most commonly during the teenage years and early adulthood with a second peak in the sixth decade.

Etiology and Risk Factors

Cause is not well-known. Both genetic and environmental factors are believed to cause the diseases.

Genetic factors

- 10% of patients with inflammatory bowel disorder have a close relative or a first degree relative with IBD.
- Family members of a patient with Crohn's disease have an increased risk of developing ulcerative colitis and vice versa.
- One susceptibility gene CARD 15 on chromosome 16 has been identified for Crohn's disease. HLA-DR 103 is associated with severe ulcerative colitis. Other additional genes are under study.
- IBD is common in Jews.

Environmental factors

- Ulcerative colitis is more common in nonsmokers and exsmokers whereas Crohn's disease is more common in smokers.
- IBD is associated with low fiber, high refined sugar diet.
- Appendectomy protects against ulcerative colitis.
- NSAIDs exacerbate the symptoms of IBD.
- Emotional factors may precipitate an exacerbation or prolong an attack of IBD.
- Some people respond well with antibiotic therapy that suggests presence of bacteria as a causative factor although no bacteria has been identified.

Pathophysiology

After an attack of a trigger the intestine is infiltrated with acute and chronic inflammatory cells and initiates abnormal inflammatory response.

Pattern of inflammatory response is different in two diseases.

Response in Crohn's disease

- Inflammation involves all four layers of intestinal wall and can occur anywhere in the gastrointestinal tract from mouth to anus but common site is terminal ileum and right side of colon.
- The entire wall of the intestine is edematous and thickened. In between there are deep longitudinal ulcers, thus the mucous membrane between them takes a classic appearance and is known as 'cobblestone'.
- Strictures at the areas of inflammation may cause intestinal obstruction.
- Inflammation extends through all the layers of intestine and penetrates the intestinal wall allowing microscopic

leak of intestinal contents into the peritoneal cavity to initiate abscess formation and fistulas.
- Inflammatory lesions are patchy, because segments of normal bowel occur between the diseased areas. The lesions separated in this way by islands of normal bowel are known as 'skip' lesions.

Inflammatory response in ulcerative colitis

- Inflammation in ulcerative colitis affects only the mucosa of the colon. The disease starts in the rectum and spreads proximally towards the cecum.
- Inflammatory lesions are continuous and diffuse.
- Multiple ulcerations followed by desquamation or shedding of the colonic epithelium occurs, resulting into bleeding.
- Inflamed mucosa unable to absorb water and electrolytes causes loss of large amounts of fluid and electrolytes.
- Areas of inflamed mucosa form pseudopolyps, tongue-like projections into the colonic lumen.

Clinical Manifestations

Both forms of IBD produce similar clinical features

- Abdominal pain, diarrhea, vomiting.
- Thirst, reduced urine output due to fluid loss through diarrhea and vomiting, fever.
- Steady and progressive weight loss.
- General appearance may be reasonably healthy (in ulcerative colitis) or wasted and malnourished (in Chrohn's disease).
- Pallor of varying degree.
- Flat or concave shape abdomen with visible peristalsis and increased bowel sounds if obstruction.
- Tenderness on the areas of inflammation.
- Hemorrhoids, perianal abscess, fistula and ulcers may be seen.

Distinguishing features in Crohn's disease

- Diarrhea is less severe than that in ulcerative colitis.
- Stool soft or semi-liquid, foul smelling and fatty.
- Urgency to evacuate may awaken the patient at night.
- Weight loss, anorexia, anemia, debility, fatigue and metabolic disturbances occur due to malabsorption of essential nutrients.

Distinguishing manifestations in ulcerative colitis

- Rectal bleeding or bloody diarrhea, 10 to 20 times more stools per day.
- Liquid stool with tenesmus, contains blood, mucus and pus.
- Feeling of urgent need to defecate.
- Mild, intermittent, colicky pain in lower left quadrant of the abdomen or severe constant pain if perforation.
- Nausea, vomiting, anorexia, fever, anemia and weight loss.

Complications

Local complications (intestinal)

Hemorrhage, strictures, perforation, fistulas, colonic dilation, toxic megacolon, increased risk of cancer in small bowel or colorectal cancers.

Systemic complications (extra intestinal)

Arthritis, ankylosing spondilitis, eye inflammations, skin lesions, e.g. erythema nodosum, pyoderma gangrenosum, thromboembolism, kidney stones, gallstones, cholangitis, osteoporosis.

Diagnostic Studies

1. Complete blood count—It reveals iron deficiency anemia from blood loss or malabsorption, elevated WBC count indicates perforation or toxic megacolon.
2. Serum albumin—Decreased level indicates protein loss from bowel or poor nutrition.
3. Serum electrolytes—Decreased level of sodium, potassium, chloride, bicarbonates, etc. found due to loss from diarrhea and vomiting.
4. Erythrocyte sedimentation rate–Elevated level indicates chronic inflammation.
5. C-reactive protein—Elevated level determines Crohn's disease activity.
6. Stool examination—It reveals presence of blood, pus, mucus, superimposed infection.
7. Sigmoidoscopy and colonoscopy—Show inflammation, ulceration, strictures, pseudopolyps.
8. Biopsy—It determines disease extent and dysplasia in patients with chronic IBD.
9. Barium studies—Strictures, skip lesions and deeper ulcers are seen in Crohn's disease. Shortened colon and pseudopolyps are seen in ulcerative colitis.
10. Plain X-ray—It severe active disease may show evidence of perforation in ulcerative colitis and evidence of intestinal obstruction or displacement of bowel loops by a mass in Crohn's disease.

Medical Management

Goals

- To control the inflammation by suppressing the inappropriate immune responses.
- To provide rest to the bowel to aid in healing.
- To improve quality of life.
- To prevent or minimize complications.

Drug therapy

1. Aminosalicylates–Sulfasalazine, a combination of 5-aminosalicylic acid (5-ASA) and sulfapyridine, reduces mild or moderate inflammation and prevents or reduces recurrences in long-term treatment regimen.
2. Mesalamine, olsalazine, balsalazide, etc. sulfa-free aminosalicylates given to people who are unable to tolerate sulfapyridine.
3. Preparations of 5-ASA as suppositories, enemas and foams are used as topical treatment to minimize the systemic effects. They are used in the treatment of ulcerative colitis and also in mild to moderate Crohn's disease when the colon is affected.
4. Antibiotics—Metronidazole, ciprofloxacin and clarithromycin may be used to treat secondary infections or in complications.
5. Corticosteroids—It is used in severe and fulminant disease to achieve remission. It is given for short time because of adverse side effects. It is not effective in maintaining remission. Topical corticosteroids, e.g. hydrocortisone enemas, suppositories or foams are used to treat disease in distal colon. Oral prednisolone is used in mild to moderate disease when patient does not respond to topical corticosteroids or 5-ASA. Intravenous corticosteroids given in severe inflammation.
6. Immunosuppressive—Azathioprine (Imuran), cyclosporine, 6 mercaptopurine, methotrexate, etc. is used when patient do not respond to 5-ASA, antibiotics or corticosteroids.

7. Immunomodulator—Infliximab (remicade) used to induce and maintain remission in patients with active Crohn's disease.

Nutritional therapy

- Low residue, high protein and high caloric diet with adequate fluids, vitamins and iron to be given to meet nutritional needs, reduce inflammation, control diarrhea and pain.
- Intravenous fluids to be given if dehydration.
- Total parenteral nutrition is given in serious cases to promote weight gain, maintain positive nitrogen balance, provide rest to the bowel and decrease fecal bulk.

Surgical therapy

- **Crohn's disease**
  - Majority requires surgery within 5 year of diagnosis.
  - Surgery is done when medical treatment fails; quality of life worsens; and complications, e.g. bleeding, perforation, obstruction occurs.

Surgical procedures are:

1. Strictureplasty—To widen narrowed bowel.
2. Resection of diseased portions of the intestine and anastomosis of the remaining intestine.

Surgery may induce remission but cannot prevent recurrence.

- **Ulcerative colitis**
  - Surgery is done when medical treatment fails; exacerbations of the disease are frequent and debilitating; complications, e.g. massive bleeding, perforation, strictures, or obstruction and suspicion of cancer appears.

Surgical procedures are:

1. Total colectomy with rectal mucosal stripping and ileoanal reservoir.
2. Total proctocolectomy with permanent ileostomy.
3. Total proctocolectomy with continent ileostomy (Kock pouch).

NURSING MANAGEMENT

Assessment

Subjective data

Diarrhea; stool containing blood, mucus, pus; tenesmus; lower abdominal pain, cramping, nausea; vomiting; anorexia; loss of weight; fatigue; malaise; history of IBD in family; use of frequent antidiarrheal medications.

Objective data

Emaciated appearance, anxious, fatigued, pale, anemic. Skin with poor turgor, dry mucous membrane, abdominal distention, hyperactive bowel sounds, tachycardia, hypotension.

Possible findings

Leukocytosis, reduced hemoglobin and hematocrit level, electrolyte imbalance, vitamin and trace metal deficiency, hypoalbuminemia, occult blood in stool, abnormal sigmoidoscopy, colonoscopy or barium study findings.

Nursing Diagnoses

1. Diarrhea related to the inflammation of the intestine as evidenced by frequent, loose or liquid stools.
2. Imbalanced nutrition, less than body requirement related to malabsorption, increased nutrient loss through diarrhea and decreased intake as evidenced by loss of body weight, anemia and fatigue.

3. Acute abdominal pain related to the inflammatory process and increased peristalsis of the intestine as evidenced by patient's verbal complains.
4. Risk for fluid volume deficit related to diarrhea, anorexia, nausea and vomiting.
5. Risk for impaired skin integrity related to diarrhea, dehydration and malnutrition.
6. Activity intolerance related to anemia as evidenced by fatigue, tachycardia and reduced hemoglobin and hematocrit level.
7. Anxiety related to the repeated attacks of diarrhea, possible social embarrassment, diagnostic tests, treatment and prognosis as evidenced by anxious look, frequent questioning about disease and prognosis.
8. Ineffective therapeutic regimen management related to chronic nature of the illness, lack of knowledge regarding the course of the disease, nutritional and drug therapy and required lifestyle changes as evidenced by repeated questioning about the disease and treatment and inability to take proper decisions regarding activities of daily living.

GOALS

1. Attainment of normal elimination pattern.
2. Maintenance of optimal nutritional status.
3. Relief of abdominal pain.
4. Prevention of fluid volume deficit.
5. Prevention of skin breakdown.
6. Promoting activity tolerance.
7. Reducing anxiety.
8. Understanding of the disease, therapeutic regimen and required lifestyle changes.

Nursing Interventions

Attainment of normal elimination pattern

- Assess the number, frequency, consistency, color, and volume of stools.
- Try to find out any precipitating factors, e.g. certain foods, activity or emotional stress as a cause of diarrhea.
- Provide the patient bedpan, commode or easy access to bathroom and take care to keep the environment odor-free.
- Keep the patient in NPO status to give rest to the bowel and encourage bed rest to decrease peristalsis.
- Administer antidiarrheal drugs as ordered and assess frequency and consistency of stools to determine the effectiveness of the medicine.
- When oral feeding resumes, encourage patient to have frequent small feedings with low residue diet to prevent irritation to the bowel.

Maintenance of optimal nutritional status

- Assess patient's body weight, hemoglobin, hematocrit level, and serum protein to assess the nutritional status of the patient.
- Administer parenteral nutrition as ordered in severe disease.
- Monitor body weight and blood glucose level daily when patient is on parenteral nutrition.
- Gradually resume oral feedings with supplemental protein, calories, iron and fluid as prescribed to maintain nutrition but minimum bowel irritation.
- Monitor body weight, hemoglobin, hematocrit and serum protein at regular intervals to assess the effectiveness of nutritional therapy.
- Instruct patient to restrict activities to conserve energy, reduce caloric requirements and intestinal hyperactivity.

Relief of abdominal pain

- Enquire from patient about the character of pain, e.g. dull, cramping, constant or intermittent and the time of occurrence, e.g. before or after foods or before elimination.
- Administer anticholinergic drugs as ordered before meal to decrease intestinal peristalsis and analgesics as ordered for pain.
- Encourage patient to change position, avoid fatigue and engage in diversional activities to reduce pain.

Prevention of fluid volume deficit

- Assess patient's skin and mucous membrane for dryness, decreased skin turgor, oliguria, elevated urine specific gravity, hypotension for fluid volume deficit.
- Administer intravenous fluids as ordered and monitor their flow rate.
- Encourage oral fluids when permitted.
- Keep accurate record of fluid intake and output, e.g. urine, liquid stool and vomitus.
- Monitor patient's daily body weight for fluid gains and losses.

Prevention of skin breakdown

- Assess patient's skin on bony prominences and perianal area every shift for dryness, redness and break in the continuity.
- Provide perianal care after each bowel movement with plain water. Dry the area with soft towel and use prescribed ointment as a skin barrier.
- Provide special care to the bony prominences with back rub and change of position at regular intervals.
- Provide pressure relieving devices, e.g. air mattress to the bedridden patient to prevent skin breakdown.

Promoting activity tolerance

- Assess patient's ability to perform activities of daily living and their effects on the patient.
- Encourage the patient to take rest periods at frequent intervals and to avoid activities that cause fatigue in order to conserve energy and reduce metabolic rate.
- Provide bed rest to the patient who is severely ill, e.g. having fever, bleeding, or frequent liquid stools.
- Encourage patient on bed rest to perform active exercises, e.g. range of joint movement and muscle setting to maintain muscle tone and prevent thromboembolism.
- Provide passive exercises if patient is unable.

Reducing anxiety

- Observe patient's verbal and nonverbal signs of anxiety.
- Encourage verbalization of patient's feelings and concerns.
- Be attentive, calm and confident to establish rapport.
- Provide information regarding the disease, treatment and prognosis to reduce anxiety.
- Plan nursing care in order to stay at patient's bedside for a longer period, when the patient is acutely ill to promote safety and reduce fear.

Understanding of the disease, therapeutic regimen and required lifestyle changes

- Assess patient's present knowledge related to the disease in order to determine his learning needs.
- Explain the disease process according to the understanding level of the patient.

- Explain the treatment regimen planned for him in order to promote compliance with treatment.
- Discuss required lifestyle changes to control the disease or prevent complications.
- Provide information on early signs of recurrence or complications and when to report to the physician.

PERITONITIS

Definition

Peritonitis is the inflammation of the peritoneum, the thin serous membrane that lines the abdominal cavity and covers the viscera.

Types

1. Primary peritonitis—It is the rare type of peritonitis, occurs when organism reaches the peritoneum through blood or lymph nodes.
2. Secondary peritonitis—It is more common type of peritonitis occurs when the organisms come into the peritoneum from gastrointestinal or biliary tract and in women reproductive tract.

Etiology

Primary

Cirrhosis with ascites. Fluid builds up in the abdomen, creating a prime environment for the growth of bacteria.

Secondary

Ruptured appendix, perforated gastric or duodenal ulcer, ruptured or gangrenous gallbladder, perforated stomach or intestine secondary to cancer or inflammatory bowel disease, bowel obstruction, diverticulitis rupture, acute pancreatitis, ischemic bowel disease, trauma, gunshot wound, knife wound, mesenteric thrombosis, peritoneal dialysis, postoperative.

Common bacteria are *E.coli, Klebsiella, Proteus, Pseudomonas.*

Risk Factors

The following factors may increase the risk for primary peritonitis

- Liver disease (cirrhosis)
- Fluid in the abdomen
- Weakened immune system
- Pelvic inflammatory disease.

Risk factors for secondary peritonitis include

- Appendicitis (inflammation of the appendix).
- Stomach ulcers.
- Torn or twisted intestine.
- Pancreatitis.
- Inflammatory bowel disease, such as Crohn's disease or ulcerative colitis.
- Injury caused by an operation.
- Peritoneal dialysis.
- Trauma.

Pathophysiology

- Leakage of contents from abdominal organs into the peritoneal cavity. The leaked contents along with bacteria irritate normally sterile peritoneum and produce an immediate chemical peritonitis. Within a few hours bacterial proliferation occurs and bacterial peritonitis develops.
- Resultant inflammatory response diverts extra blood to the inflamed area to combat the infection. The peritoneum becomes edematous. Exudation of fluid occurs.
- Fluid in the peritoneal cavity becomes turbid with increasing amounts of protein, white blood cells, cellular debris and blood. Adhesions develop to wall off the infection.

- Intestine initially reacts with hypermotility, soon paralytic ileus sets in resulting in accumulation of air and fluid in the bowel, raising pressure and increasing fluid secretion in the bowel.
- This results in depletion of circulating volume.

Clinical Manifestations

- Abdominal pain initially dull and diffused later becomes more intense, constant and localized near the area of inflammation. Movements even breathing increase pain so patient lies still and takes shallow respiration.
- Fever and chills.
- Anorexia, nausea, vomiting, thirst.
- Constipation, reduced urine output.
- Tenderness over the involved area.
- Rebound tenderness (pressing a hand on the abdomen elicits less pain than releasing the hand abruptly), muscular rigidity and spasm due to peritoneal irritation.
- Abdominal distention or ascites.
- Absent bowel sounds.
- Tachycardia, tachypnea, elevated body temperature, hypotension.
- Dry skin and mucous membrane, decreased skin turgor.

Complications

1. Hypovolemic shock
2. Sepsis
3. Intraabdominal abscess formation
4. Acute respiratory distress syndrome
5. Bowel obstruction due to adhesions.

Diagnostic Studies

1. Complete blood count reveals leukocytosis, elevated hematocrit level due to fluid shift.
2. Serum electrolyte studies show imbalance of sodium and potassium.
3. Peritoneal fluid study detects presence of blood, pus, bile, bacteria.
4. Abdominal X-ray may detect dilated loops of bowel if paralytic ileus; free air if perforation; air or fluid level if obstruction.
5. Ultrasound and CT scan show presence of ascites and abscess.
6. Peritoneoscopy allows direct examination of the peritoneum and collection of specimen for histopathological studies.

Management

Medical management

- Nil orally.
- Administration of fluid, intervenous colloid and electrolytes through IV infusion.
- Nasogastric suction.
- Analgesics.
- Antiemetics.
- Oxygen therapy.
- Intravenous administration of broad spectrum antibiotics in large doses.

Surgical management

- Surgery is performed to—
  - Locate the cause
  - Drain purulent fluid
  - Repair the damaged organ.

Surgery is performed when the patient is stable enough to withstand the stress of surgery.

Surgical procedures

1. Incision and drainage of the abscess once it is walled off.
2. Excision of appendix if ruptured appendix.
3. Resection and anastomosis of the intestine if intestinal perforation, etc.

Postoperative complications

1. Wound evisceration
2. Abscess formation
3. Acute respiratory distress syndrome
4. Sepsis, shock.

NURSING MANAGEMENT

Assessment

Subjective data

Pain in abdomen diffuse initially, later constant localized pain. Pain aggravates during movement, breathing. Anorexia, nausea, vomiting, low grade fever, thirst, history of peptic ulcer, previous surgery, peritoneal dialysis, injury, etc.

Objective data

Patient lies still, tachypnea, shallow respiration, tachycardia, low blood pressure, elevated body temperature, dry skin and mucous membrane, reduced skin turgor, oliguria, increasing abdominal distention, board-like abdomen, tenderness and rebound tenderness on palpation, abdominal guarding, absence of bowel sounds.

Possible findings

Leukocytosis, elevated hematocrit level, abnormal serum electrolyte level, presence of pus, blood, white blood cells, bacteria, etc. in perineal fluid, dilated loops of bowel or free air on X-ray, presence of ascites, abscess on CT scan.

Nursing Diagnoses

1. Acute pain related to the inflammation of the peritoneum and abdominal distension.
2. Fluid and electrolyte imbalance related to fluid shift in the peritoneal cavity secondary to the inflammatory process.
3. Anxiety related to the acute nature of the problem, uncertain cause and outcome of the condition.

GOALS

1. Relief of abdominal pain.
2. Maintenance of fluid and electrolyte balance.
3. Freedom from anxiety.

Nursing Intervention

Relief of abdominal pain

- Assess pain in abdomen, its location, severity, change in character and location of pain.
- Report physician any change in the character and location of pain.
- Administer analgesic medication as ordered. Evaluate the effectiveness of medication and report to the physician.
- Place patient in a side lying position with knees flexed to decrease tension on abdominal organs and increase comfort.
- Insert a nasogastric tube and attach it to suction to reduce pressure within the bowel and relieve pain.
- Administer broad spectrum antibiotic as ordered to control inflammation and thus reduce pain.
- Keep patient in a calm environment to promote rest.

Maintenance of fluid and electrolyte balance

- Assess vital signs, urine output, skin turgor, mucous membrane, bowel sounds, body weight, to monitor fluid and electrolyte status.
- Insert an IV line and administer fluids as ordered to replace vascular fluids lost to the peritoneal cavity.
- Administer antiemetics as ordered to prevent vomiting and thus further fluid and electrolyte losses.
- Keep patient in nil per oral status and

insert a nasogastric tube for suction to decrease distention and further leakage of bowel contents into the peritoneum
- Accurately record all intake and output.

Freedom from anxiety

- Assess verbal and nonverbal signs of anxiety, e.g. repeated questioning, apprehension.
- Carefully explain information given by the physician, in language understandable by the patient.
- Explain the treatment regimen planned for him.
- Explain preoperative care if surgery is planned for him.
- Answer all queries honestly.
- Project calm and confident approach to instill confidence in patient.
- Instruct patient to take deep breaths to promote relaxation.
- Administer sedative as ordered to reduce anxiety.

COLORECTAL CANCER

Definition

Colorectal cancer, also called colon cancer or large bowel cancer includes cancerous growths in the colon, rectum and appendix.

Incidence

It is the fourthmost common form of cancer in the United States.

It is the third leading cause of cancer-related death in the Western world.

Worldwide about 655,000 people die of colorectal cancer each year.

Etiology and Risk Factors

Major risk factors of colorectal cancer are

- Age: Risk of developing colon cancer increases with age. Most cases occur in the 60s and 70s.
- Heredity
  - Family history of colon cancer, especially in a close relative before the age of 55 or multiple relatives.
  - Familial adenomatous polyposis (FAP) carries a near 100% risk of developing colorectal cancer by the age of 40 if untreated.
  - Hereditary nonpolyposis colorectal cancer (HNPCC) or Lynch syndrome.
- Polyps of the colon, particularly adenomatous polyps, are a risk factor for colon cancer.
- History of cancer: Individuals who have previously been diagnosed and treated for colon cancer are at risk for developing colon cancer in the future. Women who have had cancer of the ovary, uterus, or breast are at higher risk of developing colorectal cancer.
- Lifestyle factors, e.g. obesity, physical inactivity, smoking, alcohol and large intake of red meat increase the risk of developing colorectal cancers and physical exercise, a diet high in fresh fruits, vegetables, grains and fish decrease the risk.
- Use of NSAIDs, e.g. aspirin and hormone replacement therapy in women seem to lower the risk.
- Low levels of selenium, folate and calcium may increase the risk.
- Constipation.
- Inflammatory bowel disease specially ulcerative colitis.
- People in industrialized countries and cities seem to have a higher risk.
- Drinking alcohol heavily may increase the risk.

Pathophysiology

- About 95% of colorectal cancers are adenocarcinoma and other rarer types include lymphoma and squamous cell carcinoma.

- Most of the adenocarcinomas begin as adenomatous polyp that arises from the mucosa lining the lumen of the colon and rectum.
- As it grows the cancer progresses from the tip of the polyp down through the body and stalk and becomes invasive and penetrates the muscularis mucosa.
- When muscularis mucosa are reached the cancer cells gain access to the regional lymph nodes and blood vessels resulting in distant metastasis. The common sites of metastasis are the regional lymph nodes, liver, lungs, peritoneum, bone and brain.
- Cancer also spreads directly to adjacent organs.
- Cancers on the right side (ascending colon and cecum) are bulky, tend to be exophytic, that is, the tumor grows outwards from one location in the bowel wall. This very rarely causes obstruction of feces, but necrosis and ulceration resulting in anemia.
- Left-sided tumors start as small button-like masses, tend to be circumferential (grows encircling the lumen), cause ulceration of the blood supply and usually obstruct the bowel.

Clinical Maifestations

The manifestations of colorectal cancer depend on the location of tumor in the bowel and whether metastasis has already taken place. Manifestations are described into local, constitutional and metastatic.

Local manifestations may appear if the tumor is located closer to the anus or on the left side of the colon

- A change in bowel habit (new-onset constipation or diarrhea in the absence of another cause).
- A feeling of incomplete defecation (rectal tenesmus).
- Reduction in diameter of stool; tenesmus and change in stool shape (ribbon shape) are both characteristic of rectal cancer.
- Rectal pain.
- Hematochezia, the passage of bright red blood in the stool or increased presence of mucus.
- Symptoms of bowel obstruction, e.g. constipation, abdominal pain, abdominal distention, and vomiting may appear when the tumor is large.
- Cancer may be felt by digital rectal examination.

Cancers on the right side of the colon may be

- Asymptomatic.
- Vague abdominal discomforts or cramps, colicky abdominal pain may be present in right-sided lesion.
- Melena, consisting of reddish brown stools may be present when the disease is located in the beginning of the large bowel.
- A feeling of mass in the abdomen.
- Palpable mass on examination.

Constitutional

- Anorexia, nausea, vomiting, weight loss, debility.
- Fatigue, palpitation, pallor due to iron deficiency anemia arising due to chronic bleeding.
- Unexplained fever.
- Paraneoplastic syndromes, e.g. deep vein thrombosis.

Complications

- Partial or complete bowel obstruction.
- Hemorrhage from extension of tumor into surrounding blood vessels.
- Perforation.
- Abscess formation.
- Peritonitis, sepsis.

Diagnostic Studies

1. Thorough personal and family history of previous cancer or colon cancer, familial polyposis, etc.
2. Physical examination reveals lump in abdomen and anemia.
3. Digital rectal examination may detect one-third of cancers of distal colon and rectum.
4. Stool test for occult blood.
5. Stool DNA test.
6. Barium X-ray studies may indicate filling defects or stricture.
7. Ultrasound, computed tomography or other imaging studies help establish tumor size and presence of metastasis.
8. Fiberoptic sigmoidoscopy or colonoscopy visualizes cancer and aids in obtaining tissue sample for biopsy.
9. Complete blood count detects iron deficiency anemia.
10. Carcinoembryonic antigen (CEA) may be elevated and the level monitored to determine the progress of the disease.

Staging

Staging of colorectal cancer is performed

- For diagnostic and research purposes
- To determine the best possible treatment options

The most common staging system is the TNM (tumors/nodes/metastasis) system, from the American Joint Committee on Cancer. This system describes:

Stage 0	$T_{is} N_0 M_0$
Stage I	$T_1 N_0 M_0$
	$T_2 N_0 M_0$
Stage IIA	$T_3 N_0 M_0$
Stage II B	$T_4 N_0 M_0$
Stage III A	$T_{1-2} N_1 M_0$
Stage III B	$T_{3-4} N_1 M_0$
Stage IV	any T any NM_1

T_{is}: Primary tumor is confined to mucosa or cancer insitu.

T_1: Primary tumor invades submucosa.

T_2: Primary tumor invades muscularis propria.

T_3: Primary tumor invades subserosa or beyond (without other organs involved).

T_4: Primary tumor invades adjacent organs or perforates the visceral peritoneum.

N_1: 1–3 regional lymph nodes are involved.

N_2: 4 or more regional lymph nodes are involved.

M_0: No distant metastasis is seen.

M_1: Distant metastasis is present.

Another method of staging colorectal cancer is Duke's classification system. Duke's classification is an older and less complicated staging system. It identifies the stages as:

A— Tumor confined to the intestinal wall.

B— Tumor invading through the intestinal wall.

C— With lymph node(s) involvement (this is further subdivided into C1 lymph node involvement where the apical node is not involved and C2 where the apical lymph node is involved).

D—With distant metastasis.

Presently the TNM system is the preferred and widely used classification system.

Medical Management

Surgical therapy

Primary treatment of colorectal cancer is surgery.

Goal is to resect the tumor with adequate margins of healthy tissue and anastomosis of the remaining bowel. Site of surgical resection depends on the site and stage of the disease:

1. Polypectomy during colonoscopy if colorectal cancer in situ.

2. Right hemicolectomy together with a segment of terminal ileum if the cancer is in cecum and ascending colon.
3. Left hemicolectomy if cancer in the descending colon.
4. Transeverse colectomy if the disease is in the middle of the transeverse colon.
5. Abdominal perineal resection with the formation of a permanent colostomy if the cancer is located within 5 cm of the anus. In this procedure the affected colon and entire rectum is excised and the anus is closed. Rectum removed through perineal incision and colon through abdominal incision.

Complications of surgery

1. Wound infection, dehiscence (bursting of wound) or hernia.
2. Anastomosis breakdown leading to abscess or fistula formation, and/or peritonitis.
3. Bleeding with or without hematoma formation.
4. Adhesions resulting in bowel obstruction.
5. Adjacent organ injury; most commonly to the small intestine, ureters, spleen, or bladder.
6. cardiorespiratory complications, such as myocardial infarction, pneumonia, arrhythmia, pulmonary embolism, etc.

Chemotherapy

- Purposes of using chemotherapy are
  - To reduce the likelihood of metastasis developing.
  - To shrink tumor size.
  - To slow tumor growth.
- Used as
  - Primary therapy when the tumor is nonresectable (for palliation).
  - Adjuvant therapy postoperatively when patient has positive lymph nodes.
  - Neoadjuvant therapy before surgery to shrink tumor.
- Commonly used drugs are
  - Combination of irinotecan, 5-FU and leucovorin, effective in metastatic cancer.
  - 5-FU, levamisole with or without leucovorin.
  - Leucovorin modulated 5-FU or capecitabine may be given to patients not suitable for triple therapy as alternative first line treatment.

Radiotherapy

Radiotherapy is not used routinely in colon cancer, as it could lead to radiation enteritis, and it is difficult to target specific portions of the colon.

It is more commonly used in rectal cancer, since the rectum does not move as much as the colon and is thus easier to target.

It is used as adjuvant therapy after surgery and chemotherapy or as a palliative measure for metastatic cancer.

Purposes of radiotherapy are to reduce tumor size and to provide symptomatic relief.

Implantation of radioactive isotopes of radium, cesium, cobalt, iridium may be used.

Biologic and targeted therapy

Three monoclonal antibodies namely cetuximab (erbitux), panitumumab (vectibix) and bevacizumab (avastin) may be used alone or with other chemotherapeutic drugs. These agents either target epithelial growth factor receptors or vascular endothelial growth factors that prevent angiogenesis.

NURSING MANAGEMENT

Assessment

Subjective data

Change in bowel habits, alternating constipation and diarrhea, urgency in defecation, rectal bleeding, mucus in stools, black tarry stools, decrease in stool caliber, increased flatus, tenesmus, rectal pain, abdominal or low back pain, weakness, fatigue, previous breast cancer or ovarian cancer, inflammatory bowel disease, familial polyposis, use of high calorie, high fat and low fiber diet.

Objective data

Pallor, cachexia, palpable abdominal mass, distention, palpable mass on digital rectal examination, positive sigmoidoscopy, colonoscopy, barium enema or CT scan. Positive biopsy.

Nursing Diagnoses

1. Imbalanced nutrition less than body requirement related to nausea and abdominal distention, anorexia as evidenced by loss of body weight, cachexia.
2. Risk for deficient fluid volume and electrolyte imbalance related to nausea, vomiting and low intake and reduced absorption as evidenced by dry mucous membrane, decreased skin turgor, concentrated urine, tachycardia, hypotension, feeble pulse.
3. Anxiety related to the diagnosis of cancer, impending surgery and prognosis as evidenced by apprehensive look, sleeplessness, frequent questioning about the disease, therapeutic intervention and prognosis.
4. Risk for ineffective therapeutic regimen management related to knowledge deficit concerning the diagnosis, the surgical procedure and self-care after discharge as evidenced by incorrect statement and repeated questioning.
5. Risk for impaired skin integrity related to the surgical incisions (abdominal, if laparotomy or abdominal and perineal both, if abdominal perineal resection), formation of a stoma and fecal contamination of peristomal skin.
6. Ineffective sexuality pattern related to abdominal perineal resection, presence of ostomy and changes in body image and self concept.
7. Risk for complications—Hemorrhage, bowel perforation, peritonitis, abscess and sepsis, thrombophlebitis.

Goals

1. Attainment of optimum level of nutrition and to prepare the patient physically for surgery.
2. Maintenance of fluid and electrolyte balance.
3. Reduction of anxiety.
4. Learning about the diagnosis, surgical procedure and self-care after discharge.
5. Maintenance of optimal tissue healing and protection of peristomal skin.
6. Adaptation and coping to the changed sexual ability and the impact of the situation on himself or herself.
7. Monitoring and managing potential complications.

Nursing Interventions

Attainment of optimum level of nutrition and to prepare the patient physically for surgery

- Provide diet high in calories, protein, and carbohydrate but low in roughage for several days before surgery.
  Provide full liquid diet 24 to 48 hours before surgery to reduce bulk.

- Encourage patient to take small amount at frequent interval to prevent nausea and vomiting.
- Monitor amount of food consumed. Monitor body weight.
- If unable to consume adequate amount orally, provide parenteral nutrition to replace the depleted nutrients, vitamins and minerals.
- Administer blood as ordered to correct severe anemia and to enhance postoperative wound healing.
- To minimize bacterial growth in the colon and to prevent wound infection administer antibiotics as ordered, e.g. neomycin, sulfonamides, cephalexin orally 12 to 48 hours before surgery, administer cathartics 12 to 24 hours before and give enemas or colonic irrigation the evening before and morning of surgery.

Maintenance of fluid and electrolyte balance

- Assess and monitor fluid intake and output and document correctly.
- Administer food and fluid in small amount and in frequent intervals to prevent vomiting.
- Administer antiemetic as ordered if nausea or vomiting.
- Observe for increasing abdominal distention, bowel sounds or pain and rigidity in the abdomen which indicate obstruction or perforation.
- When oral fluid is not tolerated insert a nasogastric tube and aspirate accumulated stomach contents to prevent abdominal distention.
- Administer intravenous fluid and electrolytes as ordered.
- Monitor serum electrolytes levels to prevent hypokalemia and hyponatremia that usually occur with gastrointestinal fluid loss.

Reduction of anxiety

- Assess patient's anxiety level and coping mechanism.
- Help patient to verbalize his concerns and doubts.
- Provide time to listen to patient and family who wishes to talk, cry or ask questions.
- Provide frank and honest explanations as much as possible.
- Provide intense emotional support if colostomy is expected.
- Teach deep breathing and relaxation technique to reduce anxiety.
- Arrange meeting with enterostomal therapist or counselor or religious guru as appropriate to reduce anxiety.
- Project a relaxed, professional and empathetic attitude to provide comfort to the patient.

Learning about the diagnosis, surgical procedure and self-care after discharge

- Assess patient's and significant family member's knowledge about the diagnosis, prognosis, surgical procedure and expected level of functioning after surgery.
- Reiterate information provided by the physician in simple language to facilitate understanding.
- Provide teaching to the patient and family member regarding preoperative preparation, e.g. cleansing and sterilization of the bowel (as explained above) and other routine preoperative care; the appearance of wound after surgery and care of wound; the technique of ostomy care if any (please see next section); pain control, dietary modification, etc.
- Refer patient to a enterostomal therapist if available.
- Introduce patient to a person who has recovered from similar illness or is managing successfully a colostomy.

Maintenance of optimal tissue healing and protection of peristomal skin

- Teach patient to splint abdominal incision during deep breathing and coughing to prevent tension on sutures.
- Assess abdominal dressing frequently during the first 24 hours after surgery for bleeding.
- Monitor pulse and respiration rate, body temperature and white blood cell counts to detect early signs of infection.
- Examine stoma (if colostomy is performed) for swelling, color (pink and red is healthy, dusky and blue indicates lack of blood supply), discharge, slight oozing (normal) and bleeding.
- Prevent fecal contamination of abdominal wound during colostomy care.
- Clean skin around stoma with mild soap and water, dry thoroughly, apply a skin barrier around the stoma before applying new colostomy pouch.
- If abdominal perineal resection, examine perineal wound for signs of hemorrhage, edema, erythema, drainage around the suture line. Examine drain or packing for amount and character of drainage (normal drainage is serosanguinous).
- Irrigate perineal wound with normal saline solution during changing of dressings.
- Change perineal wound dressings whenever soaked and keep dressings dry always.
- Once packing or drain is removed provide warm sitz baths 3 to 4 times a day for 10 to 20 minutes to increase circulation, provide comfort and help in tissue debridement.
- Teach patient to use cushion while sitting and not sit for prolonged period until healing is complete.
- Teach family member the procedure of sitz bath and management of wound.
- Refer patient to a community health nurse or a stoma clinic if possible for the management of perineal wound and stoma after discharge.

Adaptation and coping to the changed sexual ability and the impact of the situation on himself or herself

- Encourage patient to verbalize feelings and concerns about sexuality and sexual function.
- The physician or the health care members as appropriate should give time to answer patient's doubts.
- Refer patient to an enterostomal therapist or a sex counselor as appropriate or a person who is successfully managing similar situation to get practical and realistic solutions of the problems.

Monitoring and managing potential complications

- Observe for signs and symptoms of complications.
- Assess abdomen for increased and decreased bowel sounds, increasing abdominal girth, change in abdominal pain, which indicate obstruction.
- Monitor vital signs for increased temperature, pulse rate, respiratory rate, blood pressure and white blood cells count which may indicate an intraabdominal infectious process.
- Assess rectal bleeding if any and report immediately to the physician. Monitor hemoglobin and hematocrit levels and administer blood or blood components as ordered.
- Encourage patient to turn frequently from side to side every 2 hours, perform deep breathing and coughing and to get out of bed as early as possible to prevent pulmonary complications.
- Encourage patient to perform leg exercises before and after surgery to prevent thrombophlebitis which is a

common complication after abdominal perineal resection.
- Administer Injection heparin 5000 units subcutaneously every 12 hours as ordered.
- Encourage patient to wear thigh high antiembolic stockings which reduces chance of thromboembolisms.

APPENDICITIS

Definition

Appendicitis is a condition characterized by inflammation of the vermiform appendix.

Incidence

It occurs in 7% to 12% of the world's population.

The condition may occur at any age.

It is more common in 20 to 30 years of age and rare in children below 2 years of age.

Etiology

1. Obstruction of the appendix lumen by
    - Fecalith (hardened stool)
    - Foreign bodies
    - Trauma
    - Intestinal worms
    - Lymphadenitis
    - Appendicoliths (calcified deposits).
2. External occlusion of bowel by adhesions.

Pathophysiology

- Obstruction of appendix.
- Obstructed appendix fills with mucus and swells.
- Pressure rises within the lumen and wall of the appendix.
- Impaired venous drainage leads to occlusion of small blood vessels resulting in thrombosis and stasis of lymphatic drainage.
- Appendix becomes ischemic and then necrotic.
- Bacteria begin to leak out through the necrotic wall of the appendix.
- Pus forms within and around the appendix.
- If untreated, appendix eventually ruptures resulting in peritonitis.

Clinical Manifestations

- Abdominal pain, which starts in the epigastrium or periumbilical region, gradually becomes persistent and continuous. In a few hours pain localizes in McBurney's point (halfway between umbilicus and iliac crest) at right iliac fossa. Coughing increases pain.
- Anorexia and nausea.
- After vomiting pain starts.
- Low grade fever may or may not be there.
- Patient lies still, drawing the legs up, to relieve muscle tension. Straightening out the legs causes pain (Psoas sign).
- Tenderness and rebound tenderness (severe pain on suddenly releasing a deep pressure in lower abdomen).
- Muscle guarding (involuntary rigidity during palpation).
- Positive Rovsing's sign (palpation of left lower quadrant causes pain in right lower quadrant.
- Coated tongue.
- Bad breath.
- Leukocytosis.

Complications

1. Perforation leading to peritonitis, abscess formation.
2. Portal pylephlebitis (Septic thrombosis of the portal vein).

Diagnostic Studies

1. Complete blood count shows leukocytosis and elevated neutrophil count.
2. Urinalysis to rule out genitourinary problem and ectopic pregnancy in female.
3. Ultrasonography detects free fluid collection in the right iliac fossa.
4. Doppler sonography detects appendix without blood flow in color Doppler.
5. CT scan demonstrates lack of oral contrast in appendix and enlargement of appendix.

Medical Management

Uncomplicated appendicitis

- Nil orally.
- IV fluid is administered to correct dehydration.
- Antibiotic.
- Immediate appendectomy is recommended if appendicitis is diagnosed. The surgery may be done through laparotomy or laparoscopy. If the patient has not taken anything within 6 hours general anesthesia may be used. Otherwise spinal anesthesia may be used.

If perforation has already occurred:

- Surgery is delayed for at least 6 to 8 hours and antibiotic is continued.

Appendicular abscess:

- Surgical drainage of abscess is performed which is followed later by appendectomy.

Complications of Surgery

- Hernia of the incision
- Pneumonia
- Thrombophlebitis
- Bleeding
- Adhesions.

NURSING MANAGEMENT

Assessment

Subjective data

Abdominal pain starts in the epigastrium or periumbilical region, later localizes in the right iliac fossa, anorexia, nausea, vomiting, low grade fever, constipation.

Objective data

Patient lying still on bed with knees flexed, Psoas sign positive, tenderness, rebound tenderness, muscle guarding, positive Rovsing's sign, coated tongue, bad breath.

Possible findings

Leukocytosis, elevated neutrophil count, free fluid collection seen in Ultrasonography, lack of blood flow in appendix seen in Doppler sonography.

Nursing Diagnoses

1. Acute pain related to inflammation of appendix as evidenced by verbalization of patient's complain.
2. Risk for deficient fluid volume related to nausea and vomiting.
3. Risk for infection related to rupture of appendix.
4. Fear and anxiety due to sudden nature of the disease, and knowledge deficit regarding emergency surgery, preoperative preparation and prognosis.

Goals

1. Relief of pain.
2. Maintenance of fluid volume.
3. Prevention of infection or early detection of rupture leading to infection.
4. Relieving fear and anxiety by acquisition of knowledge regarding disease, treatment and prognosis.

Nursing Interventions

Relief of pain

- Assess pain by pain scale and assess change in character of pain which indicates perforation.
- Instruct patient to lie in comfortable position by drawing the legs up.
- Do not apply heat to the abdomen and do not give a laxative or an enema as these may lead to perforation.
- Reassure patient that prompt measure is being taken for surgery.
- Administer analgesic (morphine) only when surgeon evaluates the patient and prescribes it.
- Control postoperative pain by administering adequate analgesic as advised, change of positions and other comfort measures.

Maintenance of fluid volume

- Instruct patient not to take anything orally.
- Start intravenous fluids with electrolytes as ordered.
- Insert a nasogastric tube and aspirate stomach content if the patient is vomiting.
- Maintain intake and output chart.
- Postoperatively maintain intravenous fluids as ordered and start oral fluids gradually when bowel sounds are heard and patient passes flatus.

Prevention of infection or early detection of rupture leading to infection

- Monitor vital signs regularly for an increase in temperature and change in pulse and blood pressure that signify ruptured appendix.
- Assess pain closely. Generalized pain and rigid and board like abdomen indicate ruptured appendix.
- Administer antibiotic as ordered to reduce infection.
- Postoperatively monitor vital signs, respiratory status, intravenous infusion site, surgical wound and drain site for early evidence of infection.
- Provide wound care by changing dressings as per hospital protocol or whenever drainage dressings are wet.
- Assist patient in frequent change of positions and control pain adequately to facilitate deep breathing, coughing and early ambulation.

Relieving fear and anxiety by acquisition of knowledge regarding disease, treatment and prognosis

- Assess patient's knowledge regarding the disease, treatment regimen, complications and prognosis.
- Assess verbal and nonverbal signs of anxiety.
- Provide explanations of physician's statement to the patient.
- Provide explanations of procedures to be carried out and clarify patient's doubts if any.
- Explain preoperative preparation, e.g. nil orally, intravenous infusions, nasogastric tube insertion, skin preparation, etc. to the patient and obtain his cooperation.
- Teach patient deep breathing and coughing that has to be practiced postoperatively.
- Reassure patient that maximum possible care will be taken for his recovery and well-being.

HEMORRHOIDS

Definition

Hemorrhoids are perianal varicose veins.

Types

External

External hemorrhoids appear outside the anal sphincter. They are vericosities of the veins draining the territory of the inferior rectal arteries, which are branches of the internal pudendal artery.

Internal

Internal hemorrhoids appear inside the rectum above the internal sphincter. They are vericosities of veins draining the territory of branches of the superior rectal arteries.

Incidence

- It is common problem occurring in men and women of any age.
- Incidence is more in 20 to 50 years of age.
- Common during pregnancy and child birth.

Etiology and Risk Factors

Any condition that causes constipation, intraabdominal pressure or hemorrhoidal venous pressure raises the risk of hemorrhoids, e.g.

- Constipation with prolonged straining.
- Pregnancy.
- Prolonged sitting or standing.
- Obesity.
- Cirrhosis with portal hypertension.
- Congestive heart failure.
- Familial tendencies.
- Increased age.
- Absence of valves within hemorrhoidal veins.

Pathophysiology

- Hemorrhoid cushions are a part of normal human anatomy and only become a pathological disease when they experience abnormal changes. There are three cushions present in the normal anal canal.
- They are important for continence, contributing to at rest 15% to 20% of anal closure pressure and act to protect the anal sphincter muscles during the passage of stool.

Clinical Manifestations

External

- Anal itching.
- Analache or pain, specially while sitting.
- Pain during bowel movements when thrombosed hemorrhoids.
- One or more hard tender lumps near the anus.

Internal

- Bright red blood on toilet tissue, stool, or in the toilet bowl—hematochezia.
- Prolapse in severe cases or after prolonged sitting or standing and during defecation. Prolapse may return spontaneously or may be returned manually or may be present all the time.

Complications

- Bleeding
- Iron deficiency anemia
- Thrombosis
- Hemorrhoidal strangulation.

Diagnosis

External hemorrhoid is seen outside the anus. Internal hemorrhoid is diagnosed by history, digital rectal examination, proctoscopy, stool guaiac test which confirms presence of blood.

Medical Management

Conservative therapy in small uncomplicated external hemorrhoid

1. Dietary changes to prevent constipation, e.g. increasing fiber, oral fluids and stool softener viz. hydrophilic psyllium (metamucil).
2. To relieve pain
   - Cold pack in the initial stage followed by warm sitz baths 3 to 4 times a day.
   - Application of topical anesthetic or steroid preparation, e.g. lidocaine or preparation H helps relieve pain and itching.

Internal hemorrhoid may be treated by various nonsurgical procedures

1. Rubber band ligation—In this procedure proctoscope is inserted, hemorrhoid is identified and ligated with a rubber band. Rubber band around the hemorrhoid constricts the blood supply, tissue becomes necrotic, separates and sloughs off. No anesthetic is required. Aspirin or acetaminophen is given afterward to give relief from local discomfort.
2. Sclerotherapy involves the injection of a sclerosing agent, such as phenol, into the hemorrhoid. This causes the vein walls to collapse and the hemorrhoids to shrivel up.
3. A number of cautery methods have been shown to be effective for bleeding hemorrhoids. This can be done using electrocautery, infrared radiation, laser, or cryosurgery to produce local inflammation.

Surgical Management

Indication

- When medical management fails to stop excessive bleeding or pain.
- Large hemorrhoid
- Prolapse.

Surgical procedure

Hemorrhoidectomy: Hemorrhoidectomy is the surgical excision of the hemorrhoid. Surgical excision may be done by cautery, clamp or excision.

Nursing Management of Patient on Conservative Therapy

- Teach patient to avoid constipation by forming a regular bowel habit, consuming increased amount of fiber in diet and plenty of fluids to maintain adequate hydration.
- If constipation use bulk laxatives, stool softeners or mineral oils as advised by the physician.
- Monitor stool for consistency and blood.
- Teach patient not to sit on toilet for a long time.
- Teach to avoid prolonged standing or sitting.
- Encourage warm sitz baths for 15 minutes 3 to 4 times a day and apply medication.
- Report to physician if severe symptoms, e.g. pain, bleeding or prolapse.

Nursing Management of Patient after Hemorrhoidectomy

Relief of pain

- Assess pain by a pain scale.
- Administer analgesics, e.g. pethidine or any other suitable analgesics liberally as ordered as pain due to sphincter spasm is very severe initially. Later topical analgesic in the form of suppository may be administered to decrease pain.

- Monitor pain by pain scale to evaluate the effectiveness of medication and report to the physician
- Provide sitz baths 3 to 4 times a day for 10 to 15 minutes once the packing is removed, usually after 1 or 2 days to give comfort and reduce pain.
- Administer pain medication as ordered before the first bowel movement after operation to reduce pain and discomfort.

Promoting wound healing

- Assess wound for bleeding and evidence of infection.
- Change dressings with sterile technique whenever soaked. Apply a T binder or a sanitary napkin to hold the dressings in place.
- Remove pack which was inserted after operation to absorb drainage usually after 1 or 2 days.
- Provide sitz baths for comfort and keep the anal area clean at least 3 to 4 times a day and after each bowel movement.
- Encourage patient to wash the perianal area after defecation and pat it dry.
- Apply antibiotic ointment and analgesic ointment after each sitz bath.
- Maintain privacy during changing of dressings to avoid possible embarrassment.
- Teach patient to keep stool soft but formed to help prevent strictures.

VIRAL HEPATITIS

Definition

Viral hepatitis is a systemic, viral infection leading to inflammation and necrosis of liver cells and producing characteristic clinical manifestations.

Incidence

Occurs worldwide and is most common bloodborne infection.

Etiology

- Hepatitis A, hepatitis B, hepatitis C, hepatitis D, hepatitis E and hepatitis G.
- Herpes simplex.
- Cytomegalovirus.
- Epstein-Barr.
- Yellow fever adenoviruses.
- Rubella.
- Varicella.
- Retroviruses, etc. but hepatitis viruses is the most common cause of viral hepatitis. Characteristics of these viruses are shown in Table 7.1.

Table 7.1: Characteristics of different types of hepatitis viruses

Virus	Incubation period	Mode of transmission	Sign and Symptoms	Outcome
Hepatitis A (HAV)	15–50 days average 30days	Fecal-oral route, poor sanitation, poor personal hygiene, person to person contact,	Some may be asymptomatic. If symptoms, onset is acute. Preicteric phase-flu-like symptoms, headache, malaise, fever, fatigue,	Course of illness is usually mild with full recovery. Fatality rate is usually <1%. No

Contd...

Contd...

Virus	Incubation period	Mode of transmission	Sign and Symptoms	Outcome
		waterborne, foodborne, infected food handlers	anorexia. Icteric phase: dark-colored urine, jaundice of sclera and skin, tender liver.	carrier state or risk of chronic hepatitis, cirrhosis, or liver cancer
Hepatitis B (HBV)	6 weeks – 6 months	Percutaneous/ parenteral/ per mucosal exposure to blood or blood products. High risk sexual contact. Perinatal transmission from mothers to infants. Occupational hazards for health care workers	Many may be asymptomatic. Symptoms appear gradually in patients. Fever and respiratory symptoms are rare. May develop arthralgias, rash. Manifestations may be severe in nature	May be serious. Fatality rate may be 1%–10%. Carrier state possible. Increased risk of chronic hepatitis, cirrhosis and hepatic cancer
Hepatitis C (HCV)	15–160 days. Average- 50 days	Transfusion of blood and blood products, exposure to contaminated blood through equipments. Sex with infected partners	Manifestation is similar to HBV but less severe and anicteric	Frequently become chronic carrier and chronic liver disease. Increased risk of hepatic cancer
Hepatitis D (HDV)	21–140 days	Same as for HBV. Can cause infection only when HBV is present	Similar to HBV	Similar to HBV but greater likelihood of carrier state, chronic active hepatitis and cirrhosis
Hepatitis E (HEV)	15 – 65 days. Average 42 days	Fecal oral route. Contaminated water supply	Similar to HAV. Very serious outcome in pregnancy.	Same as HAV. Very severe in pregnancy
Hepatitis G (HGV)	Not known	Parenterally and sexual contact. Occurs with other infections, e.g. HBV, HCV and HIV	Asymptomatic	

Medical Surgical Nursing: Assessment and management of clinical problems Sharon L Lewis and others.

Pathophysiology

- In the liver pathophysiologic changes in various types of hepatitis is similar. Body's immune response to the virus results in pathologic changes in the hepatocytes.
- There is widespread inflammation of liver tissue with areas of necrosis. Resultant liver damage leads to impaired hepatic functions. Amount of damage depends upon the number of hepatocytes damage. Kupffer cells, the phagocytic cells present in liver sinusoids increase in number and size.
- Inflammation of the vascular and ductular tissues may interrupt circulation and bile flow (cholestasis).
- With time (3–4 months) liver cells can regenerate in an orderly manner and resume their normal appearance and function if no complications occur.

Systemic effects

- The antigen antibody complexes between the virus and its corresponding antibody produce circulating immune complex in the early phase of the disease.
- Activation of immune complex produces rash, fever, angioedema, arthritis, malaise, cryoglobulinemia (abnormal protein found in blood), glomerulonephritis and vasculitis.

Clinical Manifestations

Majority of infected persons show no clinical manifestations and the infection may not be detected in them. Manifestations if appear usually occur in two phases, e.g.

Acute phase

Anorexia, nausea, malaise, fatigue, occasional vomiting and discomfort in the right upper quadrant of the abdomen. Decreased sense of taste and smell, aversion to cigarette and strong odor, headache, low-grade fever, flulike respiratory tract infections, arthralgias, skin rashes, jaundice, pruritus, dark urine. Enlarged tender liver, splenomegally, bilirubinemia, light colored stools, weight loss.

Acute phase lasts for 1 to 4 months.

Chronic phase

Many patients with HBV infection and most of the patients with HCV infection become chronic. Many remain asymptomatic. Symptoms if appear consist of—malaise, fatigue, myalgia, arthralgias and hepatomegaly.

Complications

- Hepatitis A—Fulminant hepatic failure
No chronic stage
- Hepatitis B—Fulminant hepatic failure
Chronic hepatitis
Cirrhosis
Hepatocellular cancer
Aplastic anemia
- Hepatitis C—Liver failure
Chronic hepatitis
Cirrhosis
Hepatocellular cancer.

Diagnostic Studies

1. Stool test may reveal hepatitis A antigen.
2. Serum anti HAV IgM indicates acute infection.
3. Serum anti HAV IgG indicates previous infection or long time immunity or immunization.
4. Serum anti HBc persists during the acute phase, indicates continuing HBV infection in liver.
5. Serum anti HBs detected during con-

valescence, usually indicates recovery and development of immunity.
6. Serum anti-HBe signifies reduced infectivity.
7. Serum anti-HBxAg indicates ongoing replication.
8. Serum anti-HCV is the marker for acute and chronic infection with HCV.
9. Enzyme immunoassay used for initial screening for HCV.
10. Recombinant immunoblot assay (RIBA) is a more sensitive antibody test.
11. Serum anti-HDV is present in past or current infection with HDV.
12. HDV antigen will be present within a few days after infection.
13. Liver function test shows significant abnormalities.
    - AST and ALT—Increases in acute phase, decreases as jaundice disappears.
    - GGT—Increases
    - Alkaline phosphatase—Moderately increased.
    - Serum gamma globulin—Normal or increased.
    - Serum albumin—Normal or decreased.
    - Serum bilirubin—Increased to about 8 –5 mg/dL.
    - Urinary bilirubin—Increased
    - Urinary bilinogen—Increased
    - Prothrombin time—Prolonged.

Medical Management

1. Rest—Rest reduces metabolic demands on the liver and promotes liver cell regeneration. Since continuous rest has hazards patient should be advised to do alternating periods of activity and rest and to avoid fatigue.
2. Nutrition—A high carbohydrate, optimum protein and low fat diet helps to regenerate liver cells.
3. Maintain fluid balance.
4. Avoid alcohol and all alcoholic beverages.
5. Supplement vitamin B complex and vitamin K.

Supporting drug therapy

1. Antiemetics, e.g. dimenhydrinate (Dramamine), trimethobenzamide (Tigan)
2. Sedative, e.g. diphenhydramine (Benadryl) or chloral hydrate.

Drug therapy for chronic HBV

1. Alpha-interferon (Intron A) subcutaneous injection 3 times a week if short acting, once a week if long acting.
2. Nucleoside analogs, e.g. lamivudine (Epivir), adefovir (Hepsera), Entecavir (Baraclude) and Telvibudine (Tyzeka).
3. Hospitalization and intravenous fluid therapy when severe symptoms, e.g. nausea and vomiting.

Drug therapy for HCV

1. Combined antiviral agents, e.g. interferon (Intron A) and ribavirin (Rebetol) orally twice a week.
2. PEG Interferon injection once a week.

Prevention

- Hepatitis A—Hepatitis A vaccine for preexposure prophylaxis.
  Immunoglobulin may be given within 2 weeks of exposure.
  Combined hepatitis A and B vaccine 3 doses (0, 1 and 6 months) may be given in high risk individual, e.g. IV drug users, patient with chronic liver disease, persons requiring frequent blood

transfusions, homosexuals, etc.

- Hepatitis B— Hepatitis B vaccine, is given to children, adolescent and high-risk adults. 3 doses (0, 1 and 6 months after first). Postexposure prophylaxis (needle stick, mucous membrane contact or sexual contact)—A vaccine and hepatitis B immunoglobuline (HBIG) within 24 hours of exposure.
- Hepatitis C— No vaccine is available for HCV.
  Postexposure care—source as well as the exposed person should have anti HCV done. Follow-up testing after 4 to 6 months.
  If infected, no definite recommendation is suggested, but interferon monotherapy to treat acute HCV infection has shown some improvements.

NURSING MANAGEMENT

Assessment

Subjective data

Anorexia, nausea, change in taste (distaste for cigarettes and strong odor), vomiting, feeling of fullness in right upper quadrant, fatigue, arthralgias, myalgias, constipation or diarrhea, dark urine, light-colored stools, skin rashes, loss of body weight, history of blood transfusion, ingestion of contaminated food and water, exposure to contaminated needle, recent travel, unsanitary living conditions, exposure to hepatotoxic drugs, e.g. halothane, acetaminophen, methyldopa, use and misuse of drugs, use of IV drugs, alcohol consumption, blood and blood products transfusion, high risk sexual behavior, exposure as health care worker, resident of chronic care institution.

Objective data

Hepatomegaly, splenomegaly, lymphadenopathy, low grade fever, lethargy, rash, angioedema, jaundice, yellow sclera, multiple injection sites.

Possible findings

Abnormal liver function test results, increased serum bilirubin, decreased serum albumin, bilirubin in urine, anemia, prolonged prothrombin time, positive tests for hepatitis including anti HAV IgM, anti HBV IgM, abnormal liver scan, and positive liver biopsy.

Nursing Diagnoses

1. Imbalanced nutrition less than body requirements related to nausea, anorexia, bile stasis and altered absorption.
2. Anxiety related to uncertainty of the effects of hepatitis.
3. Activity intolerance related to fatigue and weakness.
4. Risk for disease transmission to others.
5. Ineffective therapeutic regimen management related to lack of knowledge of follow-up care and transmission of disease.

GOALS

1. Promotion of nutritional status
2. Reduction of anxiety
3. Promoting activity tolerance
4. Prevention of transmission to others
5. Effective therapeutic regimen management by acquisition of knowledge.

Nursing Intervention

Promotion of nutritional status

- Perform complete nutritional assessment to determine baseline nutritional status.
- Monitor amount of food and fluid ingested and calculate daily calorie intake to plan appropriate nursing interventions.
- Plan with dietitian regarding the type and amount of nutrients in order to provide appropriate diet.
- Provide multiple small meals, also provide candy, juice, sweetened tea and carbonated drinks to provide adequate calories.
- Provide optimum amount of protein and carbohydrate to allow recovery of injured liver cells without overfeeding. Patient with severe symptoms and at risk of hepatic encephalopathy should be given low-protein diet.
- Provide a nutritious breakfast as anorexia is less severe in the morning.
- Stimulate appetite of the patient by presenting food in attractive manner and by planning varieties of foods
- Provide oral care before each feed to stimulate appetite.
- Teach patient to avoid too hot and too cold food and fatty foods.
- Administer antiemetics as ordered if severe nausea.

Reduction of anxiety

- Encourage patient to express his feelings and concerns regarding the illness, the duration and cost of treatment, lifestyle modification, prevention of illness to others, etc.
- Explain the illness, mode of transmission to others in simple language as knowledge reduces anxiety.
- If required arrange psychosocial and financial counseling to the disturbed patient.

Promoting activity tolerance

- Provide strict bed rest when symptoms are severe.
- Initiate measures to prevent skin break down, respiratory and circulatory complications due to prolonged rest.
- Plan diversional activities, e.g. reading and music if bed rest causes anxiety and restlessness.
- Monitor symptoms of patient and liver function test results in order to plan activity schedule gradually.
- Assess patient's response to the rest and activity plan and modify it accordingly.
- Instruct patient to return to work only after physician permits.

Prevention of transmission to others

- Isolate the patient.
- Maintain strict enteric precaution if the patient is suffering from a possible A and C hepatitis virus infection.
- Maintain universal precaution for others, e.g. B, C and D infection.

Effective therapeutic regimen management by acquisition of knowledge

- Explain pathophysiology of the disease in simple manner.
- Describe rationale behind management/treatment so that appropriate follow-up care will be planned and carried out.
- Describe lifestyle changes that may be required to prevent future complications and relapse, e.g. avoidance of alcohol, over the counter drugs, promote rest and optimum nutrition.
- Instruct patient on which signs and symptoms (bleeding gums, blood in stools, delayed prothrombin time, elevated serum aminotransferase level, and sign and symptoms of hepatic encephalopathy) to report to health care

provider to enable prompt intervention.

- Instruct patient to come for follow-up visits regularly and remain under medical supervision for at least one year.
- Teach patient on measures to prevent reinfection or possible spread of infection to others:
  - For hepatitis A and E, hand washing, environmental sanitation, proper disposal of excreta, drinking safe water, maintaining proper food hygiene and immunization of family members.
  - For hepatitis B, C and D, hand washing, maintaining proper personal hygiene, avoiding sharing personal items, e.g. safety razor, needles, etc. Avoiding sexual activity until there is no chance of disease transmission, avoiding blood donation and protecting family members by immunization.

CIRRHOSIS

Definition

Cirrhosis is a chronic progressive disease of the liver characterized by degeneration and destruction of normal liver tissue and replacement with fibrous tissue and regenerative nodules leading to loss of normal liver function.

Incidence

It is the 10th leading cause of death in USA Men are doubly affected than women. Highest incidence occurs in age 40 to 60 years

Mortality is high in men and nonwhites.

Types

1. Alcoholic (Laënnec's) cirrhosis or portal or nutritional cirrhosis is associated with alcohol abuse.
2. Postnecrotic cirrhosis is a complication of viral, toxic or idiopathic hepatitis. Broad bands of fibrous tissue form in the liver. Worldwide occurrence is common. Common in women.
3. Biliary cirrhosis is associated with chronic biliary obstruction and infection. There is diffuse fibrosis of the liver with jaundice as the manifestation.
4. Cardiac cirrhosis—It is the result of long-standing severe right heart failure associated with cor pulmonale, constrictive pericarditis and tricuspid insufficiency.

Etiology

- Alcohol consumption, alcohol ingestion in presence of improper nutrition, family history of alcoholism and a hpersensitivity to alcohol is the most important cause of alcoholic cirrhosis.
- Exposure to certain chemicals, e.g. carbon tetrachloride, chlorinated napthalene, arsenic or phosphorus also may cause cirrhosis.
- Viral hepatitis specially hepatitis C and B cause postnecrotic cirrhosis.
- Intrahepatic cholestasis or obstruction of bile ducts causes biliary cirrhosis.
- Use of certain drugs, e.g. acetaminophen, methotrexate or isoniazide.
- Hepatic congestion from severe right sided heart failure, constrictive pericarditis, valvular disease, cor pulmonale, etc. cause cardiac cirrhosis.
- Alfa$_1$ antitrypsin deficiency.
- Wilson's disease.
- Hemochromatosis.

Pathophysiology

- Repeated exposure to noxious substances over a considerable period of time causes necrosis and destruction of liver cells.

- Destroyed liver cells are gradually replaced by fibrous tissue and ultimately amount of fibrous tissue exceeds the amount of normal tissue impairing normal liver function.
- Areas of residual normal tissue and regenerated liver tissue projects in between constricted fibrous tissue giving a characteristic hobnail appearance and altering the architecture of liver.
- Altered structure of the liver impairs flow of blood and lymph in the liver sinusoids and obstructs flow of bile in the bile duct channels.
- Obstruction in bile flow gives rise to jaundice.
- Impaired blood and lymph flow in the liver sinusoids ultimately raises pressure in the portal vein resulting in portal hypertension. Increased pressure in the portal vein gives rise to retrograde increase in pressure and subsequent enlargement of the esophageal, umbilical and superior rectus veins forming bleeding varices.
- Increased portacaval pressure causes hydrostatic and osmotic shift of fluid and protein in the peritoneal space to develop ascites.

Clinical Manifestations

Early

Onset is gradual.

- Gastrointestinal disturbances, e.g. anorexia, nausea, vomiting and change in bowel habits (diarrhea/constipation) due to altered metabolic function of the liver.
- Abdominal pain—Dull heavy feeling in the epigastrium, due to swelling and stretching of liver capsule.
- Fever, lassitude, slight weight loss, enlargement of liver and spleen. Palpable firm, lumpy (nodular), enlarged liver.

Late manifestations

- Jaundice.
- Peripheral edema, ascites.
- Skin lesions (due to increase in circulating estrogen as liver is unable to metabolize steroid hormones), e.g.
  - Spider angiomas (telangiectasia or spider nevi). Small dilated blood vessels with a bright red center point and spider like branches) occur on the nose, cheeks, upper trunk, neck and shoulders.
  - Palmer erythema (a red area that blanches with pressure) appears on the palms of the hands.
- Nail changes, e.g. clubbing, Terry's nails (proximal two-thirds of the nail plate appears white with distal one-third red due to hypoalbuminemia).
- Hematologic disorders, e.g. thrombocytopenia, leukopenia, anemia due to splenomegaly and coagulation disorder manifested as epistaxis, purpura, petechiae, easy bruising, gingival bleeding, or heavy menstrual bleeding as liver is unable to produce prothrombin and other clotting factors.
- Endocrine disturbances due to impaired metabolism and inactivation of adrenocortical hormones, estrogen, and testosterone manifested as gynecomastia, loss of axillary and pubic hairs, testicular atrophy, impotence with loss of libido in men; amenorrhea in younger women and vaginal bleeding in older women.
- Peripheral neuropathies may be due to dietary deficiency of thiamine, folic acid and cobalamin.
- Bone pain due to hypertrophic osteoarthropathy (chronic proliferative periostitis of the long bones).
- Hard and shrunken liver.

Complications

Portal hypertension and esophageal and gastric varices

- Structural changes in the liver due to cirrhosis cause compression and destruction of the portal and hepatic veins and sinusoids impairing normal flow of blood through the portal system.
- Stasis of blood raises pressure in the portal veins leading to portal hypertension.
- To reduce this high pressure and to improve lymphatic flow collateral channels develop. Collateral channels commonly develop in the lower esophagus, the anterior abdominal wall, the parietal peritoneum and the rectum.
- Collateral channels when united with systemic circulation develop vericosities and ultimately form esophageal and gastric varices, hemorrhoids and caput medusa (ring of varices around the umbilicus).
- These collateral vessels are very fragile as they lack in elastic tissue. Distended vessels unable to withstand high pressure bleed easily when irritated or ulcerated.
- Factors causing irritation and ulceration are alcohol ingestion, swallowing of poorly chewed course foods, regurgitation from stomach and increased abdominal pressure due to nausea, vomiting, straining at defecation, heavy lifting, coughing and sneezing.

Sign and symptoms

- Increased venous pressure in the portal circulation, splenomegaly, large collateral veins on the abdomen, ascites, systemic hypertension and bleeding esophageal and gastric varices. Bleeding from the varices may be slight oozing or massive hemorrhage. Patient may have melena or hematemesis.

Peripheral edema and ascites

- Cirrhotic liver is unable to produce adequate albumin. Decreased coloidal oncotic pressure due to hypoalbuminemia and increased portacaval pressure from portal hypertension results in peripheral edema which appears around the ankle and sacral area.
- Ascites is the accumulation of serous fluid in the peritoneal cavity and is a common manifestation of cirrhosis. Increased pressure in the liver causes protein to move out of capillaries in the lymph space. Lymphatic system is unable to carry extra protein and water. Protein and water then leak through the liver capsule to the peritoneal cavity. Oncotic pressure of the protein draws additional water in the peritoneal cavity and forms ascites.
- Ascites may also occur due to hypoalbuminemia and resultant decreased colloidal oncotic presure causing fluid shift in the peritoneal cavity.
- Another reason for ascites formation is increased level of aldosterone as damaged liver is unable to metabolize aldosterone. Hyperaldosteronism causes increased sodium reabsorption by renal tubule. Increased sodium reabsorption and increased synthesis of antidiuretic hormone results in additional water retention and ascites.

Sign and symptoms

- Abdominal distention with weight gain, umbilicus reverted in severe ascites, abdominal striae with distended abdominal wall veins.
- Signs of dehydration, e.g. dry tongue and skin, sunken eyeballs, muscle weakness, oliguria, hypokalemia.
- Risk for spontaneous bacterial peritonitis due to disturbance in immune mechanisms.

Hepatic encephalopathy

- Hepatic encephalopathy is the terminal complication of any liver disease and occurs when ammonia enters systemic circulation. Diseased liver is unable to convert ammonia (end product of protein metabolism) into urea to be excreted by the kidneys. Large amount of ammonia enters the systemic circulation, crosses blood-brain barrier and produces neurologic toxic manifestations.

Signs and symptoms

- Changes in neurologic and mental responsiveness, which ranges from sleep disturbances to lethargy to deep coma. Condition may appear gradually or abruptly.
- Early stage—Euphoria, depression, apathy, irritability, confusion, yawning, drowsiness, insomnia and agitation.
- Late stage—Slow or slurred speech, emotional lability, impaired judgment, hiccups, slow and deep respirations, hyperactive reflexes, positive Babinski's reflex.
- Terminal stage—Impending coma characterized by disorientation to time, place and person.
- Characteristic signs include asterixis/flapping tremors (bilateral asynchronous flapping of outstretched, dorsiflexed hands), difficulty in writing from left to right, apraxia (inability to construct simple figures), hyperventilation, hyperthermia, grimacing and grasping reflexes, fetor hepaticus (musty, sweet odor of the patient's breath).

Hepatorenal syndrome

- Hepatorenal syndrome is a fatal complication of cirrhosis and is characterized by functional renal failure with azotemia, oliguria, and severe ascites.
- Liver decompensation and portal hypertension results in splanchnic and systemic vasodilation and decreased arterial blood volume. Decreased arterial volume gives rise to renal vasoconstriction ultimately developing renal failure.
- The condition frequently occurs after diuretic therapy, gastrointestinal bleeding or paracentesis.

Diagnostic Studies

1. Liver function test reveals abnormal liver function. Liver enzymes, aminotransferases (AST, ALT and GGT) initially elevated due to their release from damaged liver cells but in late stage AST and ALT levels may be normal. Serum protein level and albumin level decreased, serum globulin level elevated, serum bilirubin level increased, cholesterol level decreased, and prothrombin time prolonged, alkaline phosphatase level elevated.
2. Liver ultrasound reveals irregular nodular liver.
3. CT, MRI and radioisotope liver scan provide information about liver size and hepatic blood flow and obstruction.
4. Liver biopsy confirms the diagnosis by identifying hepatocellular changes and altered lobular structure.
5. Stool test for occult blood.
6. Complete blood count reveals anemia, leukopenia and thrombocytopenia.
7. Serum electrolytes studies show hypernatremia and hypokalemia.
8. Endoscopy and upper gastrointestinal barium swallows detect esophageal and gastric varices.

Medical Management

There is no specific treatment for cirrhosis. Liver damage cannot be reversed, but treatment could stop or delay further progression and reduce complications. Treatment is usually symptomatic.

- Rest and good diet is believed to promote regeneration of liver cells by reducing the metabolic demand on the liver.
- Diet therapy for patient with cirrhosis without any complications is high in calories (3000 kcal/day with high carbohydrate, high protein content and moderate to low fat. Protein may be restricted for a very short time in patients with hepatic encephalopathy.
- Treatment for underlying cause, e.g. abstaining from alcohol (alcoholic cirrhosis), interferon for viral hepatitis, and corticosteroids for autoimmune hepatitis.
- Prevent further liver damage by avoiding use of alcohol, paracetamol, IV drug abuse and other hepatotoxic drugs.
- Provide symptomatic treatment, e.g. antacids and H_2 antagonists to decrease gastric distress and minimize the chance of gastrointestinal bleeding, antibiotics for infection, laxatives to prevent constipation, etc.
- Prevention or management of specific problems or complications, e.g.
  - Ascites is treated by salt restriction (initially 2 gm/day, in severe ascites it may be 250–500 mg/day), diuretics (e.g. spironolactone an aldosterone antagonist and potassium sparing diuretic or triamterene in combination with furosemide or thiazide drug) and fluid removal by paracentesis. Paracentesis is indicated in patients experiencing respiratory distress and abdominal pain due to severe ascites.
  - Esophageal and gastric varices.
    - Prevention of bleeding and hemorrhage—avoid ingesting alcohol, aspirin or irritating food; control cough; administration of beta blockers, e.g. Inderal.
    - Management of bleeding varices–a combination of drug therapy and endoscopic therapy is more effective.
    - Drug therapy—vasopressin (constriction of splanchnic arterial bed), beta blockers, e.g. Inderal (reduces portal venous pressure), and nitroglycerine (vasodilator and reduces side effect of vasopressin) is given to control variceal bleeding.
    - Endoscopic therapy—it comprises of sclerotherapy, ligation of varices and shunt therapy.
    - Balloon tamponade may be used if initial endoscopic therapy fails. Balloon tamponade controls bleeding by mechanical compression of the varices. Sengstaken-Blakemore tube is used for this purpose.
    - Supportive therapy during an acute hemorrhage include administration of fresh frozen plasma, packed RBCs, vitamin K, histamine (H_2) receptors blockers, e.g. cimetidine, ranitidine, proton pump inhibitors, e.g. pantoprazole, lactulose and neomycin to prevent hepatic encephalopathy from break down of blood and release ammonia in the intestine.
  - Hepatic encephalopathy is managed by administration of lactulose orally or as retention enema or via a nasogastric tube (lactulose decreases pH and thus discourages growth of bacteria in acidic medium, traps ammonia in the colon and expels ammonia by its laxative action), antibiotics, e.g. neomycin sulfate or metronidazole, vancomycin to reduce the bacterial flora in the intestine.

NURSING MANAGEMENT

Nursing Assessment

Subjective data

Weakness, fatigue, anorexia, weight loss, dyspepsia, nausea and vomiting, dull upper quadrant or epigastric pain, change in bowel habits, light colored or black stools, flatulence, decreased urinary output, dark urine, dry, yellow skin, pruritus, numbness and tingling of extremities, gum bleeding, bruising, amenorrhea or heavy menstrual bleeding, impotence. Chronic alcoholism, previous viral, toxic or idiopathic hepatitis, previous biliary obstruction and infection, right heart failure, frequent use of aspirin, acetaminophen.

Objective data

Elevated body temperature, shallow respirations, wasting of extremities, cachexia, yellow sclera, jaundice, petechiae, ecchymoses, spider angiomas, palmer erythema, alopecia, loss of axillary and pubic hair, gynecomastia, testicular atrophy, peripheral edema, abdominal distention, ascites, distended abdominal wall veins, palpable liver and spleen, hematemesis, black tarry stools, hemorrhoids, foul breath, altered mental status, asterixis, apraxia.

Possible findings

Anemia, leukopenia, thrombocytopenia, abnormal liver function studies, hypoalbuminemia, hypokalemia, elevated ammonia and bilirubin levels, abnormal abdominal ultrasound and liver scan, positive liver biopsy.

Nursing Diagnoses

1. Activity intolerance related to fatigue, general debility, muscle weakness, abdominal pain and discomfort secondary to ascites as evidenced by patients verbal complain about weakness, tachypnea and tachycardia on exertion.
2. Imbalanced nutrition less than body requirements related to dyspepsia, abdominal distention, reduced gastric motility, impaired ability of the liver to store and use nutrients and loss of nutrients from vomiting as evidenced by lack of interest in food, inability to consume adequate amount of food, cachexia and debility.
3. Impaired skin integrity related to edema, ascites and jaundice as evidenced by complaints of itching, evidence of scratch mark on skin and shiny taut skin on edematous areas and areas of skin breakdown.
4. Risk for injury and bleeding related to altered clotting mechanisms as evidenced by complaints of gum bleeding, epistaxis and delayed prothrombin time.
5. Potential complications, e.g. fluid volume excess, bleeding and hemorrhage, hepatic encephalopathy.

GOALS

1. Increased activity tolerance.
2. Improvement of nutritional status.
3. Maintaining skin integrity.
4. Reducing risk of injury.
5. Monitoring and managing potential complications: Fluid volume excess, bleeding and hemorrhage, encephalopathy.

Nursing Intervention

Increased activity tolerance

- Assess patient's ability to carry out any activity.
- Provide enough rest in bed in the acute stage to decrease the metabolic demands on the liver and increase its circulation.

- Maintain a calm and quiet environment and restrict unwanted visitors to promote rest.
- Initiate measures to prevent pressure sores, respiratory and circulatory disturbances, e.g. pneumonia and thrombophlebitis.
- As nutritional status improves plan and schedule activities gradually.
- Teach patient to rest frequently and avoid fatigue.

Improvement of nutritional status

- Provide a high calorie and high protein diet. Protein should be of high biologic value. Include vegetable protein, e.g. soya protein to decrease the chance of developing encephalopathy. Protein content should be 1 to 1.5 gm/kg of body weight. Daily calorie intake should range from 2500–3000. Vitamin B complex and minerals, e.g. potassium should be supplemented. Diet should also be low in fat and sodium (200 mg–1000 mg/day). Protein content may be restricted for a short time if the patient develops encephalopathy. Patient with severe malnutrition should be administered multivitamin supplementation through parenteral route.
- Encourage 5 to 6 frequent small meals instead of 3 large meals to ensure adequate intake by an anorexic patient. Consider patient's preferences as much as possible because a low fat and salt diet can be unpalatable.
- Monitor recorded intake for nutritional content and calories to evaluate nutritional status. Monitor patient's body weight, intake output daily.
- Provide oral care before and after each meal to provide comfort unless it stimulates nausea.
- Teach patient to use nonpharmacologic methods, e.g. distraction, music, relaxation etc. to manage nausea and to reduce use of antiemetics as they are not well metabolized by the damaged liver.

Maintaining skin integrity

- Inspect patient's skin in each shift as edematous and jaundiced skin is very susceptible to breakdown.
- Turn the very sick patient every 2 hourly to prevent pressure sores in dependent areas.
- Provide support to edematous areas with pillows under arms and legs and provide scrotal support in male patients to prevent scrotal edema.
- Trim nails short of patient to minimize injury during scratching.
- Apply calamine lotion or any other soothing lotion to minimize itching.
- Avoid alkaline or irritating soap and use of adhesive tape to prevent further irritation and injury to the skin.

Reducing risk of injury

- Provide a padded railed cot to the patient who is restless and agitated to prevent fall from bed.
- Orient the patient frequently to the time and place and explain all procedures to minimize confusion and agitation. Assist patient to get out of bed to prevent injury.
- Assess patient regularly for any injury, internal or external bleeding as the patient has impaired clotting mechanisms.
- Instruct patient to use a soft tooth brush, electric razor instead of a safety razor to prevent bleeding.
- Avoid intramuscular injections and apply pressure to venipuncture sites to prevent bleeding.
- Ensure that all hepatotoxic medications are eliminated from the treatment

regimen or their dose reduced if at all necessary. Avoid use of sedatives.
- Ensure that patient refrains from alcohol totally.
- Institute meticulous hand washing and other infection control protocol strictly as the patient is at risk of developing infection.

Monitoring and managing potential complications

Fluid volume excess
- Monitor body weight; fluid intake and output; peripheral edema, abdominal girth to evaluate the effectiveness of treatment.
- Administer prescribed diuretics to promote diuresis and prevent fluid retention.
- Provide prescribed diet low sodium, fluid restricted and no added salt to prevent fluid retention.
- Monitor laboratory values of hematocrit, BUN, protein, sodium and potassium levels in order to determine fluid and electrolyte status and effectiveness of treatment.

Bleeding and hemorrhage
- Monitor patient for bleeding by assessing epistaxis, gum bleeding, hematuria, heavy menstrual bleeding, bleeding with stool, melena, purpura, petechiae, easy bruising and bleeding from any orifices as diseased liver is unable to synthesize adequate clotting factors.
- Monitor circulatory status, e.g. pulse rate and volume, blood pressure, heart rate and rhythm, capillary refill for early detection of internal bleeding and development of hypovolemic shock.
- Gently handle patient to minimize trauma and tissue injury. Avoid injury from sharp objects.
- Use smallest gauge needle to give injections and apply firm and prolonged pressure over the injection and venipuncture site to prevent bleeding.
- Teach patient to avoid straining at stool, coughing and vigorous blowing of nose to reduce chance of bleeding at these sites.
- Administer stool softener and modify diet to prevent constipation.
- Monitor laboratory values of hematocrit, hemoglobin and prothrombin time to detect early signs of active hemorrhage, anemia and impending clotting problems.

Hepatic encephalopathy
- Assess patients for general behavior, orientation to time place and person, speech, hand writing, tremors of hand, etc. for development of encephalopathy.
- Limit physical activity to reduce production of ammonia as a by-product of metabolism.
- Administer lactulose as ordered or enemas to promote bowel elimination and decrease absorption of ammonia from the bowel.
- Restrict protein intake (controversial) to reduce ammonia production in the bowel.
- Monitor laboratory values for blood pH, electrolyte levels and ammonia level to determine the effectiveness of therapy.

ACUTE PANCREATITIS

Definition

Acute pancreatitis is the sudden inflammation of the pancreas.

Incidence

- It can occur at any age
- Most common in middle-aged people
- Both sexes are equally affected
- Mortality rate is more in aged people.

Classification

1. Mild acute pancreatitis is characterized by:
   - Edema and inflammation confined to the pancreas.
   - Presence of minimal dysfunction.
   - Return to normal function usually occurs within 6 months.
2. Severe acute pancreatitis:
   - Usually occurs in 20% of patients with a mortality of about 20%.
   - Characterized by widespread inflammation giving rise to complete enzymatic digestion of the gland and hemorrhagic necrosis.

Etiology and Risk Factors

1. Alcohol abuse.
2. Gallstone.
3. Hyperlipidemia secondary to estrogen administration, nephritis or hereditary.
4. Hypercalcemia from hyperparathyroidism.
5. Familial susceptibility.
6. Trauma, e.g. blunt abdominal trauma, intraoperative manipulation or ERCP.
7. Pancreatic ischemia during episodes of shock, cardiopulmonary bypass, visceral embolism or vasculitis.
8. Drugs, e.g. steroids, sulfonamides, azathioprine, NSAIDs, thiazide diuretics, oral contraceptives.
9. Viral infections, e.g. mumps, HIV, cytomegalovirus, Epstein-Barr virus.
10. Autoimmune disease, e.g. polyarteritis nodosa, systemic lupus erythematosis.
11. Idiopathic.
12. Other general causes, e.g. duodenal ulcer, obesity, pancreatic duct obstruction, carcinoma, scorpion venom, snake venom, peritoneal dialysis.

Pathology

- The etiologic factors, e.g. reflux of bile from the duodenum into the pancreatic duct or pancreatic duct obstruction leads to activation of lipolytic and proteolytic pancreatic enzymes. Normally, these enzymes are activated in the intestine by action of intestinal enterokinase.
- Activated proteolytic and lipolytic pancreatic enzymes damage pancreatic tissue by autodigestion. This damage or injury leads to inflammation of the pancreas.
- Inflammation of the pancreas brings about further tissue damage and enzyme activation leading to destruction of the pancreatic parenchyma.

Clinical Manifestations

- Abdominal pain
  - Located in the left upper quadrant or in the midepigastrium, radiating to back, chest, flanks and lower abdomen.
  - Onset is sudden.
  - Is severe, deep, piercing and continuous or steady.
  - Occurs after a heavy meal when the patient is lying (gallstone) or 12 to 48 hours after heavy drinking.
  - Nausea and vomiting may be present
  - Antacids do not relieve pain.
  - It may be accompanied by flushing, cyanosis, dyspnea.
  - patient assumes different positions in an attempt to relieve pain.
- Nausea, vomiting, diarrhea and loss of appetite.
- Patient appears acutely ill, anxious and distressed.
- Fever, chills, tachycardia, leukocytosis.
- Hypotension, cyanosis, cold clammy skin due to shock, mental confusion and agitation may also be there.
- Abdominal tenderness, muscle guarding, abdominal distention, reduced or absent bowel sounds.

- Ecchymosis around the umbilicus (Cullen's sign) or in the flank (Turner's sign).
- Respiratory distress, dyspnea, tachypnea, crackles in lungs, hypoxia, abnormal blood gas values.
- Myocardial depression, hypocalcemia, hyperglycemia, disseminated intravascular coagulation (DIC).

Complications

Local

- Pancreatic pseudocyst
- Pancreatic abscess
- Progression to chronic pancreatitis.

Systemic

- Acute respiratory distress syndrome.
- Pleural effusion, atelectasis, pneumonia, pulmonary emboli.
- Hypocalcemia, hyperglycemia and insulin dependent diabetes mellitus.
- Multiple organ dysfunction syndrome.
- Disseminated intravascular coagulation.

Diagnostic Studies

1. Serum amylase level elevated at early stage of the disease, and remains elevated for 24 to 72 hours.
2. Serum lipase level rises 4 to 8 hours of onset of symptoms and normalizes within 7 to 14 days of treatment.
3. Blood glucose reveals hyperglycemia.
4. Serum calcium shows hypocalcemia.
5. Serum triglyceride level reveals hyperlipidemia.
6. Abdominal ultrasound, X-ray, CT scan with contrast, may reveal the cause of pancreatitis and the status of pancreas, e.g. fluid collection, rupture, pseudocyst or abscess formation.
7. Endoscopic retrograde cholangiopancreatography, endoscopic ultrasound, magnetic resonance cholangio-pancreatography visualize pancreas and the cause of pancreatitis due to tiny gallstones etc. when the patient is allergic to contrast medium.

Medical Management

Objectives

- To relieve pain.
- Prevention or correction of hypovolemia and shock.
- Reduction of pancreatic secretion by maintaining pancreatic rest.
- Maintaining fluid, electrolyte and nutritional balance.
- Prevention or treatment of infection.
- Removal of the precipitating cause.

Pain control

- Inj. morphine or pethidine is the drug of choice.
- Antispasmodic, e.g. nitroglycerine or Papaverine may also be given to relax smooth muscle and relieve pain.

Maintain volume status, electrolyte balance

- Patient is admitted in a high dependency unit or an intensive care unit according to the severity of the condition.
- Intravenous infusion, lactated Ringer's solution and/or plasma or plasma expander is administered.
- Monitor CVP, urine output, electrolyte status.
- Vasoactive agent, e.g. dopamine if continued hypotension.
- Replace blood, if hemorrhagic pancreatitis.
- Oxygen therapy or ventilatory support if required.

Maintain pancreatic rest

- Nil orally until the patient is relieved of pain and bowel sounds are heard to reduce pancreatic secretion and thus provide pancreatic rest.
- Nasogastric suction.
- Drugs
  - Antispasmodic, e.g. propanthelin bromide (Pro-Banthine) decreases pancreatic outflow.
  - Carbonic anhydrase inhibitor, e.g. acetazolamide (Diamox) reduces volume and bicarbonate concentration of pancreatic secretion.
  - Antacids and H_2 receptor antagonists neutralize and reduce hydrochloric acid secretion (hydrochloric acid stimulates pancreatic secretion).

Nutritional support

- Nil orally in the initial period.
- Parenteral nutrition is continued till patient is relieved of pain and bowel sounds are heard.
- Postpyloric enteral feeding, via a jejunal feeding tube is started in moderate to severe pancreatitis. Enteral feeding is more physiological, prevents intestinal mucosal atrophy and is free from side effects of total parenteral nutrition. Postpyloric feeding also reduces pyloric secretion and risk of aspiration.
- Total parenteral nutrition is continued in severe pancreatitis.
- Small frequent diet with high carbohydrate content is given when oral feeds are allowed.
- Fat soluble vitamins are supplemented.

Prevention or treatment of infection

- Close observation to detect early signs of infection.
- Antibiotics at the earliest signs of infection.

Surgical Management

Indication

1. Uncertainty of diagnosis.
2. Treatment of secondary pancreatic infection, necrosis or abscess.
3. Correction of associated biliary tract disease.
4. Progressive clinical deterioration despite optimal supportive care.

Operative procedures

1. Drainage of a pancreatic abscess is performed by laparotomy with sump drainage.
2. Subtotal pancreatectomy is performed by resecting a major portion of the necrosed head of pancreas and attaching the remaining head of pancreas to the duodenum.
3. Whipple's procedure (pancreaticoduodenectomy) is performed, when pancreatitis is confined to the head of the pancreas. The procedure involves removal of distal third of the stomach, the duodenum, common bile duct, gallbladder and head of the pancreas.
4. Exploratory laparotomy to eliminate conditions, e.g. perforated organ or acute mesenteric ischemia.
5. Cholecystectomy and intraoperative cholangiography is performed in gallstone associated pancreatitis.

NURSING MANAGEMENT

Assessment

Subjective data

Severe midepigastric or left upper quadrant pain radiating to the back, aggravated by food and alcohol intake and not relieved by vomiting or antacids, etc. Nausea, vomiting, anorexia, fever, dyspnea, weakness. History of alcohol abuse, biliary tract stone, blunt trauma in abdomen, peptic ulcer, use of NSAIDs, thiazide diuretics, ERCP or any other surgery in the abdomen.

Objective data

Restlessness, anxious look, elevated body temperature, tachypnea, hypotension, tachycardia, abdominal distention, tenderness and muscle guarding, decreased bowel sounds, basilar crackles.

Possible findings

Elevated serum amylase and lipase level, leukocytosis, hyperglycemia, elevated urine amylase level after 48 to 72 hours of onset of symptoms, hypocalcemia, abnormal ultrasound and CT scan of pancreas, abnormal ERCP.

Nursing Diagnoses

1. Acute pain related to inflammation of the pancreas and surrounding tissue, biliary tract obstruction and pancreatic duct obstruction, as evidenced by verbalization of pain, restlessness, diaphoresis, changes in vital signs.
2. Risk for fluid volume deficit and electrolyte imbalance related to nausea, vomiting, nasogastric suction, nil per oral status or restricted oral intake, diaphoresis and fever.
3. Imbalanced nutrition: less than body requirement related to anorexia, nausea, vomiting, nil per oral status and nasogastric suctioning as evidenced by weight loss, weakness and fatigue.
4. Ineffective breathing pattern related to abdominal distention or ascites, pain or respiratory complications as evidenced by tachypnea, shallow respiration and basilar crackles.
5. Ineffective therapeutic regimen management related to lack of knowledge about the disease, its cause, therapeutic procedures and nursing measures.
6. Anxiety related to change in health status, hospitalization, fear of recurrence of pain and alcohol abuse withdrawal.

Goals

1. Relief of pain.
2. Maintenance of optimum fluid volume and electrolyte levels.
3. Maintenance of adequate nutritional status.
4. Maintenance of effective breathing pattern.
5. Imparting knowledge about the disease, its cause and care to be taken to prevent relapse.
6. Reduction of anxiety.

Nursing Intervention

Relief of pain

- Assess pain, its severity, location, aggravating and relieving factors if any.
- Administer prescribed analgesics and evaluate its effectiveness.
- Keep patient on nil per oral status and suction gastric contents through nasogastric suctioning to decrease pancreatic secretion, abdominal distention and thus reduce pain and promote comfort.
- Provide different comfort measures, e.g. positioning the patient on side lying and knee chest position with a pillow pressed against the abdomen or sitting up on bed with trunk flexed, back rubs, massage and quiet environment to promote comfort.
- Teach patient different nonpharmacologic measures of pain control, e.g. guided imagery, relaxation, hot and cold application, etc. and use them before, during or after any painful experience.

Maintenance of optimum fluid volume and electrolytes levels

- Monitor vital signs for changes in pulse and blood pressure due to fluid volume changes and respiration for acid base imbalances. If necessary hemodynamic monitoring should be done to detect changes in fluid and electrolyte status.
- Monitor cardiac rhythm for early signs of electrolyte imbalances.
- Administer antiemetics as prescribed to prevent vomiting and thus reduce loss of fluid volume.
- Administer fluids as ordered, e.g. lactated Ringer's solution, normal saline or blood products as indicated to maintain fluid volume.
- Monitor the patient's response to fluid administration and blood products by monitoring intake and output and assessing for edema, adventitious breath sounds, skin turgor and mucous membrane moistness.
- Monitor for neuromuscular signs of hypocalcemia, e.g. tetany, muscle spasm or cramping.
- Monitor for central nervous system changes due to hypocalcemia, e.g. personality changes, irritability, depression, anxiety, etc.

Maintenance of adequate nutritional status

- Provide parenteral nutrition and administer carbohydrate, lipids and amino acids to prevent negative nitrogen balance as long as patient is fasting.
- Assess the overall nutritional status of the patient by checking daily body weight, tissue integrity, and the presence of adequate body fat and muscle mass.
- Administer enteral feeding in small amounts via a postpyloric tube (Freka tube) as the condition of the patient improves (bowel sounds are heard and abdominal pain is absent) to reduce pancreatic stimulation and prevent intestinal mucosal atrophy.
- When oral feeds are allowed begin intake slowly by liquids only and then progress to normal diet gradually.
- Provide high caloric low fat diet to avoid overstimulation of the pancreas.

Maintenance of effective breathing pattern

- Assess patient's respiration for rate and effort, decreased lung sounds, rale or rhonchi and cyanosis.
- Administer humidified oxygen by oxygen mask. Provide ventilatory support to a very serious patient if indicated.
- Position patient in semifowler or side lying position in order to ease breathing.
- Turn patient every 2 hours, encourage deep breathing and coughing, provide incentive spirometry for optimum expansion of lungs.
- Administer analgesics to relieve abdominal pain, which may ease breathing. Schedule breathing exercises half an hour after administration of analgesics in order to get maximum cooperation from the patient.

Imparting knowledge about the disease, its cause, therapeutic procedures and nursing measures

- Assess patient's knowledge about the disease to establish baseline for teaching.
- Describe pathophysiological changes of the disease.
- Teach patient life style changes, e.g. abstinence from alcohol, avoiding tea coffee, heavy meals and spicy foods, low fat, high protein diabetic diet, regular exercise, prevention or control of

hypoglycemia, self-monitoring of blood glucose level, insulin administration, etc. that may be required to prevent future complications and/or control the disease process.
- Teach patient signs and symptoms of recurrence, e.g. steatorrhea, severe back or epigastric pain, persistent gastritis, nausea, vomiting, weight loss, elevated body temperature and evidence of hyperglycemia and instruct patient to report to the physician about these symptoms if any immediately.

Reduction of anxiety

- Assess patient's level of anxiety.
- Reassure patient that anxiety for unknown is normal.
- Explain procedure that may cause anxiety for the patient.
- Repeat explanations and instructions in simple language and direct manner as sick patient in distress has very short attention span. If possible allow significant family member to remain with patient whenever appropriate.
- Spend time with the patient to make him understand that alcohol is causing the problem.
- Recommend and encourage patient to join any supportive services available for the problem of alcoholism.

CHRONIC PANCREATITIS

Definition

Chronic pancreatitis is a long-standing inflammation of the pancreas that alters its normal structure and functions.

It can present as episodes of acute inflammation in a previously injured pancreas, or as chronic damage with persistent pain or malabsorption.

Etiology and Risk Factors

- Chronic alcoholism—It is the most common (60–80%) cause in developed countries.
- Malnutrition (lack of protein) and associated dietary factors (very high or very low fat content) are the usual cause in developing countries.
- Hereditary—Genetic factor predisposes a person to the direct toxic effects of alcohol on the pancreas even with minor drinking habits.
- Cystic fibrosis—Almost all patients with cystic fibrosis have established chronic pancreatitis, usually from birth. Cystic fibrosis gene mutations have also been identified in patients with chronic pancreatitis but in whom there were no other evidence of cystic fibrosis.
- Biliary disease such as inflammation of the sphincter of Oddi associated with cholelithiasis with resultant obstruction of pancreatic duct can cause chronic pancreatitis.
- Cancer of the ampulla of Vater, duodenum or pancreas and congenital anomalies of the pancreatic duct giving rise to obstruction may also cause chronic pancreatitis.
- Trauma of the pancreas.
- Idiopathic.
- Untreated hyperparathyroidism giving rise to hypercalcemia.

Pathophysiology

- Chronic pancreatitis may or may not follow acute pancreatitis.
- In patients with history of attacks of pancreatitis, inflammatory changes results in scarring and calcification of the pancreas causing mechanical obstruction of the pancreatic and common bile ducts and duodenum.
- Chronic alcoholism causes hyper secretion of protein in pancreatic

secretion. These proteins form plugs and calculi within the pancreatic ducts resulting into obstruction of the pancreatic ducts.
- Inflammatory changes leading scarring and calcification is irreversible and results in atrophy (loss of normal pancreatic cells) and fibrosis, which affect both endocrine and exocrine functions of the gland.
- Pseudocysts and abscesses may also develop.

Clinical Manifestations

- Abdominal pain
  - Patient has recurrent attacks of abdominal pain. Interval between pains decreases gradually and becomes constant and persistent.
  - In some patients pain diminishes as pancreas becomes fibrotic.
  - Patient describes pain as heavy, gnawing feeling or as burning and cramp like.
  - Pain increases with high protein and high fat foods and is not relieved with food intake or with antacids.
- Steatorrhea due to malabsorption of fats in food.
- Severe nausea.
- Weight loss due to malabsorption or due to reduced intake of food due to abdominal pain.
- Constipation.
- Mild jaundice with dark urine.
- Abdominal tenderness.
- Diabetes mellitus.

Complications

1. Bile duct or duodenal obstruction
2. Pancreatic pseudocyst formation
3. Pancreatic ascites
4. Pleural effusion
5. Pancreatic cancer
6. Splenic vein thrombosis
7. Pseudoaneurysms.

Diagnostic Studies

1. Serum amylase and lipase may be elevated slightly.
2. Serum bilirubin and alkaline phosphatase may be elevated.
3. ESR may be elevated.
4. Secretin stimulation test: IV secretin is administered and gastric-duodenal secretions are collected with double lumen tube. Reduced volume of secretions and bicarbonate concentrations indicate chronic pancreatitis.
5. Fecal pancreatic elastase measurement in stools detects less than 200 μg/gm and indicates pancreatic insufficiency.
6. CT scan, ultrasound, endoscopic ultrasound, MRI, ERCP and MRCP visualizes pancreatic structural changes such as, calcification, ductal dilation, pancreatic enlargement, pseudocyst formation.
7. Plain X-ray abdomen may detect pancreatic calcification.

Medical Management

Goals of management

1. Prevention and management of acute attacks:
   - Treatment of acute attacks in a patient with chronic pancreatitis is same as that of acute pancreatitis.
   - Abstinence from alcohol by a patient with alcohol related pancreatitis or endoscopy to remove pancreatic duct stone in a selected patient may prevent further attacks.
2. Relieving pain and discomfort:
   - Nonopioid analgesics in large and frequent doses are given to control pain. Opioid analgesic may also be required in later stage of disease.
   - Quitting alcohol
   - Bland diet low in fat and high in carbohydrate prevents pain.

3. Management of pancreatic exocrine and endocrine insufficiency:
   - Oral antidiabetic drugs or insulin and dietary regulations are employed for the treatment of diabetes.
   - Pancreatic enzyme replacement such as pancreatin, pancrelipase in enteric coated form is used to treat steatorrhea and malabsorption.
   - Bile salts are given to help absorb fat soluble vitamins.

Surgical Therapy

Goals

1. To correct the primary tract disease (ampullar procedure).
2. To relieve ductal obstruction (ductal drainage procedure).
3. Alleviate pain (ablative procedure).
4. Alleviate pain (denervation procedure).

- **Surgical procedures**:

1. Pancreaticojejunostomy—Side-to-side anastomosis or joining of the pancreatic duct to the jejunum, allows drainage of the pancreatic secretion in to the jejunum.
2. Pancreaticoduodenectomy(Whipple resection) is carried out when the head of the pancreas is mostly involved.

NURSING MANAGEMENT

Provide Support

- Explain patient the chronic nature of the disease as simply as possible.
- Explain the therapeutic regimen planned for him.
- Reassure patient that adherence to therapeutic regimen will help to alleviate symptoms and promote health.

Teach Self-care

- Teach patient the measures to prevent further attacks such as:
  - Adherence to a diet that is bland, low in fat and high in carbohydrates.
  - Avoid foods which cause pain and discomfort.
  - Stop taking alcohol.
  - Taking the prescribed medications such as pancreatic enzymes, bile salts, insulin or oral antidiabetic drugs regularly.
  - To observe stool for steatorrhea to determine the effect of pancreatic enzymes.
- Teach patient who has developed diabetes, blood glucose level monitoring and self administration of insulin.

CHOLECYSTITIS

Definition

Cholecystitis refers to inflammation of the gallbladder wall. It may be acute or chronic.

Incidence

Increased incidence is found in

- Obese persons
- Persons with sedentary lifestyle
- People of certain ethnic groups, e.g. Chinese, Jewish, Italians.

Etiology and Risk Factors

In majority of patients (90%) cholecystitis is caused by cholelithiasis (the presence of gallstones) or biliary sludge blocking the cystic duct directly.

Less commonly, in certain situations the gallbladder may become inflamed and infected in the absence of cholelithiasis and is known as acalculous cholecystitis, e.g.

- Tissue damage after extensive burns, trauma or recent surgery.
- Prolonged immobility, prolonged fasting and prolonged parenteral nutrition.
- Bacterial infection with *E. coli*, salmonella, or streptococci reaching gallbladder through vascular and lymphatic routes.
- Bacterial sepsis, systemic arteritis.
- Diabetes mellitus, very old and debilitated person.

Pathophysiology

- Obstruction of the cystic duct causes distention of the gallbladder impairing venous and lymphatic drainage.
- Localized inflammation possibly chemically induced initially causes mucosal damage, ultimately spreading to entire gallbladder wall.
- The inflamed gallbladder wall is edematous and thickened, areas of ischemia leading to gangrene or necrosis or rupture may be present. Functioning of gallbladder decreases when large areas of tissue are necrosed.
- Eventually bacterial infection sets in filling the gallbladder with pus.
- Inflammation often spreads to its outer covering, thus irritating surrounding structures such as the diaphragm and bowel.
- The patient might also develop a chronic, low-level inflammation which leads to a chronic cholecystitis, where the gallbladder is fibrotic and calcified.

Clinical Manifestations

- Pain in the right upper quadrant or epigastric region of the abdomen and may radiate to right shoulder and scapula. Pain starts suddenly, increases steadily and reaches peak within 30 minutes.
- Pain is accompanied by nausea, vomiting, restlessness and diaphoresis.
- Fever.
- Tenderness on right hypochondrial region.
- Abdominal rigidity, which increases on inspiration (Murphy's sign).
- Elevated body temperature.
- Leukocytosis (may be absent in elderly patients).
- Jaundice in a few patients.

Clinical manifestations in chronic cholecystitis

- History of fat intolerance, dyspepsia, heart burn and flatulence.
- Recurrent attacks of vague abdominal pain, often at night following a heavy meal.
- Nausea, belching and diarrhea.

Complications

1. Gangrenous cholecystitis
2. Subphrenic abscess
3. Pancreatitis
4. Cholangitis
5. Biliary cirrhosis
6. Fistulas, rupture of gallbladder
7. Bile peritonitis, gallstone ileus.

Diagnostic Studies

1. Ultrasonography reveals gallstones, focal tenderness over the gallbladder, thickening of the gallbladder wall and distention of the gallbladder lumen.
2. Endoscopic retrograde cholangiopancreatography (ERCP) visualizes gallbladder, cystic duct, common bile duct. Culture of bile collected during ERCP detects offending organisms.
3. X-ray abdomen and chest may show radiopaque gallstones, excludes lower lobe pneumonia.
4. Blood tests detect leukocytosis, elevated CRP (C-reactive protein), elevated serum alkaline phosphatase, elevated

serum bilirubin level if obstruction of the bile duct.

Management

Conservative therapy

- Hospitalization and bed rest.
- Morphine with atropine or any other suitable analgesics to relieve pain.
- Antibiotics, e.g. piperacillin-tazobactum (Zocin), ampicillin-sulbactum (Unasyn), cephalosporin (ceftriaxone), ciprofloxacin, metronidazole to control infection.
- Intravenous infusions to maintain fluid and electrolyte balance. Nasogastric suction if vomiting is persistent to prevent fluid and electrolyte imbalance and provide comfort.

Surgical therapy

Urgent surgery within 5 days of onset of symptoms is carried out in acute cholecystitis. Patient with chronic cholecystitis is usually advised for elective surgery.

Surgical procedure

1. Cholecystectomy—Surgical removal of the gallbladder may be accomplished by:
   - Open surgery, which is done when complications have developed or the patient has had previous surgery to the area making laparoscopic procedure technically difficult, or facilities to perform laparoscopic surgery is not available.
   - Laparoscopic procedure usually have less morbidity and a shorter recovery stay in hospital.
2. Percutaneous cholecystostomy —Insertion of a percutaneous drainage catheter into the gallbladder to drain pus. This procedure is done when patient is with severe inflammation or shock and not fit to undergo cholecystectomy.

Complications of cholecystectomy

1. Bile leak (biloma).
2. Bile duct injury.
3. Abscess.
4. Wound infection.
5. Bleeding (liver surface and cystic artery are most common sites).
6. Hernia.
7. Organ injury (intestine and liver are at highest risk, especially if the gallbladder has become adherent/scarred to other organs due to inflammation.
8. Deep vein thrombosis/pulmonary embolism.
9. Fatty acid and fat-soluble vitamin malabsorption.

Nursing Management

Please see Nursing Management of Patients with Cholelithiasis page 244 to 248.

CHOLELITHIASIS (GALLSTONES)

Definition

Presence of stones in the gallbladder is termed as cholelithiasis.

If stones migrate to the ducts of biliary tract it, is termed as choledocholithiasis.

Etiology

Actual cause of gallstones formation is unknown. Gallstones are believed to be formed by precipitation of bile constituents, e.g. cholesterol, bile salts and calcium. Precipitation of these constituents from liquid bile may occur probably due to the following reasons:

1. Change in composition of bile—Studies have shown that in patients

with cholelithiasis bile secreted by liver is supersaturated with cholesterol. Precipitation of cholesterol occurs when bile is supersaturated with cholesterol.
2. Stasis of bile in gallbladder may change the composition of bile, supersaturates bile with cholesterol and precipitates, some bile constituents. Conditions in which gallbladder stasis occurs are immobility, inflammatory or obstructive conditions of biliary system, pregnancy, total parenteral nutrition, low fat, weight reduction diet, spinal cord injury, etc.
3. Infection may predispose stone formation. Infection leading to tissue injury may alter the composition of bile. Inflammatory debris forms a point of origin around which bile constituents precipitate to form a stone.
4. Genetics and demography may influence stone formation as indicated by the higher prevalence rate of cholelithiasis in Native Americans, Northern Europeans and South Americans than in Asians.

Risk Factors

- Overweight.
- Age near or above 40.
- Female.
- Premenopausal.
- Person consuming low fiber, high cholesterol diets and diets high in starchy foods.
- Hemolytic anemias, cirrhosis and biliary tract infections may increase risk of pigment stones.

Pathophysiology

- Gallstones vary in size from as small as a grain of sand to as large as a golf ball.
- The gallbladder may contain a single large stone or numerous small stones.
- Pseudoliths or sludge (thick secretions) may be present in gallbladder either alone or in combination with gallstones.
- Composition of gallstones is affected by age, diet and ethnicity. On the basis of their compositions gallstones are mainly 3 types, e.g. (1) cholesterol stones composed of 80% cholesterol, (2) pigment stones small, dark stones composed of bilirubin and calcium found in bile, (3) mixed stones composed of cholesterol, calcium carbonate, palmitate phosphate, bilirubin, and other bile pigments.
- Most of the stones form in the gallbladder but they may also form in the common duct or hepatic ducts of the liver.
- Stones may remain in the gallbladder or migrate downward to the cystic duct or common bile duct.
- Stones may cause pain as they travel downward through the ducts or they may lodge in the ducts and produce obstruction.
- If the cystic duct is blocked, bile may flow directly from the liver to the duodenum but stasis of bile in the gallbladder gives rise to cholecystitis.

Clinical Manifestations

Manifestations vary from asymptomatic to severe symptoms.

Majority of gallstones are asymptomatic even for years and are called silent stones. Symptomatic gallstones present either as biliary colic or as cholecystitis.

The patient with biliary colic experiences:

- Pain—Intense pain in the upper right side of the abdomen:
  - It may radiate to right shoulder or between the shoulder blades.
  - Pain occurs 3 to 6 hours after a heavy meal or when the patient lies down
  - Pain steadily increases and lasts for

approximately 30 minutes to several hours.
  - Often accompanied by nausea and vomiting, tachycardia, diaphoresis and prostration. Occasionally, self induced vomiting may alleviate the manifestations.
  - When pain subsides there is residual tenderness in the right upper quadrant.
- Intolerance of fatty foods.
- Abdominal bloating, belching, flatulence, gas and indigestion.
- A positive Murphy's sign is a common finding on physical examination.

Complications

- Acute cholecystitis
- Chronic cholecystitis
- Cholangitis
- Biliary cirrhosis
- Carcinoma
- Mucocele of the gallbladder.

Diagnostic Studies

1. X-ray abdomen may reveal calcified gallstones in 15 to 20% of patients.
2. Abdominal ultrasonography detects stones in 95% of patients.
3. Oral cholecystography detects gallbladder stones and also the functioning of the gallbladder when ultrasonography is not available.
4. Percutaneous transhepatic cholangiography may be used to diagnose obstructive jaundice and to locate stones within the bile duct.
5. Endoscopic retrograde catheterization of the gallbladder (ERCG) detects gallstones especially common bile duct stones.
6. Radionuclide scanning after administration of technetium (99mTc) confirms acute cholecystitis.
7. CT and MRI detect gallstones or their complications.

Management

Nonsurgical management

1. Medical dissolution of gallstones—Oral administration of bile acid ursodeoxycholic acid or ursodiol may dissolve radiolucent gallstones not larger than 15 mm in diameter. Patient who is not obese, with no symptoms or mild symptoms may be treated by this method. The drug may have to be continued upto 2 years. The stones can recur once the drug is stopped.
2. Direct contact dissolution therapy—Cholesterol solvents, e.g. methyl tertiary terbutyl ether (MTBE) may be instilled in the gallbladder via percutaneous catheter or catheter placed at ERCP. MTBE can dissolve cholesterol stones within hours.
3. Extracorporeal shock wave lithotripsy—A biliary lithotripsor uses high energy shock waves to break stones. After the stones are broken up the small fragments pass through the common bile duct and into the small intestine. The procedure may be used in patients with normal gallbladder functions, mild symptoms and having small stones.
4. Supportive treatment—Same as cholecystitis.
   - If obstruction, replacement of fat soluble vitamins; administration of bile salts to facilitate digestion and vitamin absorption; and low fat diet.

Surgical management

Indication

- To relieve persistent symptoms
- To remove the cause of biliary colic
- To treat acute cholecystitis.

Surgical procedures

1. Cholecystectomy—Removal of gallbladder through right subcostal incision.
2. Cholecystostomy—Incision into gallbladder usually for removal of stone.
3. Choledocholithotomy – Incision into common bile duct for removal of stones.
4. Laparoscopic cholecystectomy—The most popular and commonly performed procedure is laparoscopic cholecystectomy. The gallbladder is removed through four small puncture holes made in the abdomen for camera and instruments. Due to minimal injury recovery is faster and postoperative stay in hospital is short.

NURSING MANAGEMENT OF PATIENTS UNDERGOING MEDICAL TREATMENT

Assessment

Subjective data

Moderate to severe pain in right upper quadrant of the abdomen, pain may radiate to back and scapula, nausea, vomiting, fever with chills (cholecystitis), indigestion, dyspepsia, anorexia, fat intolerance, flatulence, clay colored stools, steatorrhea, dark urine, pruritus, positive family history, obesity, sedentary lifestyle, history of weight reducing diet, prolonged fasting, use of estrogen or oral contraceptives, multiparity, pregnancy, previous abdominal surgery, previous infection, cancer.

Objective data

Right upper quadrant tenderness, palpable gallbladder, abdominal guarding, distention, splinting during respiration, diaphoresis, restlessness, elevated temperature, tachypnea, tachycardia, jaundice, yellow sclera, scratch mark on skin.

Possible findings

Abnormal gallbladder ultrasound, visible stone in abdominal X-ray, leukocytosis, elevated levels of serum liver enzymes, serum bilirubin, urinary bilirubin, etc.

Nursing Diagnoses

1. Acute pain or chronic pain related to biliary spasms as evidenced by patient's complaining of pain, restlessness, diaphoresis, tachycardia, and tachypnea.
2. Risk for fluid volume deficit and electrolyte imbalance related to vomiting and nasogastric suction.
3. Risk for injury and infection related to nonsurgical intervention for stone removal, e.g. ERCP, direct contact dissolution therapy or extracorporeal shock wave lithotripsy.
4. Inadequate health maintenance due to knowledge deficit.

GOALS

1. Relief of pain.
2. Maintenance of fluid and electrolyte balance.
3. Preventing injury and infection following interventions for stone removal.
4. Maintaining self-care.

Nursing Intervention

Relief of pain

- Assess pain with a pain scale.
- Administer prescribed analgesics as required by the patient before pain becomes more severe.
- Monitor effect of pain medication and determine amount of pain medication needed by the patient.
- Institute nursing comfort measure, e.g. providing a clean bed, quiet, environment, comfortable positioning, back rub and oral care to promote

rest and thus enhance the effects of analgesics.

Maintenance of fluid and electrolytes balance

- Introduce a nasogastric tube for suction if the patient is persistently vomiting.
- Assess patient for signs of dehydration, e.g. dry mucous membranes poor skin turgor and oliguria and document findings.
- Administer intravenous fluids as ordered to maintain hydration and electrolyte balance.
- Monitor intake output, serum electrolytes levels and report abnormalities to the physician.

Preventing injury and infection following interventions for stone removal

- Explain procedure to be undertaken for stone removal and after effect of the procedure beforehand in order to reduce stress and anxiety in patient.
- Monitor for return of gag reflex after ERCP.
- Provide bed rest for several hours and allow fluids and food only after gag reflex returns to prevent aspiration.
- Administer antibiotics as ordered to prevent infection from bacteria entering into the common bile duct from intestine.
- Assess vital signs, abdominal pain for early signs of infection, perforation or bleeding.
- If extracorporeal shock wave lithotripsy is used monitor for ecchymosis over the area of entry of shock waves and hematuria.

Maintaining self-care

- Teach patient the suggested therapeutic regimen in detail and ways to prevent recurrence.
- If oral dissolution therapy is advised educate the patient that the drug may have to be taken regularly over a period of time. Help the patient to adopt some measure to remember to take the medicine daily.
- Explain patient the side effect of medication, e.g. slight elevation in serum cholesterol and liver function test values and diarrhea.
- Teach patient to consume a low fat diet.
- Teach patient the signs and symptoms of development of complications, e.g. obstruction of the ducts and infection manifested as jaundice; pruritus; clay colored stools; dark, foamy urine; steatorrhea, fever and leukocytosis.
- Teach patient to report promptly if another attack occurs. Help patient to take decision regarding elective cholecystectomy if recurrence.

NURSING MANAGEMENT OF PATIENTS UNDERGOING SURGICAL TREATMENT

Preoperative Care

Assessment: Same as described before. Focus of assessment should be to findout presence of complications, e.g. infection or obstruction due to stone.

Assess patient's knowledge about the procedure, preoperative and postoperative care needed and the rationale for those and the level of anxiety due to the surgery.

Nursing Diagnoses

1. Knowledge deficit related to the surgery, preoperative care, postoperative expectations and recovery as manifested by frequent questioning and improper statements.
2. Anxiety related to the surgery and its outcome.

GOALS

1. Acquisition of knowledge
2. Relief from anxiety.

Nursing Interventions

Acquisition of knowledge

- Reinforce information given to the patient by the physician about the surgical procedure and its rationale. Provide written material or diagram, etc. for understanding of the patient.
- Explain patient the details of preoperative care to be carried out for the patient with rationale, e.g. nil orally after midnight; skin preparation from nipple line to midthigh, showering with antibacterial soap; enema to decrease colon mass and the chance of incontinence contaminating the operative field; nasogastric tube insertion (open cholecystectomy), etc.
- Explain patient what to expect about operation, e.g. IV fluid administration, nasogastric tube aspiration, drainage tube and T tube placement if any, postoperative pain and pain control measures, postoperative complications and ways to prevent those.
- Give verbal instruction and demonstration about postoperative exercises, e.g. turning, deep breathing, coughing, splinting wound, leg exercises, early ambulation, etc. and ensure that the patient can perform those and understand their rationale.

Relief from anxiety

- Assess patient's level of anxiety by listening and observing. Reassure patient that anxiety is normal and anything unknown is frightening.
- Thoroughly explain patient all the diagnostic and routine procedures and their rational.
- Introduce patient to other patients recovering from same surgical procedure.
- Reassure patient that all possible care will be provided to him/her.
- Display a relaxed but confident approach to the patient in order to instill confidence in him/her.

Postoperative care

Assessment: Routine postoperative assessment, e.g. vital signs, general levels of responsiveness, respiratory status, breath sounds, drainage from the biliary tubes and drainage from the incision site for amount, character and color, bowel sounds, pain near incision site, redness or swelling at the incision site, referred pain at shoulder (if laparoscopic cholecystectomy), intake, output including nasogastric suctioning and vomiting if any.

Nursing diagnoses:

1. Acute pain and discomfort related to the surgical procedure as evidenced by patient's verbal complaints.
2. Risk for pulmonary complications, e.g. atelectasis and pneumonia related to impaired gas exchange secondary to pain following high abdominal incision.
3. Risk for impaired skin integrity related to the altered biliary drainage following surgical procedure (if a T tube is placed).
4. Risk for injury related to postoperative complications, e.g. hemorrhage, fluid and electrolyte imbalance, infection, ileus, etc.
5. Risk for imbalanced nutrition less than body requirements related to inadequate bile secretion.
6. Inadequate health maintenance due to knowledge deficit about self-care activities following surgery and discharge.

GOALS

1. Relief of pain and discomfort.
2. Prevention of respiratory complications.
3. Intact skin and improved biliary drainage.
4. Early detection and control of postoperative complications.
5. Promotion of nutritional status.
6. Understanding of ambulatory and home care routines

Nursing Interventions

Relief of pain and discomfort

- Assess pain by using a pain scale.
- Administer prescribed analgesics as and when required by the patient and monitor the effect of analgesics.
- Provide a small pillow to splint the abdomen or a binder to lessen pain during coughing or movement.
- Provide comfort measures, e.g. a quiet environment, back rub, comfortable positioning to promote rest and enhance the effect of analgesics.
- Place patient to Sim's position (left side with right knee flexed) to remove the gas pocket and thus relieve referred pain to shoulder if laparoscopic cholecystectomy is performed. Encourage patient to take deep breath and also to ambulate, which facilitates movement of gas pocket away from the diaphragm.

Prevention of respiratory complications

- Encourage patient deep breathing, coughing, frequent changing of positions and early ambulation for full expansion of lungs and expulsion of accumulated secretions.
- Administer analgesics adequately to help the patient perform respiratory hygiene with ease.
- Provide incentive spirometry and steam inhalation, to encourage lung expansion and spontaneous coughing.
- Auscultate lungs for diminished breath sounds and adventitious breath sounds to monitor adequate respiratory functions.

Intact skin and improved biliary drainage

- Attach biliary drainage tube if any, to a gravity drainage bottle. Fasten tube with the patient's gown in such a manner so that there is no pull on the drainage tube.
- Observe drainage for amount, obstruction, infection or leakage in the peritoneal cavity.
- Assess patient for jaundice, pain in right upper quadrant, nausea, vomiting, clay colored stool, changes in vital signs and leakage of bile around drainage tube.
- Change dressings around drainage tube as and when necessary and if required apply skin protective cream to prevent irritation from corrosive action of bile.
- The drainage tube is removed after 7 to 14 days when amount of drainage is minimum indicating that the bile has started flowing in the intestine.

Early detection and control of postoperative complications

- Monitor vital signs and inspect surgical incisions and drains for evidence of bleeding. Also assess the patient for increased tenderness and rigidity of the abdomen. Report immediately if any of these signs occur.
- Assess body temperature every 4 hourly and check incision site, IV line, drainage or urinary drainage (if any) for evidence of infection.
- Practice meticulous hand washing and other infection control measures as per institution protocol to prevent infection.
- Monitor intake and output and maintain a strict intake output chart to prevent fluid imbalances.

- Encourage patient for early ambulation to promote circulation and thus prevent thromboembolic complications.
- Assess skin and mucous membrane integrity and provide back care and mouth care every four hours to prevent pressure sores and oral infections, e.g. parotitis.

Promotion of nutritional status

- After an open cholecystectomy the patient is not allowed anything by mouth. Fluids and foods are started gradually only after the patient starts passing flatus and bowel sound is heard.
- Continue to assess patient for abdominal distention and bowel sounds after administration of food and fluids to determine their tolerance.
- Provide patient high carbohydrate and high protein diet but low fat immediately after surgery and for a period of 4 to 6 weeks. After 4 to 6 weeks the patient usually tolerates a normal diet avoiding excessive fats.

Understanding of ambulatory and home care routines

- Patient with laparoscopic cholecystectomy is discharged early so they should be taught home health care needs and skills, e.g. wound care, medications and their administrations, dietary modifications, identifying evidence of infection or any other complications.
- Teach patient the manifestations to report, e.g. fever, chills, nausea and vomiting, jaundice, dark colored urine, clay colored stools and pruritus.
- Explain patient the dietary restrictions, e.g. low fat diet initially, gradually increasing fat contents towards normal diet, supplementation of fat soluble vitamins and avoiding alcohol to prevent pancreatitis.
- Teach patient to avoid heavy lifting and strenuous work as instructed by the physician. Return to normal activity and work after 1 week if laparoscopic cholecystectomy and after 6 weeks if open cholecystectomy.

8

Nursing Management of Patients with Disorders of Urinary System

ASSESSMENT OF PATIENTS WITH DISORDERS OF URINARY SYSTEM

Subjective Data

Chief complaints of oliguria, anuria, polyuria, frequency of urination, burning on urination, dysuria, hematuria, hesitancy, dribbling, incontinence, stress incontinence, nocturia, enuresis, retention of urine, pain in flank/ suprapubic area/urethra.

Associated symptoms of fatigue, headache, blurred vision, anorexia, nausea, vomiting, chills, itching, excessive thirst, gain of body weight, edema in face/ankle/ generalized.

Presence of diseases like—Diabetes mellitus, hypertension, multiple sclerosis, Parkinson's disease, systemic lupus erythematosis, hyperthyroidism, gout, sickle cell anemia, multiple myeloma, etc. and pregnancy.

Previous history of streptococcal infections such as impetigo, sore throat, nephrotic syndrome, viral hepatitis, tuberculosis, injury to head or back, obstetrical injury, cancer, etc.

Previous hospitalization, major surgeries, catheterization, cystoscopy, radiation therapy to pelvis and pelvic surgery.

Use of prescription drugs or over the counter drugs, nephrotoxic drugs.

Occupation such as textile workers, industrial workers, painters and exposure to chemicals like—Phenol, ethylene glycols and aromatic amines.

Habits of smoking, alcohol intake and use of recreational drugs.

Consumption of too many dairy products, high protein foods, spicy foods, carbonated beverages, caffeine, vitamin and mineral supplements and less water intake.

Sedentary work and long-term immobility.

Family history of renal or urologic problems.

Objective Data

Fatigue, lethargy, diminished alertness, puffiness on face, stomatitis, ammonia breath odor, edema in extremities, generalized edema, muscle wasting (renal failure), pallor, changes in skin turgor, bruises, rough-dry skin, yellow-gray cast on skin, excoriations, striae on abdomen and unilateral mass in abdomen.

Tenderness and palpable mass in costovertebral angle (if tumor or lesion), distended bladder on palpation, dullness over symphysis pubis on percussion (distended bladder), bruit (abnormal murmur) over costovertebral angle and upper abdominal quadrant on auscultation (impaired blood flow to kidney).

Diagnostic Studies

Urine studies

- Urinalysis provides baseline information and suggests for further tests.
- Protein determination detects presence and amounts of albumin in urine.
- Creatinine clearance is an indicator of renal function.
- Specific gravity indicates renal concentration ability.
- Urine culture detects presence of microorganisms.
- Residual urine determines amount of urine left in the bladder after voiding.
- Urine cytology detects abnormal cellular structures (bladder cancer).

Blood studies

- Blood urea nitrogen (BUN) identifies presence of kidney problems.
- Serum creatinine indicates renal function morc accurately.
- Uric acid studies determine problems with purine metabolism and also indicate kidney problem.
- Serum electrolytes studies (sodium, potassium, calcium, phosphorus, and bicarbonate) indicate renal function as these are excreted through kidneys.

Radiology and imaging

- X-ray of kidney, ureters and bladder shows size, shape and position of kidneys. Radiopaque stones and foreign bodies may also be seen.
- Intravenous pyelogram (IVP) is X-ray of the urinary tract after IV injection of a contrast medium. The presence, position, size and shape of the kidneys, ureters and bladder can be evaluated. Cysts, tumors, lesions or any obstruction may be identified. Patient with decreased renal function should not undergo IVP as contrast media may worsen renal function (nephrotoxic).
- Antegrade pyelogram (nephrostogram) is X-ray of upper urinary tract followed by injection of contrast medium percutaneously into the renal pelvis or via a nephrostomy tube. Performed to evaluate tube function or ureteral integrity after trauma or surgery in patients who are allergic to contrast media or who have decreased renal function.
- Retrograde pyelogram involves X-ray of urinary tract after introduction of contrast media into the kidney pelvis via ureteral catheters inserted through a cystoscope. Performed when patient is allergic to contrast medium or has decreased renal function.
- Renal arteriogram is visualization of renal blood vessels by fluoroscope after injecting a contrast medium in the renal artery with the help of a catheter passed through the femoral artery. Performed to diagnose renal artery stenosis, additional or missing renal blood vessels or renovascular hypertension.
- Renal ultrasound is used to diagnose renal or perirenal masses, cysts or obstruction. It is a noninvasive procedure, safely used in patients with renal failure.
- CT scan is visualization of kidneys, may be used to diagnose tumors, abscesses, suprarenal masses and obstruction.
- Magnetic resonance imaging is useful to visualize kidneys. Not useful in the diagnosis of urinary calculi or calcified tumor.
- Cystogram involves instillation of contrast medium into bladder by a cysto-

scope or by catheter, used to visualize bladder and detect vesicoureteral reflux.

- Urethrogrm is the retrograde injection of contrast media into urethra to identify strictures, diverticula or other urethral pathologic conditions.
- Voiding cystourethrogram is a voiding study of the bladder opening and urethra. The bladder is filled with contrast medium. Fluoroscopic films are taken to visualize bladder and urethra once before urination and other after urination to detect residual urine. Performed to diagnose abnormalities of the lower urinary tract such as urethral stenosis, bladder neck obstruction and prostatic enlargement.

Renal radionuclide imaging (renal scan)

The procedure involves IV injection of radioactive isotopes. The isotopes are distributed in the kidneys. Radioisotope distribution in kidneys is then scanned and mapped with the help of radiation detection probes placed over kidneys and scintillation counter. Test is useful to evaluate anatomic structures, perfusion, and function of the kidneys. Tumors abscesses and cysts appear as cold spots because of presence of nonfunctioning tissue.

Renal biopsy

It is obtaining renal tissue for examination to detect type of renal disease or to follow progress of the disease. Technique is performed by inserting a hollow needle percutaneously into the lower lobe of kidney. Needle may be inserted with CT or ultrasound guidance.

Endoscopy (cystoscopy)

It is visualization of the interior of the bladder with cystoscope, a tubular lighted scope. The instrument may also be used to insert ureteral catheters, remove stone from bladder or ureters or obtain specimens of bladder lesions for further studies.

Urodynamics

It is the urine flow study (uroflowmetry) measures amount of urine during a single voiding. Patient with a comfortably full bladder is asked to void in a special pan and to empty bladder completely. Graphic displays illustrate straining and intermittent flow pattern or other voiding disorders. The test is performed to assess the degree of outflow obstruction caused by stricture urethra or prostatic enlargement and to assess effects of bladder or sphincter dysfunction on voiding.

URINARY TRACT INFECTION

Definition

Urinary tract infections (UTI) refer to multiplication of organisms in the urinary tract. Normally urinary tract is sterile, microorganisms are confined to the lower end of the urethra.

Incidence

Occurrence of urinary tract infection is more common in women.

About one-third of all women have UTI at some time in their life.

Risk increases by 1% in each subsequent decade.

Classification

UTI is classified in several ways

1. Lower urinary tract infections, e.g. urethritis and cystitis.
2. Upper urinary tract infections, e.g. pyelonephritis, nephritis, perirenal abscess and renal abscess.

UTI may also be

1. Uncomplicated: It occurs in an otherwise normal urinary tract with normal renal function. Usually involves the bladder.
2. Complicated: It usually occurs where there is obstruction, stones or catheters, existing diabetes or neurologic diseases, pregnancy-induced changes or repeated infections.

UTI may also be described as

1. Initial/First/Isolated infection: It is uncomplicated UTI in a person who never had an infection.
2. Recurrent UTI: It is a reinfection caused by a second pathogen in a person who experienced a previous infection that was successfully cured.

Etiology and Risk Factors

Urinary tract infections are believed to cause by:

- Disturbances in mechanisms that normally maintain the urinary tract above urethra sterile, e.g. inability to empty the bladder completely; incompetence of ureterovesical junction allowing reflux and a change in the normal bacterial characteristics of urine.
- Obstruction in urine flow due to congenital abnormalities; urethral strictures; tumor in bladder; stones in kidney, ureter or bladder; compression of the urethra due to enlarged prostate.
- Decreased natural defense mechanism or immunosuppresion in elderly, persons with diabetes mellitus or HIV infection.
- Instrumentation of the urinary tract, e.g. catheterization and cystoscopic procedure.
- Injury and subsequent inflammation of the urethral mucosa.

Risk of UTI is increased in persons with

- Pregnancy.
- Diabetes mellitus.
- Multiple sex partners.
- Poor personal hygiene.
- Neurological disorders.
- Use of spermicidal agents or contraceptive diaphragm.

Pathophysiology

- Organisms from perineum gain access to the urethra and bladder most commonly via ascending route and less commonly via the blood stream or lymphatic system.
- Organisms adhere to the mucosal wall of the urinary tract and bladder to avoid being washed out with voiding.
- Organisms then defeat host defense mechanisms and colonize the epithelium of the urinary tract and initiates inflammation.

LOWER URINARY TRACT INFECTIONS

Clinical Manifestations

Uncomplicated

- Dysuria, frequent urination (more often than every 2 hours), urgency, voiding in small amounts, inability to void and incomplete emptying of the bladder.
- Cloudy urine and hematuria.
- Suprapubic pressure or discomfort and lower abdominal or flank pain.
- Abdominal distention, nausea and diarrhea may be present if ureteral involvement.
- Asymptomatic bacteriuria most commonly seen in older adults.
- If symptoms elderly adults may present with changes in mental status, fatigue,

anorexia, slight decline in body temperature and nonlocalized abdominal discomfort.

Complicated UTIs

- Manifestations may vary from asymptomatic to gram-negative sepsis with shock.
- Difficult to respond to treatment.
- Tend to recur.
- Many patients with catheter associated UTI may be asymptomatic but may develop sudden septic shock due to urosepsis.

Diagnostic Studies

1. Urine for colony counts—10^5 colony forming units per milliliter of midstream urine indicates infection.
2. Urine for cellular studies—Presence of RBCs more than 4 per high power field and more than 4 WBCs per high power field (pyuria) indicates infection.
3. Dipstick urinalysis for leukocyte esterase and nitrite activity detects bacteriuria.
4. Urine for culture and sensitivity test—It is most accurate test. Done in complicated UTIs/nosocomial infection/infection is unresponsive to empirical treatment.
5. Imaging studies, e.g. intravenous pyelography, CT scan, etc. may be carried out if obstruction is suspected as the cause for UTI.

Medical Management

Uncomplicated

- Antibiotic (according to physician's choice), e.g. trimethoprim-sulfamethonazole (bactrim, septran) or trimethoprim alone if allergic to sulfa drugs; nitrofurantoin to control infection.
- Urinary analgesic, e.g. phenazopyridine (pyridium) or combination agent, e.g. urised to relieve dysuria.
- Adequate fluid intake to flush out the urinary tract.
- Counseling about risk factors to prevent recurrence.

Complicated or recurrent UTI

- Antibiotic according to drug sensitivity results, e.g. amoxicillin, cephalosporine, fluoroquinolones, e.g. ciprofloxacin, levofloxacin, norfloxacin, ofloxacin and gatifloxacin.
- Prophylactic antibiotic therapy by a small nightly dose after voiding and before going to bed for a period of 3 to 6 months may be given if the above measure fails.
- Further investigations by imaging studies if indicated.

UPPER URINARY TRACT INFECTIONS

Pyelonephritis

Definition

Pyelonephritis is an inflammation of the renal pelvis and parenchyma.

Types

- Acute
- Chronic.

Etiology and Risk Factors

- Most common cause of pyelonephritis is bacteria, e.g. *E. coli, Proteus, Klebsiella* or E*nterobacter* species.
- Less common cause is by infections with fungi, protozoa and viruses.

Pathophysiology

- Colonization and infection of the lower urinary tract occurs due to ascent of perineal organism via the urethra.

- The organisms spread to the kidney by ascending the ureters. Vesicoureteral reflux (backward movement of urine from lower to upper urinary tract) or obstruction of the lower urinary tract facilitates upward movement of organisms through the ureters.
- Only in certain situations (about 3%) the organisms may reach the kidney through blood.
- The inflammation commonly starts in the renal medulla and spreads to the cortex. Renal pelvis is inflamed and enlarged. Small abscesses are often seen in renal parenchyma.
- With treatment as the inflammation recedes scarring develops in the interstitial tissues.
- Pregnancy-associated physiologic changes; recurring episodes of pyelonephritis can lead to a scarred, contracted poorly functioning kidney (as the nephrons are replaced by scar tissue) and chronic pyelonephritis and ultimately renal failure.

Clinical Manifestations

Acute pyelonephritis

- Sudden onset of pain in one or both loins, radiating to the iliac fossa and suprapubic area. Pain may be colicky in nature if stones are present.
- High fever with chills.
- Nausea, vomiting, malaise, headache, muscle pain and general prostration.
- History of lower urinary tract infection, e.g. dysuria, frequency of micturition and urgency for some time.
- Foul smelling, cloudy or bloody urine.
- Marked tenderness and guarding over the costovertebral angle.

Chronic pyelonephritis

Patient may not show any manifestations. The disease may be incidentally detected during diagnostic evaluation for hypertension or its complication or during an acute exacerbation of chronic infection.

Most common manifestations

- Hypertension
- Fatigue and headache
- Polyuria and excessive thirst
- Loss of appetite and weight loss.

Diagnostic Studies

- Urinalysis reveals bacteriuria, pyuria, hematuria, white blood cell casts indicating involvement of renal parenchyma.
- Blood count shows leukocytosis.
- Urine culture identifies organisms.
- Blood culture (done in severely ill and hospitalized patient) detects urosepsis.
- Ultrasonography of urinary system identifies anatomic abnormalities, hydronephrosis, renal abscesses, stones, scarring or abscesses, impaired renal function and chronic pyelonephritis.
- CT scan or MRI also evaluates kidney size, e.g. small contracted kidney in chronic pyelonephritis.
- Intravenous pyelography is not done in acute pyelonephritis but may be done in chronic pyelonephritis if ultrasound is not available.
- Blood examination may detect azotemia, low hemoglobin percentage, increased creatinine level and abnormal creatinine clearance in chronic pyelonephritis.

Medical Management

Acute pyelonephritis

- Patient with mild symptoms may be treated at home with oral antibiotics and those with severe symptoms are treated in hospital with parenteral antibiotics.

- Initially empirically selected broad spectrum antibiotics, e.g. ampicillin with gentamycin are given.
- Later antibiotics are changed according to the culture and drug sensitivity results, e.g. gatifloxacin, norfloxacin, ciprofloxacin and continued for a period of 2 to 3 weeks.
- Urinary analgesics, e.g. phenazopyri dine.
- Adequate fluid intake orally or by intravenous infusion if nausea, vomiting or dehydration.
- Antipyretic or nonsteroidal anti-inflammatory drugs to reduce fever, relieve headache or discomfort.
- Follow-up urine culture and further imaging studies if indicated.

NURSING MANAGEMENT

Assessment

Subjective data

Dysuria, burning on urination, urinary frequency, urgency, hesitancy, nocturia, suprapubic or low back pain, nausea, vomiting, anorexia, chills, malaise, previous UTI, urinary calculi, stasis, retention, multiple sex partners and use of spermicidal agents or contraceptive diaphragm.

Objective data

Tenderness at costovertebral angle, elevated temperature, chills, hematuria, cloudy urine, tender enlarged kidney, changes in mental status and deterioration of clinical status in elderly.

Possible findings

Leukocytosis, urinalysis positive for pyuria, bacteria, RBCs, WBCs, positive urine culture and abnormal findings in imaging studies, e.g. IVP and CT scan or ultrasound.

Nursing Diagnoses

1. Altered urinary elimination related to inflammation and irritation as evidenced by pain and burning on urination, urgency, hesitancy, frequency of urination, nocturia and hematuria.
2. Acute pain and discomfort related to inflammation and infection of the urethra, bladder and other urinary structures as evidenced by patient's complain of pain in flank suprapubic or lower back.
3. Inadequate therapeutic regimen management related to knowledge deficit regarding factors predisposing the patient to infection and recurrence, detection of recurrence promptly and therapeutic management.
4. Potential complication: Urosepsis.

GOALS

1. Establish normal urinary elimination pattern.
2. Relief of pain and discomfort.
3. Adequate therapeutic regimen management and self-care.
4. Prevention and early detection of complication.

Nursing Interventions

Establish normal urinary elimination pattern

- Monitor urinary elimination pattern, e.g. frequency, urgency, dysuria, amount, color, and odor of urine to determine urinary elimination status.
- Obtain midstream urine specimen for urinalysis or culture as advised to detect the pathogenic organisms and also to evaluate the effectiveness of treatment.
- Teach patient to avoid foods and drinks that may increase irritation, e.g. spicy foods and tomatoes, alcohol and caffeinated beverages, e.g. coffee, tea, chocolates and carbonated beverages.

- Teach patient to drink liberal amounts of fluids to increase renal blood flow and urine output to flush the organisms from the urinary tract.

Relief of pain and discomfort

- Assess pain thoroughly—Location, characteristics, e.g. onset, duration, frequency, quality, intensity and precipitating factors to establish history and determine baseline pain level.
- Administer prescribed analgesics, e.g. phenazopyridine and evaluate its effectiveness.
- Teach patient nonpharmacologic measures of pain relief, e.g. application of hot water bottle to lower abdomen along with drugs to supplement pain medication and increase pain relief.

Adequate therapeutic regimen management and self-care

- Assess patient's existing knowledge about the disease process, treatment regimen, and prevention of recurrence.
- Explain pathology of the disease with the help of anatomical diagrams.
- Describe rational behind the treatment regimen and importance of taking antibiotics as scheduled for the prescribed period of time and side effects of medicines, e.g. staining of urine and undergarments with phenazopyridine, pulmonary fibrosis and neuropathies with long-term use of nitrofurantoin, diarrhea and vaginal candidiasis with broad spectrum antibiotics to promote compliance with treatment.
- Teach patient
  - To take liberal amounts of fluids.
  - Proper hygienic measures, e.g. careful cleaning of perineal region with wiping from front to back after urination and cleaning with soap and water after defecation.
  - Voiding at regular intervals of 3 to 4 hours and to evacuate bladder completely.
  - Pre and postcoital voiding for women patient.
  - Avoid vaginal douches, irritating soaps, powders and sprays in the perineal area.
  - To drink lemon juice to acidify urine or to take vitamin C daily.
  - Sign and symptoms of recurrence, e.g. fever, cloudy urine, pain on urination and urgency or frequency.

Prevention and early detection of complication

- Monitor vital signs, changes in mental status in patients at increased risk of development of sepsis, e.g. elderly, patients with frequent and long-term catheter, patient with anatomic abnormalities and immunocompromised patients.
- Report any abnormality promptly, e.g. hypothermia, hyperthermia, tachycardia, tachypnea, decreased level of consciousness, hypotension and warm flushed skin as indicator of septic shock resulting from urosepsis.
- Monitor WBC counts, platelet level and coagulation function tests to detect clotting abnormality early.

ACUTE GLOMERULONEPHRITIS

Definition

Glomerulonephritis is an immunologic disorder that causes inflammation and increased cells in the glomerular capillaries.

The disease may appear in acute or chronic form.

Incidence

Acute glomerulonephritis primarily occurs in children older than 2 years of age.

But it may occur in persons of any age group.

Etiology and pathophysiology

- The disease is the result of antibody-induced injury.
- Two types of antibodies may initiate glomerular damage:
  - Antibodies specific to glomerular antigen or autoantibodies (antibodies to one's own tissue).
  - Antibodies reacting with exogenous antigens (bacteria, e.g. Beta-hemolytic streptococcus causing acute post streptococcal glomerulonephritis; virus, e.g. posthepatitis B and C glomerulonephritis; chemicals and drugs) or some nonglomerular endogenous antigens.
- In both type of antigen-antibody reactions immune complexes produced either elsewhere in the body or in the glomeruli are ultimately deposited along the glomerular basement membrane.
- Immune complex activates immune complements that attract polymorphonuclear leukocytes, histamine and other inflammatory mediators resulting in inflammation and thickening of the glomerular filtration membrane.
- Inflammation leaves scarring and damage of glomerular filtration membrane leading to decreased glomerular filtration rate and increase in the permeability of the glomerulus to larger protein molecules.

Clinical Manifestations

- Clinical manifestations vary with the severity and cause of the disease.
- Hematuria which may be microscopic or macroscopic or gross.
- Smoky urine or cola-colored urine.
- Urine contains RBCs, WBCs, casts and protein.
- Oliguria or anuria.
- Edema appears initially in face and around eyes (periorbital), later peripheral or whole body as ascites.
- Fever, chills, weakness, headache, pallor, anorexia, nausea and vomiting may be present.
- Hypertension.
- Abdominal or flank pain and tenderness over the costovertebral angle due to kidney edema and distension of the renal capsule.
- Reduced visual acuity due to retinal edema.
- Elevated BUN and serum creatinine level.
- Anemia.
  - Elderly person may exhibit.
  - Symptoms of heart failure, e.g. dyspnea, engorged neck veins, cardiomegaly and pulmonary edema due to circulatory overload.
  - Confusion, somnolence (drowsiness) and seizures.

Diagnostic Studies

1. History of past immune disorders, e.g. systemic lupus erythematosus (SLE), systemic sclerosis; exposure to drugs; immunizations; bacterial infection, e.g. Beta hemolyticus streptococcus causing sore throat or impetigo; viral infections, e.g. hepatitis B or C.
2. Urinalysis reveals hematuria, proteinuria, casts and WBCs.
3. Blood examination detects decreased hematocrit and hemoglobin , elevated BUN level, elevated creatinine level. Elevated C reactive protein and antistreptolysin O titers are found in poststreptococcal glomerulonephritis.

- Kidney biopsy confirms the disease.

Medical Management

Goals of medical management are to treat symptoms, to preserve kidney functions and to treat complications promptly and is achieved by:

- Rest.
- Fluid and salt restriction.
- Diuretics.
- Antihypertensive drugs.
- Restriction of protein if BUN and creatinine levels are elevated.
- Antibiotics if streptococcal infection is still present.
- Corticosteroids and immunosuppressants given in rapidly progressive acute glomerulonephrits.

NURSING MANAGEMENT

Nursing Assessment

Subjective data

Oliguria, anuria, cola-colored urine, smoky urine, abdominal or flank pain, fever, chills, weakness, lethargy, anorexia, nausea, vomiting, facial swelling, periorbital swelling, generalized edema, dyspnea, headache, diminished vision.

Objective data

Facial and periorbital edema, pallor, rapid bounding pulse, elevated blood pressure, rapid shallow breathing, basal crepts, ascites, edema in legs, pleural effusion, engorged neck veins.

Laboratory findings

RBCs, WBCs, casts, protein in urine; decreased hematocrit and hemoglobin level, elevated BUN and serum creatinine level. ASO titer and C-reactive protein are elevated in poststreptococcal glomerulonephritis.

Nursing Diagnoses

1. Fluid volume excess related to reduced urine output as evidenced by edema, bounding pulse, high blood pressure and basal crepts.
2. Imbalanced nutrition less than body requirement related to anorexia and restriction of diets.
3. Fatigue related to increased metabolic demand and anemia as evidenced by patient's complain of weakness, increased pulse rate and respiratory rate on exertion.
4. Risk for impaired skin integrity related to edema.
5. Risk for infection related to altered immune response secondary to immunosuppressive treatment.

GOALS

1. Maintenance of adequate fluid balance.
2. Maintenance of optimum nutritional intake.
3. Achieving balance between activity and rest.
4. Prevention of skin breakdown.
5. Prevention of infection.

Nursing Intervention

Maintenance of adequate fluid volume

- Monitor intake ouput, body weight, abdominal girth, circumference of edematous legs daily.
- Administer prescribed amount of fluid (output plus 600 mL) only throughout the day.
- Explain the rationale for restricted fluid intake to the patient and gain his cooperation.
- Teach patient to take medicine with food in order to reduce water consumption so that he is able to consume different liquids instead of water.
- Teach patient to relieve thirst by sucking ice chips, hard candy and lemon slice, etc. and to take frequent oral hygiene.

Maintenance of optimum nutritional intake

- Provide high carbohydrate, low protein and low salt diet in order to avoid protein catabolism, allow the kidneys to rest and also to control edema.
- Make the patient understand the need for restricted diet (low protein and low salt), which is usually not palatable and gain his cooperation.
- Teach patient to consume small amount at frequent intervals.
- Provide variations within the prescribed food items.
- Refer the patient to a dietician who may suggest various options with the permitted food items.
- Monitor amount of food intake, body weight, hematocrit and hemoglobin percentage, serum protein at regular intervals.

Achieving balance between activity and rest

- Provide complete rest in the acute phase.
- Encourage gradual self-care activity as the condition improves.
- Assess pulse rate, respiratory rate fatigue if any after activity.
- Teach patient to take rest in between activities.

Prevention of skin breakdown

- Assess patient's edematous areas and pressure bearing areas in each shift for redness, excoriation, etc.
- Maintain optimum skin hygiene daily and whenever required avoiding soap.
- Massage edematous skin areas and pressure bearing areas gently to increase circulation and apply moisturizing lotion to the skin to prevent drying.
- Teach patient to change his position every 2 hourly to improve circulation.
- Provide special bed to a high risk patient.

Prevention of infection

- Assess patient daily for early signs of infection, e.g. common cold and cough or sore throat.
- Restrict visitors and staff with obvious infections near patient.
- Observe infection control policy of the hospital strictly.
- Teach patient ways to prevent infections, e.g. hand washing, consuming safe drinking water, fresh foods, avoiding crowded places and taking prescribed antibiotics if any (to eradicate streptococcal infections).

ACUTE RENAL FAILURE

Definition

Acute renal failure refers to a reversible clinical syndrome characterized by rapid and almost complete loss of renal function developing over a period of hours or days with progressive accumulation of nitrogenous waste products (azotemia), e.g. blood urea nitrogen (BUN) and increasing levels of serum creatinine.

Etiology

Various causes of acute renal failure may be categorized as:

Prerenal

These are the conditions that interfere with renal perfusion and a decrease in glomerular filtration rate:
- Hypovolemia.
- Dehydration.

- Hemorrhage.
- Gastrointestinal tract losses, e.g. diarrhea, vomiting.
- Burns.
- Myocardial infarction and heart failure or cardiogenic shock.
- Vasodilation due to sepsis or shock and anaphylaxis.
- Renal artery or renal vein thrombosis.

Intrarenal

These are the conditions that damage the actual renal parenchyma of the glomeruli or kidney tubules (acute tubular necrosis:

- Prolonged prerenal ischemia.
- Nephrotoxic injury.
- Nephrotoxic drugs, e.g. aminoglycosides and amphotericin B.
- Radiocontrast agents and drug allergies.
- Severe crush injury and electric shock (myoglobin released from necrotic muscle cells).
- Hemolytic blood transfusion reaction (hemoglobin released from damaged red blood cells).
- Acute glomerulonephritis.
- Systemic lupus erythematous.
- Toxemia of pregnancy.

Postrenal

These are the conditions causing obstruction of urinary outflow due to lesion distal to the kidney:

- Benign prostatic hyperplasia or cancer.
- Bladder cancer.
- Stone in bladder or ureters.
- Strictures.
- Neuromuscular disorders from spinal cord disease.
- Trauma in back, pelvis or perineum.

Pathophysiology

Prerenal

- Decreased circulating volume decreases renal blood flow. Kidneys respond to decreased blood flow by activating renin angiotensin aldosterone system and resulting in conservation of water and sodium retention (compensatory mechanism).
- Decreased renal blood flow also decreases the capacity of the kidneys to liberate waste products that leads to a rise in BUN and serum creatinine level.
- With continued renal ischemia kidneys lose their compensatory mechanisms and intrarenal damage to kidney tissue occurs.
- Ultimate result is oliguria, increased BUN and serum creatinine level and inability to conserve sodium and excrete potassium.

Intrarenal (acute tubular necrosis)

- Prolonged hypovolemia stimulates renin angiotensin aldosterone system and results in oliguria.
- Ischemia alters glomerular epithelial cells and glomerular capillary permeability resulting in decrease in glomerular filtration rate (GFR). Decreased glomerular filtration rate reduces blood flow and causes profound tubular damage.
- Necrotic epithelial cells accumulate in the edematous damaged tubules. Tubules are obstructed, intratubular pressure increases, which further reduce GFR.
- Glomerular filtrate leaks back into the plasma through holes in the damaged tubular membranes in an attempt to decrease the intratubular pressure resulting in decrease in intratubular fluid flow.

Postrenal

- Obstruction of urinary outflow causes urine to reflux into the renal pelvis.
- Obstructed urine in the renal pelvis damages renal parenchyma and impair kidney functions.

Clinical Manifestations

The effects of ARF are manifested in every system of the body:

- **Urinary system**
  - Oliguria or anuria (polyuria or normal urine output may be found in some patients).
  - Decreased urine specific gravity and osmolality.
  - Proteinuria, casts, and increased urine sodium concentration.
- **Metabolic**
  - Increased blood urea nitrogen (BUN) and creatinine level.
  - Elevated BUN creatinine ratio (>10:1).
  - Hyponatremia, hypocalcemia, hyperkalemia, hypermagnesemia, hyperphosphatemia, acidosis, decreased bicarbonate level.
- **Cardiovascular**
  - Fluid overload, hypertension, pericarditis, pericardial effusion, dysrhythmia.
- **Hematologic**
  - Anemia, platelet dysfunction, increased susceptibility to infection, impaired wound healing.
- **Respiratory**
  - Pulmonary edema, pleural effusion, Kussmaul respirations
- **Gastrointestinal**
  - Anorexia, nausea, vomiting, diarrhea, constipation, stomatitis
- **Neurologic (uremic encephalopathy)**
  - Apathy, lethargy, impairment of recent memory, difficulty in concentrating, tremors, convulsions, stupor and coma.

Diagnostic Studies

1. History to elicit the cause of ARF.
2. Urinalysis is an important diagnostic tool. It differentiates the causes of ARF, for example:
   - Decreased specific gravity and osmolality, decreased urinary sodium and normal urinary sediment in prerenal ARF.
   - Increased urinary sodium, urinary sediment containing cells, casts and proteins in intrarenal ARF.
   - Hematuria, pyuria and crystals may be found in postrenal conditios
3. Blood—Increased serum creatinine, increased BUN level, elevated serum potassium level, decreased serum sodium level, complete blood count, pH and hemoglobin percentage.
4. Renal ultrasound reveals renal disease and obstruction.
5. Renal scan, CT scan or MRI reveals lesions and masses, obstruction, vascular abnormalities.
6. Renal biopsy detects intrarenal causes of ARF.

Prevention

Following measures may be taken to prevent ARF in hospitalized patients:

1. Maintain adequate hydration to patients at risk of dehydration.
2. Prevent and treat shock promptly with adequate fluid and blood replacement.
3. Treat hypotension promptly.
4. Ensure correct blood transfusion to prevent transfusion reactions.
5. Monitor central venous pressure, arterial blood pressure and hourly urine output of critically ill patients.
6. Continually assess kidney functions of high risk patients by hourly urine output, BUN and serum creatinine level.
7. Prevent and treat infections promptly. Prevent sepsis in patients with burns and wounds. Give meticulous catheter care to patients with indwelling catheter to prevent ascending infections.

8. Closely monitor drug dosage, duration of use and blood levels of drugs metabolized and excreted by the kidneys.

Management

Objectives

1. Prompt recognition and treatment of underlying disease.
2. Correct fluid, electrolytes and uremic abnormalities to restore homeostasis.
3. Preventing complications including nutritional deficiencies until normal kidney function is achieved.

Restoring homeostasis

- Restriction of fluids if oliguria and anuria. Fluids to be administered usually 600 mL plus previous 24 hours fluid output. Administer saline if dehydration. Monitor fluid volume status of patient by CVP (Central venous pressure monitoring).
- Diuretics, e.g. furosemide IV every 6 hourly given to induce diuresis. Initial dose may be 20 mg to 100 mg. If good result is observed in 1 hour the dose is doubled. Continuous drip of furosemide may also be given. Inj. mannitol may also be given to reduce the chance of nephrotoxicity.
- Restriction of potassium in diet to control hyperkalemia. Inj. calcium gluconate is given to reverse the neuromuscular effect of hyperkalemia leading to dysrhythmia.
- Hyperkalemia is treated by:
  - Administration of regular insulin IV along with glucose.
  - Inj. sodium bicarbonate IV.
  - Administration of sodium polystyrene sulfonate (kayexalate) orally or rectally as enema along with sorbitol.
- Sodium bicarbonate orally or IV is given to treat acidosis.
- Diet high in carbohydrate and lipids is given to reduce catabolism and level of nitrogenous waste materials. A total calorie intake of 30 to 45 kcal per kg of body weight per day is required. Protein intake should be .6 gm per kg of body weight per day. Patient on dialysis is given 1 gm to 1.5 gm protein per kg of body weight per day.
- Dialysis is indicated when:
  - Fluid overload is not corrected with diuretic therapy and uremia is not controlled.
  - Acidosis and electrolyte disturbances do not respond to pharmacologic therapy.

NURSING MANAGEMENT

Assessment

Subjective data

Oliguria or anuria, edema, nausea, vomiting, stomatitis, diarrhea or constipation, lethargy, impaired memory, past history of diarrhea, dehydration, hemorrhage, heart failure, myocardial infarction, etc. or consumption of nephrotoxic medications, malignant hypertension, severe injury, etc. history of obstruction, e.g. benign prostatic hypertrophy, bladder cancer, stone in bladder, etc.

Objective data

Distended neck vein, bounding pulse, palpitation, hypertension, Kussmaul respiration, basal crepts, pericardial friction rub, seizures, dysrhythmia, anemia, leukocytosis, low urinary output, proteinuria, low specific gravity of urine, increased urinary sodium, increased BUN and creatine level, low serum sodium, high serum potassium and other electrolytes abnormalities.

Nursing Diagnoses

1. Fluid volume excess related to inability of the kidneys to produce urine.
2. Imbalanced nutrition less than body requirement related to dietary restrictions, anorexia and altered metabolic state secondary to renal failure.
3. Risk for infection related to invasive lines, lowered resistance secondary to renal failure.
4. Risk for impaired skin integrity related to edema and poor systemic nutrition and deposition of toxins in the tissues secondary to renal failure.
5. Anxiety and apprehension regarding the sudden nature of illness and unknown outcome of disease process and therapeutic interventions.
6. Potential complication: Dysrhythmia related to electrolyte imbalance specially hyperkalemia leading to dysrhythmia.

GOALS

1. Maintenance of fluid balance.
2. Maintenance of adequate nutritional status.
3. Prevention of infection.
4. Maintenance of skin integrity.
5. Control of anxiety.
6. Prevention of complication: Dysrhythmia.

Nursing Interventions

Maintenance of fluid balance

- Monitor intake and output and record accurate findings.
- Measure daily body weight at the same time with same scale (1 kg of body weight is equivalent to 1000 mL of body fluid).
- Check vital signs, e.g. postural blood pressure, apical pulse rate, mental status skin turgor, mucous membranes, neck veins distention every 4 hours.
- Auscultate heart sounds and breath sounds.
- Administer fluid in amounts as determined and prescribed by the physician.
- Help the patient to get relief from thirst due to severe fluid restriction by frequent oral hygiene, judicious use of ice chips, lip ointment and appropriate diversional activities.
- Administer medications with meals instead of water to conserve fluid for the patient.

Maintenance of adequate nutritional status

- Monitor nutritional status of patient.
- Discuss with patient the need for dietary restrictions, e.g. salt restriction, fluid restriction and protein restriction if any.
- Collaborate with dietician and the patient to plan a more acceptable and adequate diet.
- Serve foods in small amounts and frequent intervals in an attractive manner as much as possible.
- Administer antiemetics to relieve nausea if any.
- Record amount of food taken.
- Administer parenteral nutrition as prescribed if oral intake is not adequate.

Prevention of infection

- Assess patient for early signs of infection, e.g. swelling, redness, pain, malaise and leukocytosis.
- Keep patient separated from other known infectious patient.
- Avoid indwelling catheters as these are the frequent source of infection.

- Prevent respiratory complications by frequent turning, incentive spirometry, oxygen inhalation, coughing and deep breathing.
- Practice meticulous hand hygiene and aseptic technique whenever required.

Maintenance of skin integrity

- Assess skin each shift for any signs of breakdown, excoriation, redness, etc.
- Provide skin care. Keep skin clean and well-moisturized.
- Turn frequently.
- Provide special mattress if needed.
- Keep finger nail trimmed.

Control of anxiety

- Assess anxiety level of patient as well as the relatives.
- Provide repeated explanations of therapeutic regimen as planned and told by the physician.
- Encourage patient and family members to ask questions. Clarify doubts if any in simple language. Provide written instructions whenever required.
- Provide emotional and psychological support.

Prevention of complication: Dysrhythmia

- Assess patient for the development of electrolyte imbalances specially hyperkalemia that leads to dysrhythmia.
- Assess signs and symptoms of hyperkalemia, e.g. irregular pulse rhythm, muscle weakness, abdominal cramps, flaccid paralysis and absence of deep tendon reflexes.
- Monitor ECG for conduction abnormalities, e.g. prolonged PR interval, prolonged QRS interval, peaked T wave and depressed ST segment.

CHRONIC RENAL FAILURE

Definition

Chronic renal failure or end stage renal disease (ESRD) is a progressive, irreversible loss/reduction in renal function that the kidneys are unable to maintain the body's internal environment such as metabolic, fluid and electrolyte balance.

Incidence

Varies from country to country.

Etiology

Systemic diseases

Diabetes mellitus (most common), hypertension, lupus erythematosus, polyarteritis, sickle cell disease, amyloidosis.

Local causes

Chronic glomerulonephritis, acute renal failure, repeated episodes of pyelonephritis, obstruction of the urinary tract, polycystic kidney disease, vascular disorders, nephrotoxic medications, overuse of common medications, e.g. aspirin, ibuprofen and acetaminophen or other toxic agents.

Environmental and occupational agents

Lead, cadmium mercury and chromium, some infectious diseases, e.g. hantavirus.

Pathophysiology

- Irreversible damage of nephrons leading to progressive loss of kidney function or reduced glomerular filtration rate (GFR).
- Reduced GFR leads to accumulation of serum urea nitrogen and creatinine rising their levels in blood.

- Remaining functioning nephron hypertrophy in order to filter a larger solute load and lose ability to concentrate urine and reabsorb electrolytes.
- In order to excrete a larger load of solutes a large volume of dilute urine is passed resulting in polyuria and salt wasting.
- With advancement of disease more nephron damage occurs and GFR reduces further. Body is unable to excrete waste products, excess water and salt through the kidneys.
- Accumulation of uremic toxins in the body causes uremia and ultimately death if the patient is not treated by dialysis or kidney transplant (Table 8.1).

Clinical Manifestations

- Manifestations depend upon:
  - The cause of the kidney disease
  - Degree of impairment of kidney function (stage of disease is shown in Table 8.1).
  - Age of the patient.
  - Other associated medical conditions
  - Degree of compliance with the treatment.
- Manifestations are due to build up of retained toxic and metabolic substances in the body:
  - High level of urea in the blood causes: Anorexia, bad taste in the mouth, nausea, vomiting, diarrhea, polyuria and nocturia (in the early stages), oliguria, anuria, presence of cast and protein in urine, foamy and bubbly urine, lethargy, symptoms of encephalopathy, uremic frost on skin, elevated blood urea nitrogen level.
  - High level of potassium in the blood causes: Malaise, muscle paralysis, life-threatening dysrhythmias.
  - High level of phosphates (hyperphosphatemia) causes: Itching, bone damage, nonunion in broken bones, muscle cramps associated

Table 8.1: Stages of renal failure with descriptions

Normal GFR is 125 mL/min		
Stage I	GFR> or = 90 mL/min	Patient remains asymptomatic, no laboratory abnormality, normal or increased GFR
Stage II	GFR = 60-90 mL/min	Mild decrease in GFR, patient may be asymptomatic, but may develop laboratory abnormalities and hypertension
Stage III	GFR 30-59 mL/min	Moderate decrease in GFR, patient may be asymptomatic but may develop hypertension and laboratory abnormalities in various organ systems
Stage IV	GFR 15-29 mL/min	Severe decrease in GFR, symptoms of kidney failure appear
Stage V	GFR<15 mL/min	Full blown clinical manifestations of uremia appear

Medical Surgical Nursing: Assesment and management of clinical problems. Sharon Lewis and olthers.

with hypocalcemia and hyperparathyroidism in late stage.
- Fluid volume overload leads to: Edema in legs, ankles, feet, face and hands; shortness of breath due to pulmonary edema; high blood pressure, congestive heart failure.
- Decreased synthesis of erythropoietin leading to anemia results in: Fatigue, difficulty concentrating, disturbance in memory, dizziness, headache.
- Metabolic acidosis causes: Severe diarrhea, deep and rapid breathing.
- Back pain may be a presenting symptom, if polycystic kidney disease is the cause of renal failure.

Diagnostic Studies

1. Urinalysis— Reveals proteinuria, RBCs, WBCs, casts and glucose
   — Albumin to creatinine ratio = more than 300 mg per 1 gm of creatinine.
2. Blood test reveals elevated blood urea nitrogen and creatinine level, altered serum electrolytes level, decreased hematocrit and hemoglobin concentration.
3. Renal ultrasound—It reveals obstruction and determines size of kidney.
4. Renal scan, CT scan reveals obstruction or lesion.
5. Renal biopsy detects interstitial disease of kidney.

Medical Management

Conservative therapy

- Carried out for patients with stage 1 to stage 4 disease.
- To slow down the progression of the disease to stage 5 and thus delay the need for dialysis or renal transplant.
- To treat the signs and symptoms as much as possible and to prevent complications.
- To provide an optimal quality of life for patient and significant others.

1. Control and treatment of hypertension by:
   - Change of lifestyle, e.g. reduction of body weight, exercise, avoidance of alcohol and smoking, low fat and low salt diet, antihypertensive drugs and drugs to correct dyslipidemia, e.g. statins.
2. Slow the progress of the disease:
   - Angiotensin converting enzyme inhibitors (ACEIs) or angiotensin II receptor antagonists (ARBs).
3. Control and treatment of hyperkalemia:
   - Intravenous administration of regular insulin and glucose.
   - Inj. sodium bicarbonate if acidosis
   - Sodium polystyrene sulfonate (kayexalate) by mouth or retention enema.
   - Inj. calcium gluconate in advanced cardiac diseases.
   - Low potassium diet.
4. Nutritional therapy to control metabolic waste:
   - Restriction of protein .6 to .8 gm/kg of body weight/day for patient not undergoing dialysis and 1.2 to 1.3 gm/kg of ideal body weight for patient undergoing dialysis. 50% protein intake should be of high biological value.
   - Provide adequate calorie from carbohydrate and fat to minimize catabolism of body protein.
   - Vitamin supplementation.
   - Low sodium and potassium diet.
   - Low phosphate diet, e.g. diary products.

5. Control of hypervolemia:
   - Fluid is restricted to 600 mL plus the amount of urine output of previous day.
6. Correction of anemia:
   - Administration of erythropoietin (epoetin alfa or epogen).
   - Iron and folic acid supplementation
7. Control of hyperphosphatemia:
   - Restrict phosphate rich foods, e.g. dairy products.
   - Administer calcium rich phosphate binders, e.g. calcium carbonate and calcium acetate.
   - Supplement vitamin D and calcium.
   - Treatment of hyperparathyroidism if any.
8. Treatment of stage 5 disease:
   - Dialysis
   - Renal transplantation.

NURSING MANAGEMENT

Nursing Assessment

Subjective data

Polyuria, frequent urination, nocturnal urination, less frequent urination, oliguria, anuria, nausea, vomiting, diarrhea, loss of weight, anorexia, bad taste in the mouth, lethargy, fatigue, edema, gain of weight, itching, muscle cramps, pain in back, shortness of breath, poor memory, difficulty in concentrating, diabetes, use of over the counter medications or nephrotoxic medications, past history of any renal disease and history of kidney disease in the family.

Objective data

Dry frosted skin, edema at ankles, legs, feet and face, hypertension, bounding pulse, anxious look, rapid shallow breathing, presence of cast, protein, blood in urine, elevated blood urea nitrogen, elevated serum creatinine, decreased hemoglobin, pancytopenia, reduced size of kidney in ultrasonography, abnormal finding in renal scan.

Nursing Diagnoses

1. Fluid volume excess related to the inability of the kidney to excrete fluid and excessive fluid intake as evidenced by edema, weight gain, bounding pulse, hypertension, and shortness of breath.
2. Nutritional deficits related to altered metabolic activity, dietary restrictions of nutrients, e.g. protein and salt, nausea, vomiting as evidenced by refusal of food and loss of body weight.
3. Activity intolerance related to fatigue, anemia, retention of waste products and dialysis procedure.
4. Risk for infection related to depressed immune functions secondary to chronic kidney failure, vascular access sites for dialysis and malnutrition.
5. Risk for impaired skin integrity related to edema, dry skin, pruritus and uremic frost secondary to chronic kidney failure.
6. Risk for injury related to altered metabolism of calcium secondary to chronic kidney disease.
7. Grieving and anxiety related to loss of kidney function, therapeutic plan, e.g. commencement of dialysis or plan for kidney transplant.

GOALS

1. Maintenance of fluid balance.
2. Maintenance of adequate nutritional intake.
3. Participation in activity within tolerance limit.
4. Prevention of infection.
5. Maintaining optimum skin integrity.
6. Prevention of injuries.

7. Adequate coping and understanding about the disease and therapeutic procedure.

Nursing Intervention

Maintenance of fluid volume

- Monitor fluid status by daily weight, intake and output balance, pulse volume, skin turgor, edema, neck vein distention, respiratory effort and rate.
- Limit fluid intake to prescribed volume.
- Explain to patient and family the rationale for fluid restriction.
- Help patient and family to identify the sources of fluid, e.g. foods and fluids taken with medications.
- Provide low salt and low fat diet to control edema and hypertension.
- Help patient to cope with the discomfort associated with fluid restriction, e.g. using lip balms performing frequent oral hygiene, eating ice chips, or using spray bottles rather than drinking.
- Monitor administration rate of IV fluids carefully if any.
- Monitor fluid status during dialysis by monitoring the vital signs, postural blood pressure, pulse rate, intake and output.

Maintenance of adequate nutritional intake

- Monitor nutritional status by changes in body weight, serum protein, albumin, hemoglobin and hematocrit levels.
- Assess for anorexia, nausea and vomiting or unpalatable diet contributing to inadequate intake.
- Provide patient's food preferences within dietary restrictions.
- Explain patient the need for dietary restrictions and their relationship to urea and creatinine level.
- Provide a written list of food items that are allowed and ways to enhance their taste without the use of sodium or potassium.
- Arrange for dietary consultation with a dietician if available.

Participation in activity within tolerance limit

- Assess factors contributing to activity intolerance, e.g. anemia, fluid and electrolyte imbalances, depression, etc.
- Encourage patient in self-care activities as much as possible with frequent rest periods in between the activities.
- Monitor fatigue, increase pulse rate or dyspnea for activity intolerance.

Prevention of infection

- Monitor for localized and systemic signs of infection, e.g. redness and swelling at IV site or vascular access site, dysuria, hematuria, cloudy urine, chills and fever for early detection and appropriate intervention.
- Teach patient to avoid crowded places and persons with infection.
- Restrict visitors and hospital personnel with infections.
- Ensure aseptic technique during all invasive procedures.
- Follow meticulous hand washing before and after each patient care and infection control protocol of the hospital.
- Teach patient and family members early signs of infection in order to obtain prompt treatment.

Maintaining optimum skin integrity

- Assess skin every shift for dryness, areas of poor circulation, breakdown and infection.
- Keep skin clean. Eliminate use of soap when skin is dry. Use moisturizing oil in the bath water or apply moisturizer directly on the skin.
- Avoid use of alcohol or perfumes as these are drying.

- Teach patient to keep nails trimmed.
- Release continuous pressure from the skin by frequent change of positions if edema is present.
- Assess feet of diabetic patient daily and teach them foot care.

Prevention of injuries

- Monitor serum calcium level at regular Interval.
- Monitor electrolyte levels associated with hypocalcemia, e.g. hyperphosphatemia, hypomagnesemia and alkalosis in order to detect the degree of bone demineralization.
- Administer prescribed calcium preparations to prevent and treat hypocalcemia.
- Administer prescribed phosphate binders to prevent and treat hyperphosphatemia that causes hypocalcemia.
- Provide adequate intake of vitamin D supplements to facilitate GI absorption of calcium to promote bone mineralization.
- Teach patient lifestyle changes, e.g. fall risk reduction, avoiding unsafe practices that may result in traumatic or pathologic fractures.

Adequate coping and understanding about the disease and therapeutic procedure

- Assess patient's psychological status.
- Listen to patient's expression of grief due to the loss of kidney function.
- Convey a caring attitude and provide emotional support to build a relationship with patient.
- Discuss with patient and relatives the ways of handling the situation. Encourage them to actively plan and decide on the future treatment plan, e.g. dialysis or renal transplant together.
- Encourage family members to provide support when the patient is grieving.
- Refer patient to community support group or peer group for counseling.

DIALYSIS

Definition

Dialysis is defined as the movement of fluids and molecules through a semipermeable membrane from one compartment to another.

Clinically dialysis is defined as a technique in which certain substances in the blood move across a semipermeable membrane to the dialysis solution called dialysate.

Purposes

1. To correct fluid and electrolyte imbalances.
2. To remove waste products from the body when the kidneys fail to do so.
3. To remove certain medications and other toxins from the blood in medication overdose or poisoning.

Methods

1. Peritoneal dialysis
2. Hemodialysis.

Principles of Dialysis

The following principles are used to accomplish the goals of dialysis

Diffusion is the passage of solutes or particles from an area of high concentration to an area of low concentration through a semipermeable membrane. In renal failure, urea, creatinine, electrolytes and uric acid move from the blood to the dialysate and thus lower their concentration in blood.

Osmosis is the movement of fluid from an area of lesser solute concentration to an area of greater solute concentration.

Glucose is added to the dialysate to create an osmotic gradient across the semipermeable membrane so that excess fluid in blood is pulled out.

Ultrafiltration refers to removal of water or fluid from the blood either by producing osmotic or hydrostatic gradient. In peritoneal dialysis, osmotic gradient is produced by adding glucose in the dialysate and in hemodialysis, gradient is created by increasing the pressure (positive pressure) in the blood compartments or by lowering pressure in the dialysate compartment (negative pressure).

Peritoneal Dialysis

In peritoneal dialysis, dialysate solution is instilled repeatedly in the peritoneal cavity through an abdominal catheter and is removed after allowing some time for exchange of substances (dwell) between the blood and dialysate.

Advantages

- It is relatively easy to use.
- May be performed in community settings or at home without sophisticated equipments that are necessary for hemodialysis.
- It allows greater mobility and more independence to the patient than that of hemodialysis.

Indication

- Patients with severe cardiovascular system diseases, in whom rapid changes in fluid and solutes concentration that occur with hemodialysis are harmful.
- Diabetic patients with the potential to develop retinal hemorrhage due to heparin use during hemodialysis.
- To achieve good glucose control in diabetics.
- Treatment of choice for children (it does not hamper growth, like hemodialysis).

Contraindication

- Obesity.
- History of multiple abdominal surgical procedures, chronic abdominal disease, e.g. diverticulitis and pancreatitis, recurrent episodes of peritonitis, abdominal malignancies.
- Respiratory disease, e.g. obstructive pulmonary disease.
- Recurrent abdominal or inguinal hernia.
- Severe vascular disease.
- Back pain.

Types of peritoneal dialysis

- **Most common types of peritoneal dialysis are**:

1. Continuous ambulatory peritoneal dialysis.
2. Automated peritoneal dialysis.

- **Continuous ambulatory peritoneal dialysis**:
  - This procedure is carried out by exchanging 1.5 to 3 liter of dialysate (usually 2 liter) at least 4 times daily with dwell times of 4 to 10 hours.
  - The dialysate solution is instilled in to the peritoneal cavity from a collapsible plastic bag through a disposable plastic tube for the prescribed period of time and then drained by gravity flow and a new bag of dialysate solution is instilled.
  - Major advantages of this procedure are:
    1. Continuous exchange process closely resembles normal kidney function resulting in easy maintenance of homeostasis.
    2. There is no need of machinery, electricity and water source.
    3. The patient can perform any desired activity during dialysis.
- **Automated peritoneal dialysis**:
  - Automated peritoneal dialysis requires use of an automated devise

called cycler to deliver the dialysate. The cycler times and controls the fill, dwell and drain phases. The machine cycles 4 or more exchanges at night (when the person is sleeping) with 1 to 2 hours per exchange.
  - In the morning the machine is disconnected. Fluid is usually left in the abdomen during daytime. To ensure adequate dialysis in the daytime 1 or 2 manual exchanges may also be prescribed.
  - Disadvantage of this procedure is that it is difficult to achieve desired clearance of solute and fluid with only nighttime dialysis.
- **Complications of peritoneal dialysis are:**
  1. Exit site infection.
  2. Peritonitis.
  3. Displacement and obstruction of the abdominal catheter.
  4. Abdominal pain.
  5. Lower back pain.
  6. Hernias.
  7. Hypotension or overhydration manifested as pulmonary edema and heart failure.
  8. Hypoalbuminemia.
  9. Hyperglycemia in diabetics.
  10. Encapsulating sclerosing peritonitis and loss of ultrafiltration development of a thick fibrous membrane that surrounds and compresses the bowel for unknown reasons.

Nursing Management

- Explain the patient and the family about the procedure and obtain an informed consent.
- Assess and record baseline vital signs, body weight and serum electrolyte levels.
- Encourage to empty bladder and bowel in order to prevent their injury by catheter insertion.
- Administer antibiotics as ordered.
- Assess anxiety of the patient and provide emotional support and instruction, by remaining with the patient.
- Assemble required administration set, tubing and other articles as required and help the physician in inserting the abdominal catheter.
- Maintain strict aseptic technique during the procedure and during addition of medications to the dialysate as ordered, e.g. heparin, insulin, etc.
- Warm dialysate to body temperature to prevent abdominal pain and discomfort and to dilate the vessels of the peritoneum that increases urea clearance. Do not overheat.
- Teach patient on long-term peritoneal dialysis the care of the catheter, exit site care, exchange procedure, consuming high protein diet (protein is lost with peritoneal dialysis) and adequate fluid intake.

Hemodialysis

Indication

- Acute renal failure requiring short-term dialysis.
- End stage renal disease requiring long-term or permanent therapy.
- Patients with fluid and electrolyte disturbances.
- Remove toxic substances, e.g. overdose of barbiturates from the body.

Procedure

In this procedure patient's blood, rich with toxins and nitrogenous wastes is diverted into a machine, a dialyzer, (artificial kidney) cleaned and then returned to the patient. The dialyzer serves as a synthetic semipermeable membrane, replacing the renal glomeruli and the tubules as the filter for the impaired kidneys. While the blood is circulating in the dialyzer, a mechanical proportioning pump causes dialysis fluid or dialysate to flow on the other side of the semipermeable membrane. Toxins and nitrogenous wastes diffuse across the membrane from the blood to the dialysate. Excess water is removed from the blood by the process of ultrafiltration, which is achieved by applying negative pressure or a suctioning force to the dialysis membrane.

In order to draw blood from the patient and send to the dialyzer vascular access is created. Several types of vascular access used are:

Dialysis catheter: Dialysis catheter is double-lumen large bore catheter that is inserted into internal jugular, subclavian or femoral vein. This is used when immediate access to the bloodstream is required. Catheter may be placed at bedside and may be used immediately after placement. It cannot be used longer than 3 weeks and is associated with infection, thrombosis and venous stenosis.

Arteriovenous fistula: Arteriovenous fistula is the method of choice for long-term dialysis. It is created surgically by joining an artery in the arm to a vein. The resultant fistula between an artery and a vein is allowed to heal and mature (usually for a period of 4–6 weeks) and then used for dialysis. During dialysis 2 large-bore needles are placed in the fistula, one in the arterial side for arterial flow to the dialyzer and the other in the venous segment for reinfusion of the dialyzed blood.

Arteriovenous graft: Arteriovenous graft is created by surgically placing an artificial vein of synthetic or biological material under the skin in the arm, thigh or chest area. This procedure is used when arteriovenous fistula cannot be created. Graft can be used 2 weeks after insertion. Infection, thrombosis and aneursyms are common problems of the graft.

Complications

1. Hypotension due to rapid removal of fluid during dialysis.
2. Painful muscle cramps due to rapid removal of sodium and water from extra-cellular space.
3. Loss of blood due to accidental separation of blood tubing, dislodgement of needles, heparinization and blood being not completely rinsed from the dialyzer.
4. Dysrhythmias resulting from electrolyte and pH changes and by removal of anti-arrhythmic medications during dialysis.
5. Hepatitis B and C may occur due to lack of precautionary measures needed during blood transfusion.
6. Sepsis of vascular access site and bacterial endocarditis may occur due to frequent and prolonged access to the vascular system.
7. Disequilibrium syndrome occurs due to very rapid changes in the composition of the extracellular fluid than in the composition of cerebrospinal fluid. This creates a high osmotic gradient in the brain resulting into fluid shift in the brain, causing cerebral edema. Signs and symptoms of this condition include nausea, vomiting, restlessness, confusion, headache, decreased level of conscious, twitching, jerking and seizures.
8. Air embolism.

NURSING MANAGEMENT

- Explain patient about the procedure.
- Assess patient's body weight, blood

pressure, peripheral edema, heart sounds and lung sounds in order to determine his fluid status before dialysis.
- Assess condition of skin, vascular access site and body temperature for evidence of any infection.
- During dialysis continuously monitor patient's vital signs every 30 minutes in order to detect rapid changes in blood pressure that may occur.
- Provide comfort measures as required as the procedure may continue for 3 to 5 hours.
- Teach patient about dietary modifications and fluid intake according to his condition.
- Provide some recreational equipments, e.g. books, television or music to remove boredom during treatment.
- Assess emotional status of the patient on long-term hemodialysis.
- Encourage patient to ventilate his problem and provide reassurance and support in order to live a productive life as long as possible.

URINARY CALCULI

Definitions

Urinary calculi (urolithiasis) commonly called stones are calcification or crystal aggregations formed anywhere in the urinary system.

Incidence

- More common in men.
- Occurs in 3rd to 5th decades of life.
- Recurrence within 5 years of life in 50% of patients.
- Incidence of kidney stones seems to increase in industrialized countries whereas incidence of bladder stones is more in developing countries.

Classification

Urinary calculi are classified according to their location and chemical composition.

As per location

- Nephrolithiasis refers to stones in the kidney.
- Calyceal refers to stone in the major or minor calyx.
- Ureterolithiasis refers to stones in the ureters.
- Cystolithiasis refers to stones in the urinary bladder.

As per chemical composition

- Oxalate calculus (calcium oxalate)—It is the most common type of stones worldwide. These stones are irregular in shape and covered with sharp projections, which tend to cause bleeding. These stones are radiopaque. Oxalate stones are associated with primary hyperoxaluria.
- Phosphate calculus—A phosphate calculus (calcium phosphate often with ammonium magnesium phosphate or struvite stone) is smooth and dirty white.This type of stone is usually associated with urinary tract infection by urea-splitting bacteria. Commonly seen in women and in persons predisposed to urinary tract infections. These stones grow rapidly and are usually of large size and fill most of the collecting system forming a staghorn calculus. Easily seen in radiographs because of its large size.
- Uric acid and urate stone—These stones are hard, smooth and often multiple. Color varies from yellow to reddish brown. Uric acid-stones are associated with conditions that cause hyperuricosuria (excessive amount

of uric acid in urine) with or without hyperuricemia (excessive amount of uric acid in the serum) and disorder of acid base metabolism resulting in excessively acidic urine. They are radiolucent but may cast a faint radiological shadow if they contain calcium.
- Cystine stone—These stones are associated in people with some inborn errors of metabolism that leads to cystinuria. Hexagonal, translucent, white crystals of cystine appear only in acid urine.

Etiology

Supersaturation of urine

Stones are believed to be formed when urine is supersaturated with poorly soluble crystalloids which may result from—
- Increased solute load.
- Fluid depletion.
- Deficiency of substances that normally prevent crystallization in the urine (inhibitor substances, e.g. citrate, magnesium).
- Abnormal urinary pH (higher pH or alkaline urine predisposes to calcium stones and low pH or acidic urine predisposes to uric acid and cystine stones.

Urinary obstruction, stasis and infection

Urinary tract infections with urea splitting bacteria, e.g. *proteus, Klebsiella, Pseudomonas, Staphylococcus* make urine alkaline and facilitates stone formation. Infected stones are frequently seen in patients with:
- External urinary diversion
- Long-term urinary catheter
- Urinary retention
- Neurogenic bladder
- Bladder neck obstruction
- Prolonged immobilization.

Risk Factors

1. Hot and humid climate leading to dehydration.
2. Immobility, sedentary lifestyle increasing stasis of urine.
3. Metabolic disturbances that increase amount of calcium, uric acid, oxaluric acid, citric acid and other ions in urine.
4. Diet high in animal proteins (increase uric acid excretion), tea or fruit juices (increase urinary oxalate level) and low in calcium and fluids.
5. Excessive intake of calcium supplements, vitamin D, vitamin C.
6. Family history of stone formation, gout.
7. Previous history of urinary calculi.
8. Recurrent urinary tract infections.
9. Metabolic disorders, e.g. renal tubular acidosis, hyperparathyroidism, primary hyperoxaluria, etc.
10. People living in areas where there is excessive fluorine level in water.

Clinical Manifestations

Urinary stones produce variable symptoms

- Silent stone—Stones in the kidney may remain asymptomatic. Large bilateral stones producing no symptoms for long-time may cause destruction of renal parenchyma and uremia or urinary tract infection may be the first manifestation.
- Pain is the most common symptom in persons (75%) with urinary stones.
  - Fixed renal pain located posteriorly in renal angle and anteriorly in the hypochondrium, worse on movement particularly during climbing stairs.
  - Renal colic or ureteric colic is severe agonizing pain passing from loin to groin, penis, scrotum or labium as the stone passes down the ureter or

obstructs a ureter. Pain comes in waves lasting 20 minutes to 60 minutes.

- Nausea and vomiting may be associated with pain.
- Mild shock with cool, moist skin and tachycardia due to severe pain.
- Tenderness on gentle palpation of kidney at costovertebral angle in the affected side.
- Hematuria, pyuria, dysuria and oliguria (if obstruction).
- Elevated body temperature if associated with infection.

Diagnostic Studies

1. Urinalysis—It detects urinary pH, red blood cells, bacteria, leukocytes, urinary casts and crystals.
2. Urine culture detects infecting organisms in the urinary tract and sensitivity to determine the susceptibility of these organisms towards antibiotics.
3. 24 hour urine collection to measure total daily urinary volume, magnesium, sodium, uric acid, calcium, citrate, oxalate and phosphate.
4. Collection of stones by straining urine and analysis of the stones to detect their composition.
5. Complete blood count detects neutrophilia.
6. Renal function test may detect abnormally high blood calcium levels.
7. X-ray of kidney, ureter and bladder detects calcium oxalate, calcium phosphate and magnesium phosphate stones which are radiopaque.
8. Intravenous pyelogram or a retrograde pyelogram (injection of contrast agent followed by a X-ray of kidney, ureter and bladder) confirms the diagnosis.
9. CT scan if available can detect almost all types of stones and gives a clearer idea of the size and location of the stone.
10. Ultrasound imaging of the kidneys gives details about the presence of hydronephrosis which suggests that the stone is blocking the outflow of urine. It also reveals presence of radiolucent stones which are not detected by CT or plain X-ray of KUB.

Management

Medical management

- When stones are small and not causing considerable obstruction or associated infection various nonsurgical measures may be employed to facilitate the passage of the stones and to prevent stone recurrence:
- Analgesics—It is intravenous administration of NSAIDs or opioids or acetaminophen are given to control the acute attack of pain. Analgesics may be administered orally in less severe pain.
- Antispasmodic agents may also be given to control colic pain resulting from spasms of the ureter.

Medications

- Thiazide diuretics inhibit the formation of calcium containing stones by reducing urinary calcium excretion.
- Acetazolamide (diamox) alkalinizes (increasing the pH) the urine and prevents formation of uric acid stone.
- Certain dietary supplements, e.g. sodium bicarbonate, potassium citrate, sodium citrate and magnesium citrate alkalinizes urine and prevents uric acid stone formation. Increased citrate concentration also reduces the aggregation of calcium oxalate stones.
- Allopurinol is used in the treatment of uric acid stone in persons in whom hyperuricosuria and hyperuricemia persists despite the use of urine alkalinizing agents.

- Antibiotics administered for long-term to prevent struvite stone formation.

Dietary modifications

- Increased fluid intake of 3 to 4 liters per day to maintain a urine output of 2 to 3 liters facilitates passage of small stones, prevents formation of new stones by decreasing the concentration of solutes and also prevents infection. The kind of fluid depends on dietary restrictions of the patient but at least 50% of fluid should be water.
- Increased intake of dietary calcium, reduced intake of protein and sodium is believed to prevent calcium stone formation.
- Avoid high oxalate foods, e.g. tomatoes, tea, cola drinks, beer, spinach, cabbage, chocolate, peanuts, apples, grapes, etc. and a high intake of supplemental vitamin C to prevent oxalate stones.
- Avoid high purine diet, e.g. wine, bony fish and organ meat to reduce the risk of uric acid stones.

Surgical management

Most urinary calculi can be treated nowadays by minimal access techniques. More invasive open surgery may also be required where facilities or expertise for such techniques are lacking.

Percutaneous nephrolithotomy: Through the soft tissue of the loin a hollow needle is inserted into the renal parenchyma through which nephroscope is passed to visualize the stone. Small stones may be grasped under vision and extracted whole and larger stones are fragmented by an ultrasound, electrohydraulic or laser probe and removed in pieces. A nephrostomy drain is left in place to decompress the kidney and to allow repeated access if stone particles remain.

- Complications
  - Profuse bleeding from punctured renal parenchyma.
  - Perforation of the collecting system.
  - Perforation of the colon or pleural cavity during placement of the hollow needle.

Extracorporeal shock wave lithotripsy (ESWL): A lithotriptor machine is used to deliver externally-applied, focussed, shock waves or high intensity pulses of ultrasonic energy to fragment the stone over a period of 30 to 60 minutes. Since shock-waves are poorly transmitted through air both the patient and the shock-wave generator are placed over a bath of water. Fragmented stones are passed down the ureters if ESWL is successful.

- Complications
  - Acute trauma resulting in internal bleeding and subcapsular hematoma.
  - Infection from bacteria released from fragmented stone.
  - Ureteric colic and obstruction from a bulky stone fragment.

Open surgery

Operations for removal of kidney stones are usually performed via a loin or lumbar approach.

Pyelolithotomy: Involves incision into the renal pelvis for the removal of stone from the kidney pelvis. Incision is given directly on the stone and the stone is removed with gallstone forceps taking care not to break it. If there is no infection pelvic incision is closed with absorbable sutures. If infection, a drain is placed through nephrostomy to drain the system.

Nephrolithotomy: Involves incision into the kidney parenchyma to remove a stone.

It is indicated when a complex calculus branching into the most peripheral calyces (staghorn stone).

Partial nephrectomy: Removal of a part of the kidney may be necessary when the stone is present in the lowermost calyx and there is associated damage to the surrounding parenchyma.

Nephrectomy: Removal of a kidney may be indicated when the kidney is destroyed with infection and obstruction associated with stone disease.

Ureterolithotomy: It is the incision into the ureter to remove a stone.

Cystolithotomy: Involves incision into the bladder to remove a stone.

NURSING MANAGEMENT

Assessment

Subjective data

Acute, severe, colicky pain in flank, back, abdomen passing down to groin or genitalia, nausea, vomiting, fever, chills, decreased urinary output, blood in urine, urinary urgency, frequency, feeling of fullness in bladder, burning, dysuria.

Chronic urinary tract infection, urinary obstruction, enlarged prostate, prolonged bed rest, gout, previous urinary stones, hyperparathyroidism, chronic diarrhea, intake of excessive animal proteins, oxalates, excessive calcium supplementation, low intake of dietary calcium, low fluid intake.

Objective data

Tenderness, guarding on palpation in the renal areas, fever, dehydration, warm flushed skin or cool moist skin and pallor, oliguria, hematuria, passage of stones in urine.

Possible findings

RBCs, WBCs, pus, casts, crystals, bacteria on urinalysis. Elevated levels of uric acid, calcium, phosphorus, oxalate, or cystine values in 24 hour urine sample, increased blood urea and serum creatinine level, anatomic abnormality or presence of stone in intravenous pyelogram or on X-ray of KUB.

Nursing Diagnoses

1. Acute pain related to irritation and spasms from stone movement in the urinary tract as evidenced by patient's verbal complaints, restlessness.
2. Altered urinary elimination related to trauma, infection or blockage in the urinary tract from stones as evidenced by hematuria, oliguria, dysuria and frequency.
3. Ineffective therapeutic regimen management related to knowledge deficit regarding prevention of recurrent stone formation as evidenced by questioning about self-care to cure from disease and further attack.
4. Fear and anxiety regarding the planned surgical methods of stone removal if any as evidenced by anxious look, insomnia and frequent questioning about prognosis.
5. Risk for injury related to the surgery and postoperative complications.

GOALS

1. Relief of pain.
2. Achieving optimum urine flow.
3. Understanding of disease process and preventive measures.
4. Alleviating fear and anxiety about the surgical procedures.
5. Prevention and early detection of injury and postoperative complications.

Nursing Interventions

Relief of pain

- Perform a thorough assessment of patient's pain, the severity, location and type. Use a pain scale and record data for future evaluation.
- Administer analgesics, antispasmodics and antiemetics as ordered by the physician.
- Administer analgesics on a regular schedule and do not allow pain to become severe.
- Teach patient to use relaxation technique, e.g. guided imagery, therapeutic or healing touch along with pain medication to achieve better pain relief and to reduce the dose of medication.

Achieving optimum urine flow

- Monitor urine for amount, frequency, dysuria, odor, hematuria, and passage of stone to determine the status of urinary function and also to evaluate the effect of treatment if any.
- Encourage patient to drink at least 2 to 3 liters of fluid per day to maintain hydration, increase volume of urine and passage of small stones and bacteria if any.
- Encourage patient to ambulate as ambulation promotes passage of stones.
- Teach patient the sign and symptoms of infection and obstruction and report immediately if any.

Understanding of disease process and preventive measures

- Assess patient's existing knowledge about the disease, treatment regimen planned for him and self-care in order to plan an effective teaching program.
- Teach patient the disease process, help him to identify any precipitating factors for stone formation, e.g. sedentary lifestyle, immobility, low intake of water, low calcium and oxalate containing diet, metabolic diseases, etc. to prevent recurrence of stone formation.
- Describe the rationale behind treatment regimen, e.g. use of analgesics and antispasmodics, Thiazide diuretics, allopurinol or any surgical intervention for better compliance.

Alleviating fear and anxiety about the surgical intervention

- Discuss with patient about the surgical procedures planned for him. Reinforce information provided by the physician.
- Discuss preoperative care, operative and postoperative expectations, e.g. flank incision, placement of nephrostomy tube, etc. with the patient.
- Reassure patient that all possible care will be taken for the patient.
- Introduce him with patients recovering from surgeries for urinary stones.

Prevention and early detection of injury and postoperative complications

- Encourage patient to increase fluid intake after surgical intervention to wash out possible stone fragments.
- Assess patient's vital signs for evidence of internal bleeding and urine for amount, color, odor, stone fragments, etc. to detect any injury caused by the surgical intervention.
- Monitor drainage from the nephrostomy/ureterostomy/suprapubic and urethral catheters if any for amount, color, consistency and chemical sediment. Monitor the patency of all drain-

age tubes and record the output of every individual catheter every hour for the first 24 hours and then every 4 to 8 hours until removal.

- Report a total urine output of .5 mL/kg/hour or a lack of output from urethral catheters for more than 15 minutes immediately.
- Take care so that the catheters are not dislodged by securing the tube with patient's skin with tape.
- Maintain strict asepsis while checking the patency of the tubes or during irrigation of the tubes if ordered.
- Teach and encourage patient to take deep breaths 10 to 20 times each hour to prevent respiratory complications if the patient has undergone an open operation.

9

Nursing Management of Patients with Disorders of Endocrine System

NURSING ASSESSMENT OF PATIENT WITH ENDOCRINE DISORDERS

Subjective Data

During an assessment ask the patient about any general state of health, if there are any specific changes.

Medications

Ask about use of medications, the drug, dose, and the length of time taken. Patient should be specifically asked about the use of hormone replacements such as insulin, thyroid, or corticosteroid, e.g. corticosteroid may cause glucose intolerance in the susceptible patient by increase glycogenolysis and insulin resistance.

Surgery or other treatment

Enquire about previous hospitalization, surgery, and chemotherapy and radiation therapy. Surgery of the brain or a severe blow to the head could have resulted in pituitary or hypothalamic alternations.

Nutritional and metabolic pattern—a major function of the endocrine system is regulating metabolism and maintaining homeostasis, the patient with endocrine dysfunction will often experience alternations in nutritional metabolic pattern. Report changes in appetite and weight can indicate endocrine dysfunction. Weight loss with increase appetite may indicate hyperthyroidism or DM (Type I). Weight loss with decrease appetite may indicate hypopituitarism, hypocortisolism. Difficulty in swallowing or change in neck size may indicate a thyroid disorder or inflammation. Hair loss can indicate hypopituitarism, hypothyroidism, and hypoparathyroidsm.

Elimination

Ask about increase thirst and urination that can indicate diabetes mellitus or insipidus. Ask the patient about the frequency and consistency of bowel movements. Frequent defecation may indicate hyperthyroidism. Constipation is seen in patients with DM, hypothyroidsm, hypoparathyroidism and hypopituitarism.

Activity and exercise

Ask history of fatigue hyperactivity are two common problems associated with endocrine problems.

Sleep

Rest obtain a detailed history. Sleep disturbances are frequently seen in endocrine dysfunction.

Objective Data

On physical examination.

Vital signs

Variations in temperature may be associated with thyroid function. Tachycardia, bradycardia, hypotension or hypertension may be seen in variety of endocrine related problems.

Height and weight

Growth patterns abnormalities suggest problems associated with growth hormone. Changes in weight also may be associated with endocrine dysfunction.

Mental emotional status

Assess patient's orientation, alertness, memory, affect, personality, anxiety and appropriateness of dress and speech. Endocrine disorders can cause changes in mental and emotional status.

Integument

Note the color and texture of the skin, hair hand nails. Inspect the skin for pigmentation and positive ecchymosis. Hyperpigmentation is a classic finding but also seen in ACTH producing tumors and acromegaly. Palpate the skin for texture and presence of moisture.

Hair

Should be examined for texture and appearance. Dull or brittle, hair, excessive hair growth, hair loss may indicate endocrine dysfunction.

Head

Inspect the size and contour of the head. Facial features should be symmetric. Inspect the eyes for position, symmetry, shape, eye movements, opacity over the lens, lid lag and edema. Puffiness of face periorbital edema.

Neck

Generalized enlargement of the thyroid gland. Localized enlargement of the thyroid gland.

Diagnostic Tests

Laboratory studies used to diagnose endocrine problems that include direct measurement of the hormone level or they may involve an indirect indication of the gland function by evaluating blood or urine components affected by the hormone.

Pituitary studies

- Growth hormone (somatotrophin) evaluates GH secretion. Identify GH deficiency or excess.
- Gonadotrophin levels—Follicle-stimulating hormone (FSH), luteinizing hormone (LH) useful in distinguishing primary gonadal problems from pituitary insuffic iency.
- Prolactin levels—Decreased levels in postpartum women.
- Radiology: MRI—Useful in identification of tumors involving the hypothalamus or pituitary.

Thyroid studies

- Serum studies—Thyroid-stimulating hormone (TSH). The most sensitive method for evaluating thyroid disease.
- Thyroxine (T4) Total—Measures total serum level of T4, useful in evaluating thyroid function and monitoring thyroid therapy.

- Triiodothyronine (T3)—Measures serum level of T3. Helpful in diagnosing hyperthyroidism if T4 levels are normal.
- Radiology: Ultrasound—It evaluates thyroid nodules to determine if fluid filled (cystic) or solid tumor.
  - Radioactive iodine uptake (RAU) provides direct measurement of functional activity of solitary thyroid.
  - Thyroid scan Used to evaluate nodules of the thyroid.
  - Parathyroid hormone Measures PTH level in serum.

Parathyroid studies

Total serum calcium—to help to detect bone and parathyroid disorders. Hypercalcemia indicate primary hyperparathyroidism and hypocalcemia can indicate hypoparathyroidism.

Adrenal studies

- **Serum studies**
  - Cortisol—It evaluates status of adrenal cortex function.
  - Aldosterone—It evaluates hyper aldosteronism.
  - Adrenocorticotrophic hormone (ACTH), corticotrophin— Measures thc plasma level of ACTH.
  - ACTH suppression (dexamethasone suppression)—Assess adrenal function and specially helpful if hyperactivity is suspected. Useful in evaluation of Cushing's syndrome.
- **Urine studies**
  - 17 ketosteroids—Measures androgen metabolites in urine and evalutes adrenocortical and gonadal function.
  - Aldosterone—Measures urinary aldosterone level evaluate adrenal function. Useful in determining therapy for hypertension.
  - Free cortisol—Measures free (unbound) cortisol. Preferred test to evaluate hypercortisolism.
- **Radiology**
  CT scan—Abdominal CT scan is the radiologic examination of choice for the adrenal gland. Used to detect tumor and size of tumor mass or metastatic spread.

Pancreatic studies

- **Serum studies**
  - Fasting blood glucose level—Measures circulating glucose level.
  - Oral glucose tolerance. The 2 hour test is used to diagnose diabetes mellitus if fasting blood sugar is equivocal. Patient drinks 75 gm of glucose; samples for glucose are drawn immediately and at 30,60 and 120 minutes.
  - Capillary glucose monitoring—It is used to give immediate glucose oxidase or electrochemical methods.
  - Glycosylated Hb%—Measures degree of glucose control during previous 3 months.
- **Urine studies**
  - Glucose—It estimate amount of glucose in urine.
  - Ketones—Measures amount of acetone excreted in urine as a result of incomplete fat metabolism. Normal value is negative or trace ketone. Positive result can indicate lack of insulin and diabetic acidosis.
- **Radiology**
  CT scan—Abdominal CT scan is used to identify tumors or cysts.

DIABETES MELLITUS

Definition

- Diabetes mellitus is a group of metabolic diseases characterized by high blood sugar (glucose) levels, which result from defects in insulin secretion, or action, or both.
- Diabetes mellitus, commonly referred to as diabetes was first identified as a

disease associated with 'sweet urine,' and excessive muscle loss in the ancient world. Elevated levels of blood glucose (hyperglycemia) leads to spillage of glucose into the urine, hence the term sweet urine.

Causes

- Insufficient production of insulin (either absolutely or relative to the body's needs), production of defective insulin (which is uncommon), or the inability of cells to use insulin properly and efficiently leads to hyperglycemia and diabetes.
- The condition affects mostly the cells of muscle and fat tissues, and results in a condition known as 'insulin resistance.' This is the primary problem in type 2 diabetes.
- The absolute lack of insulin, usually secondary to a destructive process affecting the insulin producing beta cells in the pancreas, is the main disorder in type 1 diabetes.
- In type 2 diabetes, there is a steady decline of beta cells that adds to the process of elevated blood sugars. Essentially, if someone is resistant to insulin, the body can, to some degree, increase production of insulin and overcome the level of resistance. After time, if production decreases and insulin cannot be released as vigorously, hyperglycemia develops

Etiology and Classification

- There are two major types of diabetes, called type 1 and type 2.
- Type 1 diabetes is also called insulin-dependent diabetes mellitus (IDDM), or juvenile onset diabetes mellitus.
- In type 1 diabetes, the pancreas undergoes an autoimmune attack by the body itself, and is rendered incapable of making insulin.
- Abnormal antibodies have been found in the majority of patients with type 1 diabetes. Antibodies are proteins in the blood that are part of the body's immune system. The patient with type 1 diabetes must rely on insulin medication for survival.
- Exposure to certain viral infections (mumps and Coxsackie viruses) or other environmental toxins may serve to trigger abnormal antibody responses that cause damage to the pancreas cells where insulin is made.
- Type 1 diabetes tends to occur in young, lean individuals, usually before 30 years of age, however, older patients do present with this form of diabetes on occasion.
- This subgroup is referred to as latent autoimmune diabetes in adults (LADA). LADA is a slow, progressive form of type 1 diabetes. Of all the patients with diabetes, only approximately 10% of the patients have type 1 diabetes and the remaining 90% have type 2 diabetes.
- Type 2 diabetes was also referred to as noninsulin dependent diabetes mellitus (NIDDM), or adult onset diabetes mellitus (AODM).
- In type 2 diabetes, patients can still produce insulin, but do so relatively inadequately for their body's needs. In many cases this actually means the pancreas produces larger than normal quantities of insulin. A major feature of type 2 diabetes is a lack of sensitivity to insulin by the cells of the body (particularly fat and muscle cells).
- Diabetes occurs much more frequently in women with a prior history of diabetes that develops during pregnancy (gestational diabetes). Diabetes can occur temporarily during pregnancy. Significant hormonal changes during pregnancy can lead to blood sugar elevation in genetically predisposed individuals.

- 'Secondary' diabetes refers to elevated blood sugar levels from another medical condition. Secondary diabetes may develop when the pancreatic tissue responsible for the production of insulin is destroyed by disease, such as chronic pancreatitis, trauma, or surgical removal of the pancreas.
- Diabetes can also result from other hormonal disturbances, such as excessive growth hormone production (acromegaly) and Cushing's syndrome.
- Certain medications may worsen diabetes control, or 'unmask' latent diabetes. This is seen most commonly when steroid medications (such as prednisone) are taken and also with medications used in the treatment of HIV infection (AIDS).

Clinical Manifestations

- Polyuria, polyphagia and polydipsia.
- Elevated blood sugar levels and loss of glucose in the urine.
- Weight loss despite an increase in appetite.
- Fatigue, nausea and vomiting.
- Patients with diabetes are prone to developing infections of the bladder, skin, and vaginal areas.
- Fluctuations in blood glucose levels can lead to blurred vision. Extremely elevated glucose levels can lead to lethargy and coma.

Diagnostic Tests

1. Fasting blood glucose (sugar)
   - After the person has fasted overnight (at least 8 hours), a single sample of blood is drawn and sent to the laboratory for analysis.
   - Normal fasting plasma glucose levels are less than 100 milligrams per deciliter (mg/dL).
   - Fasting plasma glucose levels of more than 126 mg/dL on two or more tests on different days indicate diabetes.
2. A random blood glucose test can also be used to diagnose diabetes. A blood glucose level of 200 mg/dL or higher indicates diabetes.
3. When fasting blood glucose stays above 100 mg/dL, but in the range of 100 to 126 mg/dL, this is known as impaired fasting glucose (IFG).
4. The oral glucose tolerance test:
   The oral glucose tolerance test (OGTT) is a gold standard for making the diagnosis of type 2 diabetes.
   - With an oral glucose tolerance test, the person fasts overnight (at least eight but not more than 16 hours).
   - Then first, the fasting plasma glucose is tested. After this test, the person receives 75 gm of glucose (100 gm for pregnant women).
   - Blood samples are taken at specific intervals to measure the blood glucose.
   - The classic oral glucose tolerance test measures blood glucose levels five times over a period of three hours. A baseline blood sample taken followed by a sample two hours after drinking the glucose solution.
   - In a person without diabetes, the glucose levels rise and then fall quickly. In someone with diabetes, glucose levels rise higher than normal and fail to come back down as fast.
5. Glycosylated hemoglobin: The term HbA1c is referred to as an A1c. The A1c is an average blood glucose level measured over the previous 3 months.
6. Glycosylated albumin: The concentration of glycosylated albumin (fructosamine) represents the average blood glucose level over the previous 7 to 10 days.
7. Ketonuria: Presence of ketones in the urine indicates that the body is using

fat as a major source of energy, which may result in ketoacidosis.

Management

Goals

Restoring and maintaining blood glucose levels to as near normal as possible by balancing diet, exercise and the use of oral hypoglycemic agents or insulin.

1. Regulate blood glucose—Promote proper nutrition.
   - Specific goals are—
     - Improving blood glucose and lipid levels.
     - Providing consistency in day to day food intake.
     - Facilitating weight management.
     - Providing adequate nutrition for all stages of life.
2. Promote regular physical activity—Exercise lowers blood glucose by increasing CHO metabolism, fosters weight reduction and maintenance, increase insulin sensitivity, increase HDL, decrease triglycerides, lowers BP and redness stress and tension.
3. Administer medications—**Oral anti-diabetes Agents**: Pharmacologic interventions should be considered when the client cannot achieve normal or near normal blood glucose levels with nutrition and exercise therapies.

- Indications—
  - RBS levels less than 300 mg/dL
  - Fasting blood sugar less than 250 mg/dL
  - Inadequate control after exercise and diet therapies.
- Medications—
  - Sulfonyl urea (OHA)
  - Megutinedes (OHA)
  - Biguanides (insulin sensitizers)
  - Thiazolidinediones(insulin sensitizers).
- Insulin therapy—
  - Clients with type 1 DM do not produce enough insulin to sustain life.
  - They depend on exogenous insulin administration on a daily basis.
  - In contrast, clients with type 2 DM are not dependent on exogenous insulin for survival.
- Sources—
  - Pork pancreas
  - Made chemically by recombinant DNA technology (rapid, short, intermediate and long-acting).
- Action Insulin works to lower blood glucose by promoting the transport of glucose into cells, and by inhibiting the conversion of glycogen and amino acids to glucose.
- Rapid acting—Insulin lispro (humalog) and insulin aspart(novolog) are used in the management of clients with type 1 and type 2DM.
  - Humalog and novolog are available as premixed insulin containing both rapid acting and an intermediate acting component.
  - Humalog mix 75/25 contains 75% insulin lispro in a crystalline protamine form (intermediate-acting, and 25% soluble (rapid-acting) insulin lispro.
  - Novomix 70/30 contains a mixture of 70% insulin as part as the crystalline protamine form (intermediate-acting) and 30% soluble (rapid-acting) insulin aspart.
  - Administration of a mixture of insulin produces a more normal glycemia in clients than use of single insulin.
  - When rapid acting insulin is mixed with an intermediate or long-acting insulin, the insulin should be injected within 15 minutes before a meal.
  - Insulin dosage: A simple regimen with fixed doses may be used at first. The starting dose of insulin is 0.5 unit/kg/day. 2/3rd of the dose is commonly given in the morning and 1/3rd is given in the evening.

Complications

Acute complications

1. Diabetic ketoacidosis (DKA) referred to as diabeteic acidosis and diabetic coma, is caused by a profound deficiency of insulin and is characterized by:
   - Hyperglycemia
   - Ketosis
   - Acidosis
   - Dehydration
   - Common in patients with Type I DM but may also be seen in type 2 in conditions of severe illness or stress when the pancreas cannot meet the extra demand for insulin.

Precipitating Factors

- Illness and infection
- Inadequate insulin dosage
- Undiagnosed type 1 DM
- Poor self-management
- Neglect.

Pathophysiology

- When the circulating supply of insulin is insufficient, glucose cannot be properly used for energy so that the body breaks down fat stores as a secondary source of fuel.
- Ketones are acidic by products of fat metabolism that can cause serious problems when they become excessive in the blood.
- Ketones alters the pH balance, causing metabolic acidosis to develop. Ketonuria is a process that begins when ketone bodies are excreted in the urine.
- During this process, electrolytes become depleted as cations are eliminated along with the anionic ketones in an attempt to maintain electrical neutrality.
- Insulin deficiency impairs protein synthesis and causes excessive protein degradation.
- Insulin deficiency also stimulates the production of glucose from amino acids (from protein) in the liver and leads to further hyperglycemia.
- As there is a deficiency of insulin, the additional glucose cannot be used and the blood glucose level rises further adding to the osmotic dieresis.
- Untreated condition leads to severe depletion of Na^+, K^+, Cl^-, Mg^{++}, PO_4^-.
- Vomiting caused by the acidosis results in more fluids and electrolytes losses. Eventually, hypovolemia followed by shock will occur.
- Renal failure may eventually occur from hypovolemic shock. This causes the retention of ketones and glucose and the acidosis progress.
- Untreated condition leads to dehydration, electrolyte imbalance,and acidosis.
- If the condition is not treated, death is inevitable.

Clinical Manifestations

- Dry mouth
- Thirst
- Abdominal pain
- Nausea and vomiting
- Gradually increase restlessness
- Confusion
- Lethargy
- Flushed dry skin
- Sunken eyes
- Breath odor of ketones
- Kussmaul's respiration.

Laboratory Findings

- Blood glucose level: More than 300 mg/dL.
- ABG: pH: less than 7.3, $NaHCO_3$: 15 mEq/L
- Ketones present in blood and urine.

Management (Table 9.1)

See Table 9.1 for management of acute complication of diabetes mellitus.

Table 9.1: Management of acute complications of diabetes mellitus

Emergency management	Ongoing monitoring
• Ensure patent airway • Administer oxygen via nasal cannula or a nonbreather mask • Establish IV access with a large bore cannula • Begin fluid resuscitation with 0.9% NaCl solution 1 L/hour until BP increases and urinary output 30–60 mL/hr • Begin continuous regular insulin drip 0.1 U/kg/hr • Identify history of DM, time of last food, and time/ amount of last insulin injection	• Monitor vital signs, level of consciousness, cardiac rhythm, O_2 saturation and urine output • Assess breath sounds for fluid overload • Monitor serum glucose and serum K^+ • Administer K^+ to correct hypokalemia • Administer $NaHCO_3$ if severe acidosis (pH<7.0)

2. A hyperosmolar coma usually occurs in elderly patients with type 2 diabetes. Like diabetic ketoacidosis, a hyperosmolar coma is a medical emergency. Immediate treatment with intravenous fluid and insulin is important in reversing the hyperosmolar state.
3. Hypoglycemia
   - In patients with diabetes, the most common cause of low blood sugar is excessive use of insulin or other glucose-lowering medications.
   - When low blood sugar levels occur because of too much insulin, it is called an insulin reaction.
   - Blood glucose is essential for the proper functioning of brain cells. Therefore, low blood sugar can lead to central nervous system symptoms such as: dizziness, confusion, weakness and tremors.

Chronic Complications

- Diabetes complications are related to blood vessel diseases and are generally classified into small vessel disease; microvascular complications), such as those involving the eyes (diabetic retinopathy), kidneys (diabetic nephropathy) and nerves (diabetic neuropathy).
- Large vessel disease involving the heart and blood vessels (macrovascular complications). Diabetes accelerates (atherosclerosis) of the larger blood vessels, leading to coronary heart disease (angina or heart attack), strokes, and pain in the lower extremities because of lack of blood supply (claudication).

NURSING MANAGEMENT

Nursing Assessment

Subjective data

Past history of mumps, rubella, coxsackievirus or other viral infections, recent trauma, infection or stress, pregnancy, cushing's disease, family history of type 1 and type 2 diabetes mellitus. Use of and compliance with insulin or oral hypoglycemic drugs.

History of any recent surgeries, obesity weight loss (type 1), weight gain (type 2), thirst, hunger, nausea, vomiting. Complain of constipation or diarrhea, frequent urination, nocturia, skin infections. Presence of muscle weakness, fatigue, abdominal pain, headache, blurred vision, numbness, frequent vaginal infections, depression, irritability.

Objective data

- Eye: Soft, sunken eyeballs, vitreal hemorrhage, cataracts.
- Integumentary: Dry, warm inelastic skin, pigmented lesions; ulcers, loss of hair or toes.
- Respiratory: Rapid, deep respirations.
- Cardiovascular: Hypotension; weak rapid pulse.
- Gastrointestinal: Dry mouth, vomiting, fruity breath.
- Neurologic: Altered reflexes, restlessness, confusion, stupor, coma.
- Musculoskeletal: Muscle wasting.

Nursing Diagnoses

- Imbalanced nutrition more than body requirements related to intake in excess of activity expenditure as evidenced by hyperglycemia, weight gain.
- Ineffective therapeutic regimen management related to insufficient knowledge as evidenced by continued hyperglycemia inaccurate statements regarding diabetes and its management.
- Risk for injury related to decrease tactile sensation, episodes of hypoglycemia.
- Risk for peripheral neurovascular dysfunction related to vascular effects of diabetes.

PLANNING OUTCOMES/GOALS

- Maintains a balance of nutrition.
- Describes self-care measures that may prevent or decrease progression of chronic complications.
- Experiences no injury resulting from decreased sensation in feet.
- Implements measures to increase peripheral circulatory status.

Nursing Interventions

Maintains a balance of nutrition

- Monitor nutritional intake along with blood glucose, urine ketones and daily weight.
- Plan a diet for the patient with the primary goal of glucose control.
- Give small meals at frequent interval.
- Assess the signs of hypoglycemia.
- Monitor signs of diabetic ketoacidosis if there is prolonged elevated glucose levels, laboratory values and patient's physical condition.

Describes self-care measures that may prevent or decrease progression of chronic complications

- Educate the patient to monitor blood glucose at regular intervals.
- Advice the patient to take prescribed insulin or oral hypoglycemic drugs as ordered.
- Prescribe diabetic diet plan.
- Encourage the patient for regular exercise and rest.
- Educate the patient to monitor and report high blood glucose level to prevent chronic complications.

Experiences of no injury resulting from decreased sensation in feet

- Assess the skin daily for any dryness or breaks.
- Give foot care with warm water and soap.
- Keep the feet dry and advice him to wear soft shoes to prevent any cut.
- Elevate the foot end of the patient having history of neuropathy to improve venous return.
- Treat dermal ulcers as indicated and prescribed.
- Promote optimal blood glucose control in patients with skin breakdown.

Implements measures to increase peripheral circulatory status

- Assess the peripheral pulses.
- Check any discoloration of the skin or presence of dermal ulcer.
- Elevate the foot end of the patient with peripheral neuropathy. Administer insulin or oral hypoglycemic agents as indicated.
- Report prolonged hyperglycemia to prevent further complications.

PITUITARY DISORDERS

The pituitary gland is a tiny organ, the size of a pea, found at the base of the brain. As the master gland of the body, it produces and secretes many hormones that travel throughout the body, directing certain processes stimulating other glands to produce different types of hormones. The pituitary gland controls biochemical processes important to our well-being.

The pituitary gland makes these types of hormones:

Prolactin

Prolactin stimulates milk production from the breasts after childbirth to enable nursing. It also affects sex hormone levels from ovaries in women and from testes in men.

Growth Hormone (GH)

GH stimulates growth in childhood and is important for maintaining a healthy body composition and well-being in adults. In adults it is important for maintaining muscle mass as well as bone mass. It also affects fat distribution in the body.

Adrenocorticotropic Hormone (ACTH)

ACTH stimulates the production of cortisol by the adrenal glands. Cortisol, a so-called 'stress hormone' is vital to our survival. It helps to maintain blood pressure and blood glucose levels.

Thyroid-stimulating Hormone (TSH)

TSH stimulates the thyroid gland, which regulates the body's metabolism, energy, growth, and nervous system activity. This hormone is also vital to our survival.

Antidiuretic Hormone (ADH)

ADH, also called vasopressin, regulates water balance. If this hormone is not released properly, it can lead to too little hormone (called diabetes insipidus), or too little hormone (called syndrome of inappropriate ADH).

Luteinizing Hormone (LH)

LH regulates testosterone in men and estrogen in women.

Follicle-stimulating Hormone (FSH)

FSH promotes sperm production in men and stimulates the ovaries to enable ovulation in women. Luteinizing hormone and follicle-stimulating hormone work together to cause normal function of the ovaries and testes.

Pituitary Tumors

- Cause of pituitary disorders is pituitary gland tumors. The pituitary gland is made of several cell types. Sometimes these cells grow too much or produce small growths.
- These growths are called pituitary tumors, and they are common in adults. These are not brain tumors and are not a form of cancer. Pituitary tumors can interfere with the normal formation and release of hormones.

Types of Tumors

- Secretory and nonsecretory tumors.
- Secretory tumors produce too much of a hormone, creating an imbalance of proper hormones in the body.
- Nonsecretory tumors cause problems because of their large size or because they interfere with normal function of the pituitary gland.

Pathophysiology

Hypersecretion

- Too much of any hormone secreted into the body is usually caused by a secretory pituitary gland tumor.
- Many secretory tumors make too much prolactin, the hormone that triggers milk production in new mothers. Other tumors may affect the adrenal glands, making too much of the hormones that stimulate them and causing a hormone imbalance.
- Tumors also can make excess growth hormone or too much of the hormone that stimulates the thyroid gland leading to overproduction of thyroid hormones.

Hyposecretion

- Too little of any hormone secreted into the body is usually caused by a nonsecretory pituitary gland tumor, which interferes with the ability of the normal pituitary gland to create hormones.
- It can also be caused by a large secretory tumor. Hyposecretion can also happen with surgery or the radiation of a pituitary gland tumor.

Tumor mass effects

- As a pituitary gland tumor grows and presses against the normal pituitary gland or other areas in the brain, it may cause headaches, vision problems, or other health effects related to hyposecretion.
- Tumor mass effects can be seen in any type of pituitary tumor that grows large enough. Injuries, certain medications, and other conditions can also affect the pituitary gland.

Secretory Tumors

- Prolactinoma—A prolactinoma is the most common, accounting for about 40% of pituitary gland tumors.
  - This is a tumor on the pituitary gland that produces too much prolactin, the milk hormone.
  - While excess milk discharge from breasts is one of the symptoms of a prolactinoma, there are many other signs of this kind of tumor.

Symptoms

- Changes in menstrual cycle or complete loss of periods.
- Headaches.
- Infertility.
- Milk discharge from breasts that is unrelated to giving birth.
- Problems with vision.
- Vaginal dryness or pain during intercourse.
- Reduced sex drive.
- Osteoporosis or bone loss.
- Inadequate function of the testes in males leading to the inability to get or maintain an erection.
- Infertility.

Treatment

- About 80%–90% of prolactinoma patients can be treated successfully with a dopamine agonist drug.

- The use of this drug eliminate or reduce symptoms of a high prolactin level, return prolactin levels to normal, help restore normal function to the pituitary, and usually reduce the pituitary gland tumor size.
- Radiation therapy is rarely used with large tumors.
- Some patients with very small tumors, which are stable in size and do not have any associated symptoms, may be monitored carefully without treatment.

Acromegaly and Gigantism

- Acromegaly is a rare disease caused by a noncancerous tumor in the pituitary gland.
- The disease is caused by the hypersecretion of growth hormones and the ensuing hormone imbalance.
- It affects metabolism, affects the cardiac system, glucose metabolism, joints, and bones.
- Symptoms of acromegaly may evolve slowly, overtime.
- Indications of acromegaly usually begin between the ages of 30 and 50 and give rise to changes in physical appearance.

Gigantism is similar to acromegaly but occurs in children. When the condition begins at a young age, before a child's growth plates have closed, that child may grow to be unusually tall. Puberty may be delayed in children with this disorder.

Symptoms

- Interrupted menstrual cycle.
- Deepening of the voice.
- Impotence or the inability to get or maintain an erection.
- Oily skin or acne.
- Coarser facial features such as a noticeably large nose.
- Excessive sweating.
- Teeth that are spreading out.
- Enlarged hands, feet, head, nose, and jaw.
- Enlarged tongue and sleep apnea, which is interrupted breathing while sleeping.
- Small growths of skin that are called skin tags.
- Memory loss or not being able to think clearly.
- Thicker flesh on the palms and feet.
- High blood pressure.
- Fatigue.
- Headaches.
- Carpal tunnel syndrome resulting in achy wrists and hands.
- Osteoarthritis or bone loss.
- Colon polyps or growths
- Peripheral vision defects causing an inability to see well at the edges of your vision.
- Reduced sex drive.

Treatment

a. Surgery is done through a procedure called transsphenoidal microsurgery. The surgery is performed through the sinus passages behind the nose. Removing or reducing the pituitary tumor that causes acromegaly will reduce growth hormone levels and relieve the pressure caused by the tumor mass. A craniotomy may be required on very rare occasions to remove a tumor that cannot be removed through a transsphenoidal method.If there is still tumor left or hormone levels are not yet normal, medicine and/or radiation therapy may be given.

b. The medication of choice is octreotide, which is given most often by a monthly intramuscular injection. This therapy may be given to control overproduction of growth hormone after noncurative surgery, or in patients who are not surgical candidates.

c. A new medication called pegvisomant has now been approved for acromegaly. Instead of eliminating the extra growth hormone by the pituitary tumor, it works to stop the hormone from acting on the body. It is given by a daily injection.

Cushing's Disease

Cushing's disease occurs when a pituitary tumor is associated with hypersecretion of pituitary ACTH, causing too much cortisol by the adrenal glands. While Cushing's disease is uncommon, it is significant in that it affects as many as 4,000 people each year in the United States.

Symptoms

- Muscle weakness.
- Purple stretch marks.
- Rapid and unexplained weight gain with a rounder face and abdomen often with thin legs or extremities.
- Increased fat in your neck and above your collar bone and upper back.
- Memory loss or not being able to think clearly.
- Menstrual cycle disorders.
- Skin changes and red cheeks.
- Osteoporosis.
- Depression.
- Mood and behavior disorders.
- High blood sugar levels.
- Hypertension or high blood pressure.

Treatment

a. A combination of medication, surgery, and radiation is used. The first line therapy is surgical and cure rates with an experienced neurosurgeon are more than 90%. A patient will typically have transsphenoidal microsurgery through the nasal sinuses.
b. When surgery does not work, radiation therapy may treat any remaining tumor mass.

TSH-Secreting Tumors

A TSH-secreting pituitary gland tumor secretes too much thyroid-stimulating hormone, which then causes the thyroid gland to become overactive and make too much thyroid hormone, causing hyperthyroidism. These tumors are very rare.

Symptoms

- Heart palpitations
- Fast heart beat
- Irregular menstrual cycle
- Headaches
- Visual disturbances
- Difficulty sleeping
- More frequent bowel movements
- Inability to tolerate heat
- Excessive sweating
- Fatigue
- Weight loss
- Nervousness.

Treatment

a. The first treatment for these tumors is usually transsphenoidal microsurgery, through the nasal sinuses. Unless the tumor is large, surgery alone can typically provide a complete cure.
b. If surgery does not remove the entire tumor, octreotide is an effective medication.
c. Radiation therapy also may be prescribed. The radiation will destroy the remaining tumor, but the process is slow.

Nonsecretory Tumors

Nonfunctioning adenoma

- Some tumors of the pituitary are troublesome because they secrete too many hormones that upset the balance of good health, other tumors of the pituitary do not secrete hormones. Instead, they cause health problems because of their size and location. A nonfunctioning adenoma is one example.

- This nonfunctioning adenoma may cause headaches and vision problems. This type of pituitary gland tumor also may cause hyposecretion, so the pituitary does not produce enough of the hormones necessary for good health. The symptoms of nonfunctioning adenomas fall into two categories—tumor mass effects or hyposecretion effects.

Tumor mass effects

- Visual field disturbances, most commonly loss of peripheral vision, at the edges of vision range.
- Headaches.
- Abnormal control of eye movements.

Hyposecretion effects

- Loss of appetite.
- Weight loss or weight gain.
- Fatigue.
- Irregular menstrual cycle.
- Infertility.
- Reduced sex drive.
- Impotence or failure to get or maintain an erection.
- Inadequate function of the ovaries or testes.
- Frequent urination during night.
- Joint pains.
- Dizziness.
- Low blood pressure.

Treatment

a. Transsphenoidal microsurgery, through the nasal sinuses. After surgery, visual field problems improve in the majority of patients.
b. Hormone replacement may be necessary to correct the hormone imbalance and restore normal hormone levels.

HYPOTHYROIDISM

Definition

Hypothyroidism is a condition characterized by abnormally low thyroid hormone production.

- Thyroid hormone regulation—The chain of command

Hypothalamus – TRH
↓
Pituitary – TSH
↓
Thyroid – T4 and T3

Causes

- Hashimoto's thyroiditis.
- Lymphocytic thyroiditis (which may occur after hyperthyroidism).
- Thyroid destruction (from radioactive iodine or surgery).
- Pituitary or hypothalamic disease.
- Medications.
- Severe iodine deficiency.

Clinical Manifestations

- Fatigue
- Depression
- Modest weight gain
- Cold intolerance
- Excessive sleepiness
- Dry, coarse hair
- Constipation
- Dry skin
- Muscle cramps
- Increased cholesterol levels
- Decreased concentration
- Vague aches and pains
- Swelling of the legs.

Complications

- Myxedema coma
- Cardiomyopathy
- Heart failure
- Pleural effusion.

Diagnostic Tests

- History taking and physical examination: Clinical symptoms—fatigue, cold intolerance, constipation, and dry, flaky skin.

- Blood for thyroid hormone—T3 and T4 may be normal in early hypothyroidism. Sr TSH levels help determine the cause of hypothyroidism. If the level of TSH is high, the defect is in the thyroid and low when it is in the pituitary or hypothalamus.

Management

Medical management

1. Levothyroxine (levoxyl, synthroid) a form of T4 . The average dose is approx 1.6 micrograms/kg/day.
2. Liotrix is a synthetic mix of levothyroxine (T4) and liothyronine (T3) in a 4:1 combination.

NURSING MANAGEMENT

Nursing Assessment

Subjective data

Ask the patient about the problem of excessive sleepiness, fatigue, constipation. History of any major diseases in the past is to be focused.

Objective data

Assess for weight gain, fatigue, slowed or slurred speech, cold intolerance, skin changes, constipation, dyspnea. Assess for bradycardia, distended abdomen, dry, thick or cold skin, thick brittle nails, paresthesias, and muscular aches and pains.

Nursing Diagnoses

- Imbalanced nutrition more than body requirements related to calorie intake in excess of metabolic rate as evidenced by hypometabolism and weight gain.
- Constipation related to gastrointestinal hypomotility as evidenced by irregular, hard stools.
- Activity intolerance related to decreased metabolic rate, and mucin deposits in joints and interstitial spaces as evidenced by generalized weakness and muscle and joint stiffness.
- Disturbed thought process related to hypometabolism as evidenced by forgetfulness,memory loss, somnolence and personality changes.

Planning Outcomes/Goals

- Maintains low caloric diet that meets nutritional needs.
- Experiences, regular, soft formed stools that are easy to pass.
- Participates in self-care activities of daily living with minimal discomfort and fatigue.
- Demonstrates cognitive orientation with correction of hormone deficiency.

Nursing Interventions

Maintains low caloric diet that meets nutritional needs

- Assess the weight and nutritional status of the patient.
- Monitor and record intake for nutritional content and calories.
- Instruct the patient how to plan appropriate meals(e.g. low calorie).

Experiences, regular, soft formed stools that are easy to pass

- Encourage increased fluid intake (e.g. 2–3L/ day) to maintain soft stool.
- Instruct patient/family on high fiber diet.
- Monitor bowel movements, including frequency, consistency, shape, volume and color.
- Administer laxative/stool softener as ordered to stimulate GI motility.

Participates in self-care activities of daily living with minimal discomfort and fatigue

- Monitor patient for evidence of excess physical and emotional fatigue.
- Monitor patient's oxygen response (e.g. pulse rate, cardiac rhythm, respiratory rate) to determine effect of activities and plan increase activity.
- Encourage alternate rest and activity periods to prevent fatigue.
- Promote bed rest/activity limitation to improve patients' tolerance and comfort level.

Demonstrates cognitive orientation with correction of hormone deficiency

- Monitor changes in sensation and orientation to determine appropriate interventions.
- Inform patient of person, place and time to decrease confusion.
- Use environmental cues (e.g. signs, pictures, clocks, calendars) to maintain orientation to time and day.
- Explain all procedures, including sensations likely to be experienced during the procedure, to reduce anxiety and frustration.

HYPERTHYROIDISM

Definition

Hyperthyroidism is the term for overactive tissue within the thyroid gland causing an overproduction of thyroid hormones (thyroxine or 'T4' and/or triiodothyronine or 'T3').

- Hyperthyroidism is thus a cause of thyrotoxicosis, the clinical condition of increased thyroid hormones in the blood.

Causes

- Most often, the entire gland is overproducing thyroid hormone. This is called Graves disease.
- Less commonly, a single nodule is responsible for the excess hormone secretion, called a "hot" nodule.
- Thyroiditis (inflammation of the thyroid) can also cause hyperthyroidism. Functional thyroid tissue producing an excess of thyroid hormone occurs in a number of clinical conditions.

The major causes in humans

- Graves' disease an autoimmune disease usually, the most common etiology with 50%–80% worldwide.
- Toxic thyroid adenoma thought to be atypical due to a low level of dietary iodine in this country).
- Toxic multinodular goiter.

High blood levels of thyroid hormones (most accurately termed hyperthyroxinemia) can occur for a number of other reasons

- Inflammation of the thyroid is called thyroiditis. There are several different kinds of thyroiditis including Hashimoto's thyroiditis (immune-mediated), and sub acute thyroiditis (dequervain). These may be initially associated with secretion of excess thyroid hormone, but usually progress to gland dysfunction and, thus, to hormone deficiency and hypothyroidism.
- Oral consumption of excess thyroid hormone tablets is possible, as is the rare event of consumption of ground beef contaminated with thyroid tissue, and thus thyroid hormone (termed 'hamburger hyperthyroidism').
- Amiodarone, an antiarrhythmic drug is structurally similar to thyroxine and may cause either under- or over activity of the thyroid.

- Postpartum thyroiditis (PPT) occurs in about 7% of women during the year after they give birth. PPT typically has several phases, the first of which is hyperthyroidism. This form of hyperthyroidism usually corrects itself within weeks or months without the need for treatment.

Clinical Manifestations

- Weight loss.
- Anxiety.
- Intolerance to heat.
- Hair loss.
- Muscle aches.
- Weakness.
- Fatigue.
- Hyperactivity.
- Irritability.
- Hypoglycemia.
- Apathy.
- Polyuria.
- Polydipsia.
- Delirium.
- Tremor.
- Pretibial myxedema and sweating.
- Patients may present with a variety of symptoms such as palpitations and arrhythmias (atrial fibrillation), shortness of breath (dyspnea), loss of libido, amenorrhea, nausea, vomiting and diarrhea.
- Long-term untreated hyperthyroidism can lead to osteoporosis. These classical symptoms may not be present often in the elderly.
- Neurological manifestations can include tremors, chorea, myopathy, periodic paralysis.
- Minor ocular (eye) signs, which may be present in any type of hyperthyroidism, are eyelid retraction ('stare'), extraocular muscle weakness, and lid-lag.
- In hyperthyroid stare (Dalrymple sign) the eyelids are retracted upward more than normal (the normal position is at the superior corneoscleral limbus, where the 'white' of the eye begins at the upper border of the iris). Extra-ocular muscle weakness may present with double vision.

Complications

- Thyrotoxic crisis (or thyroid storm) is a rare but severe complication of hyperthyroidism, which may occur when a thyrotoxic patient becomes very sick or physically stressed.
  - Symptoms can include: an increase in body temperature to over 40°C Celsius (104°F), tachycardia, arrhythmia, vomiting, diarrhea, dehydration, coma, and death.
  - Thyroid storm requires emergency treatment and hospitalization.
  - The main treatment is to decrease the circulating thyroid hormone levels and decrease their formation.
  - Propylthiouracil and methimazole are two agents that decrease thyroid hormone synthesis and are usually prescribed in fairly high doses.
  - To inhibit thyroid hormone release from the thyroid gland, sodium iodide, potassium iodide, and/or Lugol's solution can be given. Beta-blockers such as propranolol (inderal, inderal LA, innopran XL) can help to control the heart rate, and intravenous steroids may be used to help support the circulation.

DIAGNOSTIC TESTS

- Measuring the level of thyroid-stimulating hormone (TSH), produced by the pituitary gland (which in turn is also regulated by the hypothalamus's TSH-releasing hormone) in the blood is typically the initial test for suspected hyperthyroidism.
- Measuring specific antibodies, such as anti-TSH-receptor antibodies in Graves disease, or antithyroid peroxidase in Hashimoto's thyroiditis—a common

cause of hypothyroidism—may also contribute to the diagnosis.

- Blood tests that show a decreased thyroid - stimulating hormone (TSH) level and elevated T4 and T3 levels confirm the diagnosis of hyperthyroidism.
- Thyroid scintigraphy is a useful test to characterize hyperthyroidism. This test procedure typically involves two tests performed in connection with each other: an iodine uptake test and a scan (Imaging) with a gamma camera. The uptake test involves administering a dose of radioactive iodine (radioiodine), typically Iodine-123 ,which is the most suitable isotope of iodine for the diagnostic study of thyroid diseases is an almost ideal isotope of iodine for imaging thyroid tissue and thyroid cancer metastasis.

Management

Temporary medical therapy

- Thyrostatics (antithyroid drugs)
  - Thyrostatics are drugs that inhibit the production of thyroid hormones, such as carbimazole and methimazole and propylthiouracil.
  - Thyrostatics are believed to work by inhibiting the iodination of thyroglobulin by thyroperoxidase, and, thus, the formation of tetraiodothyronine (T4).
  - Propylthiouracil also works outside the thyroid gland, preventing conversion of (mostly inactive) T4 to the active form T3.
  - Because thyroid tissue usually contains a substantial reserve of thyroid hormone, thyrostatics can take weeks to become effective, and the dose often needs to be carefully titrated over a period of months.
- Beta-blockers
  - Beta-blockers, typically used to treat high blood pressure, are a class of drugs that offset this effect, reducing rapid pulse associated with the sensation of palpitations and decreasing tremor and anxiety. Thus, a patient suffering from hyperthyroidism can often obtain immediate temporary relief. Propranolol and metoprolol are most frequently used to augment treatment for hyperthyroid patients.

Permanent treatments

Surgery as an option predates the use of the less invasive radioisotope therapy (radioiodine 131 thyroid ablation), but is still required in cases where the thyroid gland is enlarged and causing compression to the neck structures, or the underlying cause of the hyperthyroidism may be cancerous in origin.

Surgery—Surgery (to remove the whole thyroid or a part of it) is not extensively used because most common forms of hyperthyroidism are quite effectively treated by the radioactive iodine method, and because there is a risk of also removing the parathyroid glands, and of cutting the recurrent laryngeal nerve, making swallowing difficult, and even simply generalized staph infection as with any major surgery.

Radioactive isotope

- In iodine-131 (radioiodine) radioisotope therapy, radioactive iodine-131 is given orally (either by pill or liquid) on a one-time basis, to severely restrict, or altogether destroy the function of a hyperactive thyroid gland.
- This isotope of radioactive iodine used for ablative treatment is more potent than diagnostic radioiodine (iodine-123), which has a biological half-life from 8 to 13 hours.
- Iodine-131, which also emits beta-particles that are far more damaging to tissues at short range, has a half-life of approximately 8 days.

- Patients not responding sufficiently to the first dose are sometimes given an additional radioiodine treatment, at a larger dose.
- Iodine-131 in this treatment is picked up by the active cells in the thyroid and destroys them, rendering the thyroid gland mostly or completely inactive.
- Since iodine is picked more readily (though not exclusively) by thyroid cells, and (more important) is picked up even more readily by over-active thyroid cells, the destruction is local, and there are no widespread side-effects with this therapy.
- The principal advantage of radioiodine treatment for hyperthyroidism is that it tends to have a much higher success rate than medications.
- As radioactive iodine treatment results in destruction of thyroid tissue, there is often a transient period of several days to weeks when the symptoms of hyperthyroidism may actually worsen following radioactive iodine therapy.

NURSING MANAGEMENT

Subjective Data

Collect health history and examination focus on the occurrence of symptoms related to increased metabolism. Ask the patient to report changes in emotional status and stress with the coping strategies.

Objective Data

Weight loss, anxiety, intolerance to heat, hair loss, muscle aches, weakness, fatigue, hyperactivity, irritability, hypoglycemia, apathy, polyuria, polydipsia, delirium, tremor, palpitations.

Nursing Diagnoses

- Altered nutrition related to accelerated metabolic rate, excessive appetite, and increased gastrointestinal activity.
- Ineffective coping related to irritability, hyperexcitability, apprehension, and emotional instability.
- Disturbances in self-esteem related to changes in appearance, excessive appetite and weight loss.

Planning outcomes

- Maintain nutritional status
- Improve coping ability
- Improve sel-esteem.

Nursing interventions

Maintain nutritional status

- Assess the weight and nutritional status.
- Select appropriate foods and fluids to replace fluid loss through diarrhea and diaphoresis.
- Encourage the patient for high protein and high calorie food.
- Serve the meal in a quiet environment which will aid in digestion.

Improve coping ability

- Assess the stress factors for the patient.
- Use a calm, unhurried approach to the patient.
- Encourage the patient to ventilate his feelings.
- Provide a calm, noise-free and relaxing environment.
- Explain every procedure to the patient before doing.
- Repeat the instructions if needed.

Improve self-esteem

- Convey an understanding of the patient's concern for his problems.
- Educate the patient and family members about the disease and its treatment.
- Give positive feedback towards prognosis of the disease.

10

Nursing Management of Patients with Disorders of Reproductive System

NURSING ASSESSMENT OF PATIENTS WITH REPRODUCTIVE DISORDERS

Assessment

Subjective data

Complaints of amenorrhea, dysmenorrhea, polymenorrhea, menorrhagia, metrorrhagia, pelvic pain, pain in back, vaginal discharge, feelings of something coming down from vagina, dyspareunia, itching in vagina, frequency of urination and loss of control of bladder and bowel.

Past history of sexually transmitted diseases, rubella, major operations and operations on reproductive tract.

Current health status, presence of any acute or chronic health problems like diabetes, hypothyroidism, hyperthyroidism, cancer, anemia, hypertension, angina and thrombophlebitis.

Use of medications prescribed or over the counter such as antihypertensive, diuretics, hormones, oral contraceptives, herbal drugs, etc.

History of allergy to any drugs specially sulfonamides, food and latex or rubber.

Habits of smoking, use of recreational drugs and alcohol.

Age at menarche, menstrual cycle, duration of menstrual period, last menstrual period.

Sexual practices, number of sex partners, number of pregnancies, outcomes of pregnancies.

Family history of cardiovascular diseases, and diabetes, cancers of the reproductive organs.

Objective data

Physical examination of women with reproductive disorders involves examination of the breasts, abdomen (see Chapter 7), and genitalia.

Inspection of breasts for size, symmetry, shape, skin color, vascular patterns, presence of lesion and dimpling of skin over breasts.

Palpation of breasts for mass and nipple for mass and discharge.

Inspection of genitalia for contour, hair distribution, skin characteristics, lesions, evidence of inflammation, swelling and discharge.

Speculum examination for walls of the vagina and cervix for evidence of inflammation, polyp, suspicious growth and discharge.

Palpation of the cervix for consistency, mobility, size, and position; uterus for size, mobility, and contour.

Diagnostic Studies

1. Urine test for
   - Human chorionic gonadotropin (hCG) detects pregnancy and hydatidiform mole.
   - Follicle-stimulating hormone to determine gonadal functions.
2. Blood studies
   - Serum hCG detects pregnancy.
   - Prolactin level for unexplained galactorrhea.
   - Serum estradiol and progesterone to assess ovarian function.
   - Serologic test for syphilis VDRL (venereal disease research laboratory).
   - Fluorescent treponemal antibody absorption test detects syphilis with accuracy.
3. Cultures of discharges from vagina, endocervix, rectum detects Treponema pallidum (syphilis), Nisseria gonorrhea, *Clamydia* and *Trichomonas* infection.
4. Gram stain of smears obtained from vagina for detection of gonorrhea and chlamydia.
5. Cytologic studies
   - Pap (Papanicolaou) test studies abnormal cells obtained from endocervix and ectocervix. It is a screening test for cancer.
   - Nipple discharge test identifies infection or cancer.
6. Radiologic studies
   - Mammography detects masses in breast before they are palpable.
   - Ultrasound (pelvic) obtains images of the pelvic organs.
   - Transvaginal ultrasound detects pregnancy, ectopic pregnancy, ovarian cysts and other pelvic masses.
   - Breast ultrasound detects fluid filled masses in breast.
   - CT scan and MRI detects primary and metastatic tumors in the pelvis.
   - Hysterosalpingogram involves injection of contrast medium through cervix into uterine cavity followed by X-ray. It detects abnormal uterine shape, blockage of fallopian tubes, and adhesions near ovary.
7. Laparoscopy allows visualization of pelvic structures with fiberoptic scopes inserted through small abdominal incision.
8. Biopsy from breast, cervix endometrium, etc. confirms cancer.

PERIMENOPAUSE AND MENOPAUSE

Definition

Menopause is defined as permanent physiological cessation of menstruation associated with loss of ovarian follicular activity.

Perimenopause is a normal life transition that begins with the first signs of change in menstrual cycles and ends after cessation of menses.

Age at Menopause

- Menopause usually occurs at 45 to 55 years of age.
- Average is 50 years.
- Menopause may occur earlier than this. The reasons of early menopause may be due to illness, surgical removal of ovary or uterus, side effect of radiation therapy or cancer chemotherapy, malnutrition, cigarette smoking, obesity, etc.

Pathophysiological Changes

- Regression of ovarian follicles starts at puberty and increases after age 35 years. Elderly women possess a fewer

follicles that are responsive to follicle-stimulating hormone.
- As ovarian function decreases, levels of estrogen progesterone decline.
- Levels of follicle-stimulating hormone and luteinizing hormone rises 10 to 20 folds due to negative feed back process and may take several years to return to premenopausal level.
- Reduced estrogen level causes decreased frequency of ovulation and changes in the reproductive organs and tissues.

Clinical Manifestations

Some women remain asymptomatic, but in some women symptoms appear.
- Initially irregular menses later on cessation of menses.
- Vasomotor symptoms 'Hot flush' is experienced by some women (hot flush is described as sensation of warmth in the upper part of the chest, neck and face followed by profuse sweating; sensation may last for several seconds to 5 minutes; occur most often at night resulting into disturbed sleep. Sensation of hot flush is triggered by hot weather, hot meal, alcoholic beverage, stress and warm clothing).
- Atrophic vaginal epithelial changes lead to infection, vaginal bleeding upon minimum trauma, dryness, pruritus, leukorrhea and dyspareunia.
- Atrophic lower urinary tract changes cause decrease in bladder capacity and loss of tone of bladder and urethral tissue giving rise to urgency, frequency, dysuria, recurrent urinary tract infections, urge and stress incontinence.
- Risk of ischemic heart disease, coronary artery disease and strokes increases.
- Breast tenderness and atrophy of breast tissue.
- Psychologic changes that include increased frequency of anxiety, headache, insomnia, irritability, dysphasia, depression, dementia, mood swing and inability to concentrate.
- Thinning, loss of elasticity and wrinkling of the skin due to decrease of collagen, purse string wrinkling around mouth, crowfeet around eyes, loss of some pubic and axillary hair and balding.
- Redistribution of fat, a tendency to gain weight, muscle and joint pain and risk of osteoporosis.

Diagnostic Studies

1. History of cessation of menstruation for consecutive 12 months during climacteric.
2. Appearance of menopausal symptoms such as hot flush and night sweats.
3. Vaginal cytology reveals low estrogen.
4. Serum FSH and LH level elevated.
5. Serum estradiol level lowered.

Management

Nonhormonal treatment

Counseling—Explaining the woman that it is a normal physiologic process and does not indicate pregnancy or cancer. This will remove fear and minimize anxiety, insomnia, and depression.

Nutritional therapy—Advise woman to take balanced diet with adequate protein, calcium and other vitamins. Include soya protein in diet.

Supplement calcium and vitamin D—Daily intake of 1 to 1.5 gm calcium along with 400 to 800 IU/day of vitamin D is required to prevent osteoporosis and fracture.

Exercise—Daily weight bearing exercises, walking, jogging reduces bone resorption and osteoporosis.

Mild tranquilizers to relieve, anxiety, insomnia and depression.

Hormone replacement therapy (HRT)

- **Indication**
  1. Severe menopausal symptoms.
  2. High risk of osteoporosis, heart disease, and Alzheimer's disease.
  3. Woman who demand a quality of life in menopausal years.
  4. Woman with premature menopause or surgical or radiation menopause.
- **Contraindication**
  1. Liver and gallbladder disease.
  2. Breast cancer, uterine cancer or family history of cancer.
  3. Previous history of thromboembolism.
- **Advantages of HRT**
  1. Improvement of vasomotor symptoms.
  2. Increase in bone mineral density and prevention of osteoporosis.
  3. Possible cardioprotective effect.
  4. Reduced risk of colorectal cancer.
- **Drugs for HRT**
  1. Estrogen therapy with conjugated estrogen in the dose of 0.625 to 1.25 per day or micronized estrogen 1 to 2 mg per day is given commonly.
  2. Progestins such as medroxyprogesterone acetate in the dose of 2.5 to 5 mg per day or micronized progesterone in the dose of 100 to 300 mg per day is added with estrogen in women with intact uterus to prevent endometrial hyperplasia.
- **Route of administration**
  - Oral
  - Subdermal implants
  - Percutaneous gel
  - Transdermal patch
  - Vaginal cream.
- **Duration of treatment**
  1. Short-term therapy for a period of 3 to 6 months is given to women with menopausal symptoms.
  2. Long-term therapy for a period of 3 to 5 years may be given to delay osteoporosis and reducing the risk of cardiovascular disease in menopausal women.
- **Other drugs used in menopause**
  a. Raloxifene, a selective estrogen receptor modulator 60 mg daily given to prevent osteoporosis; reduces LDL cholesterol and increases HDL; reduces risk of endometrial and breast cancer. But it does not improve hot flush.
  b. Biphosphonates (alendronate) increases bone mineral density by preventing osteoclastic bone resorption.
  c. Clonidine, a imidazoline derivative, with a dose of .2 to .4 mg daily reduces severity and duration of hot flushes.
  d. Calcitonin inhibits bone resorption. Calcitonin nasal spray or injection along with calcium and vitamin D supplementation increases bone mineral density and prevents fracture.
  d. Soya protein acts as selective estrogen receptor modulator, is found to reduce vasomotor symptoms.

NURSING MANAGEMENT

Relief from Anxiety, Sleeplessness and Depression

- Teach patient that menopause is a normal physiological process, not pregnancy or cancer.
- Reassure patient that with time she will be able to adjust with the physiological changes associated with menopause.
- Listen to patient's concern in order to remove misconception of the woman and clarify her doubts in simple terms.

Improving Vasomotor Symptoms

- Explain patient that vasomotor symptoms are commonly experienced by majority of women.
- Teach patient to use loose cotton clothing especially at night. Keep environment cool.
- Reduce intake of alcohol and coffee as these increase vasomotor symptoms.
- Apply cold compress during hot flush.
- Teach patient to record frequency and duration of hot flushes.
- Teach patient to take drugs if prescribed by the physician.
- Explain patient the advantages and disadvantages of hormone replacement therapy and also the side effects of the drugs prescribed for him.

Prevention of Complications: Osteoporosis; Cardiovascular Disease, Genitourinary Infections, Dyspareunia, Urinary Frequency, etc.

- Teach the woman to take a balanced diet with adequate protein, calcium.
- Encourage woman to take supplemental calcium with vitamin D as prescribed regularly.
- Encourage the woman to perform regular weight bearing exercises, walking, jogging to reduce bone resorption and also to reduce LDL cholesterol and increase HDL cholesterol that prevents coronary artery diseases.
- Teach patient to practice meditation or to engage into social work that relieves anxiety, depression and promote a well-being.
- Teach patient to perform Kegel exercises that would promote control of bladder and bowel.
- Teach patient perineal hygiene, meticulous hand washing after defecation and urination.
- Encourage patient to report if dyspareunia. Apply estrogen cream to vagina as ordered to prevent vaginal dryness.
- Encourage regular follow-up and participate in cancer screening programs such as pap test and breast examination.

DISORDERS OF MENSTRUAL CYCLE

Dysmenorrhea

Definition

Dysmenorrhea is abdominal cramping pain or discomfort of varying intensity associated with menstrual flow.

Types

Primary dysmenorrhea

- It occurs in the absence of any identifiable pelvic pathology.
- It begins in the few years after menarche.
- It usually gets cured after pregnancy and vaginal delivery.

Secondary dysmenorrhea

- It is the result of some pelvic pathological conditions.
- It occurs after adolescence.
- Common age of its occurrence is 30 to 40 years.

Etiopathology

Primary dysmenorrhea

1. The condition is believed to be due to excessive production of prostaglandins or/and an increased sensitivity of the myometrium to its normal production.
   - During menstruation degeneration of endometrium releases prostaglandins.
   - Prostaglandins cause painful contraction of the uterus and constriction of small blood vessels supplying the endometrium.

- Increased uterine contractions and vasospasms give rise to tissue ischemia and increased sensitization of the pain receptors leading to menstrual pain.

2. Psychological factors such as anxiety and tension during adolescence may also lower pain threshold.
3. Certain anatomical defects of uterus such as narrowing of cervical canal, stenosis of the internal os, septate or bicornuate uterus or hypoplastic uterus may also cause dysmenorrhea.

Secondary dysmenorrhea

Pelvic pathology such as endometriosis, chronic pelvic inflammatory disease, uterine fibroids, etc. contribute to secondary dysmenorrhea.

Clinical Features

Primary dysmenorrhea

- Pain starts 12 to 24 hours before the menstruation or just with the onset of menstruation.
- Severity of pain usually lasts for a few hours on the first day of menstruation or just with the onset of menstruation.
- Pain is described as crampy lower abdominal pain often radiating to the lower back and medial aspect of thighs.
- Pain is often associated with nausea, vomiting, diarrhea, headache, fatigue, and light headedness.
- Pallor, cold sweats, occasional fainting and rarely syncope or fainting may occur.

Secondary dysmenorrhea

- Pain may be unilateral, usually constant in nature.
- Pain starts several days before menstruation and usually continues longer than in primary dysmenorrhea.
- Depending upon the underlying pathology other symptoms such as dyspareunia, painful defecation or irregular bleeding may accompany.

Diagnostic Studies

Complete health history including menstrual, gynecological history

It reveals age of onset of dysmenorrhea.

Pelvic examination

It detects presence of abnormal pathology.

Ultrasonography

It detects pelvic pathology.

Management

- Application of heat to lower abdomen and back.
- Regular exercise decreases endometrial hyperplasia and thus reduces prostaglandins synthesis.
- NSAIDs (naproxen, mefenamic acid, ibuprofen, indomethacin) started at the first sign of menstruation and continued 4 to 8 hours to inhibit prostaglandin activities.
- Aspirin (prostaglandins inhibitor) every 4 hours.
- Oral contraceptive reduces hyperplasia of the endometrium.
- Acupuncture and transcutaneous nerve stimulation for clients who do not like medication.

NURSING MANAGEMENT

Nursing care focuses on educating the patient about controlling and preventing pain.

Controlling Pain

- Explain patient the etiopathology of the condition as well as the rational for treatment regimen.

- Teach patient self-care measures to minimize pain such as:
  - To take rest during acute pain and lying down for short periods.
  - Drinking hot drinks.
  - Taking warm baths.
  - Applying heat to the lower abdomen and back.
  - Taking NSAIDs as ordered before pain becomes severe or practicing noninvasive pain relief strategies such as distraction and guided imagery.

Preventing Pain

- Reassure patient that this is a very common condition for women. The condition usually gets cured after marriage and child birth.
- Encourage patient to perform regular physical exercises since exercise reduces endometrial hyperplasia and thus reduce release of prostaglandins.
- Teach patient to develop proper nutritional habits such as taking well balanced diet and a lot of fibers to prevent constipation.
- Encourage patient to maintain proper body mechanics.
- Teach patient to eliminate stress and fatigue specially before menstruation.

Premenstrual Syndrome

Definition—Premenstrual syndrome (PMS) is a disorder in women in which a group of physical and psychological symptoms occur during the last few days of the menstruation cycle and before the onset of menstruation.

There is cyclic appearance of a large number of symptoms during the last 7 to 10 days of the menstrual cycle.

The symptoms can be severe enough to interfere with usual activities and to disturb interpersonal relationships.

In a type of PMS woman have a severe mood disorder in addition to PMS and is known as premenstrual dysphoric disorder (PMD-D).

Etiology—Exact cause is not understood. The following factors may play a role:

1. Alteration in the level of estrogen-progesterone ratio.
2. Decreased synthesis of serotonin is observed in women with PMS.
3. Psychological and psychosocial factors.
4. Genetic predisposition.
5. Alteration in the level of other hormones such as Thyrotropin releasing hormone, prolactin, prostaglandins, renin, aldosterone.
6. Nutritional factors such as deficiencies of pyridoxine and magnesium.

Clinical Manifestations

Clinical manifestations vary from woman to woman and for an individual woman, from one cycle to another.

Physical symptoms

- Breast discomfort or tenderness.
- Peripheral edema.
- Sensation of weight gain.
- Feeling of abdominal fullness.
- Headache, fatigue, heart palpitations, and dizziness.
- Low back pain.

Behavioral symptoms

- Irritability, anxiety, tension and restlessness.
- Depression, mood swings, tearfulness.
- Fear of losing control.
- Increased appetite.
- Confusion, forgetfulness.

Diagnostic Studies

1. Thorough medical history to rule out possible causes of symptoms.
2. Maintenance of a diary recording symptoms for 2 or 3 menstrual cycles.
3. Administration of goserelin (zoladex), GnRH analogue subcutaneous depot every month for 3 months—relief of symptoms along with amenorrhea suggests the diagnosis of PMS.

Collaborative Management

No single treatment is available. Goals of management are:
1. To relieve the severity of symptoms
2. To enhance the quality of life and woman's sense of control.

Nonpharmacologic strategies

1. Explanations and reassurance
2. Stress management and relaxation therapy by yoga, meditation, imagery, and biofeedback training.
3. Dietary changes:
   - To reduce refined carbohydrates intake.
   - Avoid caffeine, alcohol.
   - Supplement vitamin B_6, magnesium and calcium.
   - Limit salt intake before menstruation.
4. Exercises:
   - Perform regular physical exercise, e.g. aerobic exercises.
   - Limit exhaustion by taking extra rest in premenstrual phase.

Pharmacologic strategies

Drug therapy may be given to reduce symptoms such as:
1. Diuretics (aldactone, spironolactone)—to relieve fluid retention.
2. Prostaglandin inhibitors (ibuprofen—to reduce cramping pain, backache and headache.
3. Vitamin B_6 supplementation—to improve mood.
4. Calcium and magnesium supplementation—It may alleviate physiologic and psychologic symptoms.
5. oral contraceptives—To suppress ovulation and thus to maintain uniform hormonal balance.
6. Tranquilizers (alprazolam, buspirone)—It relieves psychologic symptoms
7. Antidepressants (fluoxetin, tricyclic antidepressants, sertraline)—It provides relief in severe PMS.

ABNORMAL UTERINE/VAGINAL BLEEDING

Abnormal uterine or vaginal bleeding is a common gynecological problem and manifests in following ways:

Oligomenorrhea

Definition

When menstrual bleeding occurs at regularly long intervals, generally more than 35 days apart is known as oligomenorrhea.

Causes

1. During adolescence and menopause due to anovulation.
2. obesity
3. Hormonal disturbances such as hyperthyroidism, hyperprolactinemia
4. Tubercular endometritis
5. Ovarian or adrenal tumor producing androgen.

Hypomenorrhea

Definition

When menstrual bleeding is scanty and lasts for less than 2 days is called hypomenorrhea.

Causes

1. Endometrial tuberculosis
2. Malnutrition
3. Premenopausal period
4. Thyroid dysfunction.

Menorrhagia

Definition

Menorrhagia is defined as cyclic bleeding at normal intervals but continued either for a long duration (more than 7 days) or in excessive amount (more than 80 mL) or both.

Causes

1. Pelvic diseases such as fibroids, adenomyosis, pelvic endometriosis, tubercular endometriosis.
2. Intrauterine contraceptive devices in utero.
3. Systemic diseases such as liver diseases, severe hypertension, congestive cardiac failure, hypothyroidism and hyperthyroidism.
4. Blood disorders such as leukemia, idiopathic thrombocytopenic purpura.
5. Emotional upset.

Diagnostic Studies

Thorough clinical evaluation to find out the cause.

Management

- Treatment of underlying disease causing menorrhagia.
- Treatment of the effect of menorrhagia, i.e. anemia by providing high protein and iron containing diet; supplementation of iron orally or parenterally and by giving blood transfusion in severe anemia.

Polymenorrhea/Epimenorrhea

Polymenorrhea is defined as the cyclic bleeding where the cycle is reduced to less than 21 days and remains constant at that frequency.

The term epimenorrhea is used when frequent cycles are associated with excessive or/and prolonged bleeding.

Causes

1. Hyper-stimulation of the ovary by the pituitary hormones as in adolescence and preceding menopause, following delivery and abortion.
2. Ovarian hyperemia such as pelvic inflammatory disease or ovarian endometriosis.

Metrorrhagia

Definition

Metrorrhagia/Spotting Breakthrough bleeding is described as irregular acyclic bleeding from the uterus or bleeding between menstrual periods.

In menometrorrhagia bleeding is so irregular and excessive that the menstrual period cannot be identified.

Causes

Dysfunctional uterine bleeding—during adolescence, following abortion or child birth, and preceding menopause.

Pelvic diseases such as submucus fibroid, uterine polyp, carcinoma cervix, endometrial carcinoma.

Dysfunctional Uterine Bleeding (DUB)

Definition

DUB is defined as a state of abnormal uterine bleeding in absence of any pelvic pathology.

Causes

1. Alteration in the ratio of endometrial prostaglandins, which is responsible for hemostasis during menstruation.
2. Incoordination in the hypothalamo-pituitary ovarian axis. It is more prevalent in extremes of reproductive period such as adolescence and premenopause.
3. Emotional influences, worries, anxieties and sexual problems may also disturb the normal hormonal balance.
4. Hormonal imbalances following childbirth and abortion.

Clinical manifestations

- Uterine bleeding that may be abnormal in frequency or amount or duration or combination of three.
- Anemia.
- Enlargement of the size of uterus.

Diagnostic studies

1. History of bleeding from vagina not from urethra or rectum.
2. History of use of steroids, oral contraceptives and presence of IUCD in utero.
3. Assessment of bleeding by number of pads used, size and number of clots passed and duration of bleeding; nature of menstrual bleeding—cyclic and acyclic; relation to age.
4. Blood for complete hemogram to find out the effect of bleeding and to rule out blood dyscrasias.
5. Blood for TSH, T3 and T4 to rule out thyroid disorders.
6. D and C to rule out organic disorders.

Management

1. General measures—Rest during bleeding. Assurance and sympathetic handling. Correction of anemia.
2. Hormone therapy to correct hormonal imbalance such as progestin, dydrogesterone, Norethisterone acetate, combined estrogen progestogen.
3. Nonhormonal therapy such as
   - Antifibrnolytic agents (Tranexamic acid), counteracts the endometrial fibronolytic system.
   - Ethamsylate, reduces endometrial capillary fragility.
   - Mefenamic acid, inhibits prostaglandins synthesis, reduces menstrual blood loss.
4. Surgical therapy is performed when other measures fail.
   - Uterine curettage is performed to remove the necrosed and unhealthy endometrium.
   - Hysterectomy is performed when hormonal therapy fails; blood loss impairs health of patient and for patients who have completed family.
   - Endometrial ablation may be performed as an alternative to hysterectomy when hysterectomy is contraindicated. Through a hysteroscope laser is administered to destroy endometrial tissue which produce amenorrhea.

NURSING MANAGEMENT

Providing Emotional Support and Reassurance

- Explain patient that abnormal uterine bleeding is a common problem among the women in reproductive age group.
- Reassure patient that you will be always present with her whenever she will be examined by a doctor or during any diagnostic or therapeutic procedures.
- Explain in simple language about the diagnosis and therapeutic intervention planned by the physician.
- Explain patient about the drug therapy, need for compliance of the treatment, side effect of the drugs and need for regular follow-up.

- Discuss with patient along with the partner the consequence of hysterectomy if planned by the physician.

Teaching Patient Self-care

- Encourage patient to take some extra rest during the period of active bleeding in order to avoid fatigue.
- Teach hygienic measures such as use of sanitary napkins, perineal care after defecation and micturition, proper disposal of pads and meticulous hand washing.
- Explain the importance of optimum nutritional intake such as high protein foods with plenty of green leafy vegetables to combat anemia due to excessive blood loss.

(Nursing management of patients undergoing hysterectomy is discussed in later section).

INFERTILITY

Definition

Infertility is defined as the inability to conceive after at least 1 year or more years of regular coitus without contraception.

Incidence

- 20% of women remain infertile after 1 year.
- 10% of women remain infertile after 2 years.

Types

1. Primary infertility means when the woman never conceives.
2. Secondary infertility denotes failure to conceive subsequently after the first pregnancy.

Etiology

Infertility may be caused by the factors inherent in the male, female, both male and female or by unknown factors.

Female factors

Female factors of infertility are described in the following categories:

1. Ovarian factors or factors associated with ovulation such as anovulation, oligoovulation, corpus luteum insufficiency and luteinized unruptured follicular syndrome.
2. Tubal obstruction or dysfunction resulting from pelvic infections causing peritubal adhesions or endosalpingeal damage; previous pelvic surgery or sterilization; tubal endometriosis, polyps within tubal lumen and tubal spasms.
3. Uterine or cervical factors such as uterine hypoplasia, inadequate secretory endometrium, fibroid uterus, tubercular endometritis, congenital malformations of uterus, congenital elongation of the cervix, second degree uterine prolapse, polyp in cervical canal.
4. Vaginal factors such as atresia vagina or transverse vaginal septum.
5. General factors such as advanced age of the wife beyond 35 years, lack of knowledge of coital technique.

Male factors

Male factors of infertility described as:

1. Pretesticular or hormonal causes such as hormonal disturbances from pituitary and adrenal tumors, thyroid disorders, cirrhosis of liver, etc.
2. Testicular causes such as vericocele, big hydrocele or filariasis; hypoxia of testes caused by tight undergarment, congenital anomalies of testes, e.g. undescended testes; genitourinary infections affecting testes, e.g. mumps,

sexually transmitted organisms, tubercular infections; effects of medications on testes, e.g. chemotherapeutic drugs, beta blockers, antihypertensives, antidepressants, anticonvulsants and anabolic steroids; effects of thermal factors on testes, e.g. working in hot environment; and effects of malnutrition, debilitating diseases, heavy smoking, alcohol abuse, exposure to agricultural, industrial or warfare agents.

3. Posttesticular causes include congenital blockage of vas deferense, epididymitis; surgical trauma, e.g. herniorrhaphy or vasectomy; and gonococcal and tubercular infections of efferent ducts; erectile dysfunction and ejaculatory defect such as retrograde, premature or absence of ejaculation and hypospadius.

Diagnostic Studies

1. History from both the partners is obtained to determine the need for specific diagnostic studies. History should include medical, nutritional, psychosocial functioning, sexual, reproductive, occupation, lifestyle, habits and addiction.
2. Physical examination of both the partners to find out general health status, any anatomical abnormalities, presence of hydrocele, vericocele, sexually transmitted diseases, etc.
3. Routine urine and blood examination to detect presence of any associated illness such as diabetes, liver disease, thyroid disorders, etc.
4. Basal body temperature recording for the woman to detect whether there is regular ovulation.
5. Serum hormone levels, e.g. FSH, LH, prolactin to detect hypogonadotrophic hypogonadism.
6. Urinary LH and serum progesterone to detect ovulation.
7. Hysterosalpingogram to detect tubal patency.
8. Postcoital studies to determine whether cervical mucus membrane is favorable for the sperms.
9. Endometrial biopsy to detect ovulation and functioning of the corpus luteum.
10. Semen analysis to determine sperm count, morphology, motility, viability, etc.
11. Transrectal ultrasound to detect prostate, seminal vesicles and ejaculatory ducts obstruction.
12. Testicular biopsy to differentiate primary testicular failure from obstruction as a cause for severe oligospermia or azoospermia.

Management

Management depends on cause of infertility

1. Counseling of both partners to reduce stress, remove misconception, myths, and improve sexual practices.
2. Drugs:
   - Follicle-stimulating hormone recombinant, progesterone, human chorionic gonadotrophin and gonadotrophin releasing hormone may be given to stimulate ovulation.
   - Clomiphene citrate may be given to stimulate spermatogenesis.
3. Surgery:
   - Surgical procedure may be undertaken to correct hydrocele, obstruction of vas deferense or undescended testes.
   - Removal of ovarian tumor or uterine fibroids, release of blockage of fallopian tube.
4. Intrauterine insemination—Sperm from the partner or donor is collected and introduced into uterine cavity.

5. Assisted reproductive therapy (ART) includes:
   - In vitro fertilization (IVF) and embryo transfer.
   - Gamete intrafallopian transfer.
   - Zygote intrafallopian transfer, etc.

NURSING MANAGEMENT

- Assessment of couple experiencing infertility by collection of detail history to find out the probable cause of infertility.
- Teaching the couple regarding physiology of reproduction.
- Counseling to remove stress, anxiety, avoidance of abusive substances, etc.
- Explaining and preparing the couple for undergoing different diagnostic tests and treatment.

ABORTION

Definition

Abortion is the expulsion or extraction from its mother of an embryo or fetus weighing 500 gm or less, when it is not capable of independent survival (WHO).

The expelled embryo or fetus is called abortus. The term miscarriage is also used for spontaneous abortion or unintended loss of a pregnancy.

Incidence

10%–20% of all pregnancies end in abortion.
10% are induced illegally.

Classification

1. Spontaneous or unintentional abortion
   a. Threatened
   b. Inevitable
   c. Complete
   d. Incomplete
   e. Missed
   f. Recurrent or habitual
   g. Septic (less common).
2. Induced or elective
   a. Legal
   b. Illegal
   c. Septic.

Etiology

Common causes of abortion

a. Genetic factors—50% of abortions are due to fetal chromosomal abnormalities.
b. Endocrine disorders such as diabetes, thyroid abnormalities, deficient progesterone secretion by the corpus luteum.
c. Immunological disorders.
d. Maternal medical illnesses and infections.
e. Anatomic abnormalities such as cervical incompetence, bicornuate uterus, septate uterus, uterine fibroid, and intrauterine adhesions.
f. Unknown.

Pathophysiology

- In early weeks of abortion the ovum dies first. The dead ovum surrounded by decidual covering expelled out as a whole mass.
- In later weeks of abortions the death fetus is expelled first. The placenta and membrane may remain totally attached to the uterine wall or a part of it gets separated leading to hemorrhage.

THREATENED ABORTION

Definition

Threatened abortion is a clinical entity where the process of abortion starts but does not progress to a state from where recovery is impossible.

Clinical Manifestations

- Painless vaginal bleeding. Bleeding may be slight, spotting, brownish or red in color. Bleeding usually stops spontaneously.
- Backache or dull pain in lower abdomen may occur.

Diagnosis

1. Ultrasonography reveals viable fetus.
2. A gentle per vaginal examination by the physician (if ultrasound is not available) detects gravid uterus, height of uterus corresponds to period of amenorrhea, os is closed.

Management

1. Complete rest in bed till bleeding is stopped.
2. Diazepam may be given to promote rest and also to relieve abdominal discomfort.
3. After bleeding stops limited activities may be permitted and is advised to avoid heavy work, stimulant and coitus.
4. To come for follow up after 3 to 4 weeks.

Prognosis

In two-third of patients pregnancy may continue beyond 28 weeks but preterm labor, intrauterine growth retardation and fetal anomalies are common.

In one-third of cases pregnancy terminates either as inevitable or missed abortion.

INEVITABLE ABORTION

Definition

It is the clinical type of abortion where the process of abortion has advanced to a stage from where continuation of the pregnancy is not possible.

Clinical Manifestations

- History of pregnancy or a period of amenorrhea.
- Vaginal bleeding increases gradually with lower abdominal colicky pain.
- Per vaginal examination reveals dilated internal os through which product of conception is felt.

Management

1. Injection methergin is given to control bleeding.
2. IV fluid and blood transfusion is given to correct fluid loss.
3. Dilatation and evacuation (D and E) followed by curettage is done if pregnancy is less than 12 week.
4. After 12 weeks of pregnancy, Inj oxytocin 10 units in 500 mL of normal saline infused at a rate of 40 to 60 drops per minute to hasten the process of abortion. Retained placenta is separated and removed manually under GA.

COMPLETE ABORTION

Definition

In complete abortion the products of conception are expelled totally.

Clinical Manifestations

- History of pregnancy or a period of amenorrhea.
- Sudden vaginal bleeding along with cramping abdominal pain and expulsion of a fleshy mass per vagina.
- After expulsion of fleshy mass abdominal pain and vaginal bleeding reduce.
- Per vaginal examination reveals uterine

size smaller than period of gestation, os is closed and bleeding is less.
- On examination the expelled fleshy mass is found to be complete.

Management

Patient does not require any treatment when the abortion is complete.

Transvaginal ultrasound may be performed to ensure complete expulsion of fetus.

INCOMPLETE ABORTION

In incomplete abortion the product of conception is not expelled totally, but a part is retained within the uterus.

Clinical Features

- History of expulsion of a fleshy mass per vagina followed by:
  - Pain in lower abdomen.
  - Persistent vaginal bleeding.
  - Per vaginal examination reveals height of the uterus smaller than period of gestation, patulous cervical os, which admits examiner's tip of finger.
  - Expelled abortus found to be incomplete.

Complications

- Hemorrhage
- Sepsis
- Placental polyp.

Management

- Intravenous fluid is administered to correct the volume deficit caused by hemorrhage.
- Dilatation and evacuation of the uterus under general anesthesia to remove the retained product.
- Histological examination of the removed product in late cases.

MISSED ABORTION

When the fetus is dead and retained in the uterus for a variable period of time, it is called missed abortion.

Clinical Features

- Symptoms of threatened abortion occur initially.
- Later brownish vaginal discharge continues.
- Symptoms of pregnancy disappear gradually.
- Height of the uterus stops increasing, becomes smaller in size.
- Test for pregnancy is found to be negative.
- Ultrasonography detects empty fetal sac, absence of fetal cardiac movement.

Complications

- Psychological problem
- Infection
- Coagulation disorder.

Management

If the pregnancy is less than 12 weeks

- Expectant treatment—Wait for a period of time for spontaneous expulsion of the conceptus.
- Prostaglandin E1 (misoprostol) 800 mg administered vaginally. It may be repeated after 24 hours if needed. Product is expelled usually within 48 hours.
- Suction evacuation or dilatation and evacuation.

If pregnancy is more than 12 weeks, any of the following methods used for evacuation

- Prostaglandin E1 200 microgram vaginally every 4 hours for 5 such if needed.
- Oxytocin drip (10–20 units in 500 mL

normal saline) 30 drops per minute started. The flow may be increased if no result.

- Surgical dilatation and evacuation is performed if medical treatment fails.

RECURRENT ABORTION (HABITUAL)

Recurrent or habitual abortion is defined as three or more successive, spontaneous abortions before 20 weeks.

Etiology

Cause of recurrent abortion is complex. One or multiple causative factors of abortion may be present.

Management

Before pregnancy

- After two consecutive abortions woman should be referred for genetic testing and counseling and to explore other possible causes of abortions.
- Appropriate treatment to be carried out according to the cause if any.

During pregnancy

- Supportive counseling and tender loving care to be provided to remove stress and instill confidence in patient that successful pregnancy is possible.
- Monitor fetal viability ultrasonographically at 8 to 9 weeks of pregnancy.
- Advise to take extra rest and to avoid sexual intercourse, strenuous activities, travelling, heavy meals, constipation etc. to prevent spontaneous abortion.
- Antibiotics if infection is suspected.
- Progesterone to support the endometrium.
- Cervical circlage operation if dysfunctional or incompetent cervix. It involves placing a purse-string suture around the cervix at the level of the internal os to prevent the cervix dilate prematurely. The procedure is done at about 14 weeks of pregnancy and the suture must be removed 2 to 3 weeks before term or the onset of labor. Cervical circlage operation may be performed by two different methods:
  1. Shirodkar operation
  2. McDonald's operation.

SEPTIC ABORTION

Clinical evidences of infection of the uterus and its content associated with any abortion is termed as septic abortion.

Incidence

- About 10% of all hospital admissions with abortions are septic.
- Majority of septic abortion occurs following illegally induced abortion.

Etiology

- Infection usually caused by endogenous organisms (present in vagina) such as anaerobic streptococci, *Clostridium welchii, Tetanus bacillus* and *aerobic Escherichia coli, Klebsiella, Staphylococcus, Pseudomonas,* etc.
- Organisms enter in the uterus due to absence of aseptic technique, incomplete evacuation of the uterus and injury to the genital tract occurring during abortion procedure.

Clinical Features

- History of illegal termination of pregnancy.
- Fever with chills and rigor if septicemia.
- Hypothermia occurs in endotoxic shock.
- Rising pulse rate.

- Pain in abdomen.
- Internal examination reveals a tender uterus, patulous os or boggy feel of the uterus and offensive purulent vaginal discharge.

Diagnostic Tests

1. Cervical or high vaginal swab for culture detects offending organism and sensitivity of the organism to antibiotic.
2. Blood for Hb%, blood cell counts, ABO and Rh-grouping.
3. Urine analysis and culture.
4. Ultrasonography of pelvis and abdomen reveals retained products, intrauterine and intraabdominal free fluid in the peritoneal cavity or pouch of Douglas.
5. Blood culture, if chills present, to detect septicemia.
6. Serum electrolytes and coagulation profile.
7. Plain X-ray abdomen if bowel injury suspected.
8. Chest X-ray to detect pulmonary complications, e.g. atelectasis.

Complications

1. Hemorrhage
2. Injury to uterus and adjacent structures
3. Generalized peritonitis
4. Endotoxic shock
5. Acute renal failure
6. Thrombophlebitis.

Prevention

- Prevent unwanted pregnancies, encourage family planning practices among eligible couple.
- Rigid enforcement of legalized abortion.
- Use of antiseptics and aseptic techniques during internal examination or during operation for spontaneous abortion.

Treatment

- Admit patient in hospital and keep patient isolated.
- Immediate administration of broad spectrum antibiotics later on selection of antibiotics may be done according to sensitivity result.
- Analgesics and sedatives administered as required.
- Antitetanus serum and antigas-gangrene serum to be administered if illegal. induced abortion.
- Blood transfusion to correct anemia.
- Evacuation of the uterus at least 24 hours after starting antibiotic therapy.

INDUCED ABORTION (ELECTIVE ABORTION)

A voluntary termination of pregnancy either by medical or surgical method before the viability of the fetus is called induction of abortion or elective abortion.

Type

- Legal
- Illegal or criminal.

In India induced abortion has been legalized by 'Medical Termination of Pregnancy Act', 1971 and enforced from 1972. According to the provision of the Act induction of abortion is permitted under the following circumstances by a licensed medical practitioner:

1. Continuation of pregnancy involves serious physical and emotional risk of mother.
2. Risk of the child being born with serious physical and mental abnormalities making the child handicapped for life.
3. Pregnancy caused by rape.
4. Pregnancy caused by failure of a contraceptive device.

Methods of Induction of Abortion or Termination of Pregnancy

Medical

Mifepristone—A progesterone antagonist that prevents implantation of the ovum. When administered orally within 10 days of an expected menstrual period produces medical abortion in most patients. Combined with prostaglandin (PGE1) misoprostol either orally or by vaginal suppository success rate is increased (95%). It is effective when used within 49 days of last menstrual period.

Methotrexate and misoprostol—Methotrexate a teratogenic substance administered at a dose of 50 mg/square meter followed by 7 days later misoprostol vaginally is highly effective if given within 56 days of gestation.

Oxytocin—High dose oxytocin used with intravenous saline is effective in 80% cases of second trimester abortion.

Surgical

Vacuum aspiration—It is done up to 12 weeks with minimal cervical dilatation and aspirating the uterine content by a uterine aspirator in an outpatient department.

Suction evacuation—It is an improved method, which uses a suction machine fitted with a canula of various sizes. It is effective in terminating pregnancy within 10 weeks.

Dilatation and evacuation—In this method dilatation of the cervix is performed either by using metal dilators (rapid method) or by using laminaria tent (hygroscopic osmotic dilators) (slow method) and then evacuating the uterus.

Intrauterine instillation—Intrauterine instillation of hypertonic saline (20%) or hypertonic urea (40%) administered through abdominal route results in uterine contractions.The procedure is used less commonly.

Hysterotomy—Hysterotomy is performed (rarely) when D and E cannot be performed safely; uterine anomalies or fibroid in the lower uterine segment; or attempt of medical termination of pregnancy has failed. The procedure is combined with sterilization operation.

NURSING MANAGEMENT

- Explain the patient about the procedure in detail, what to expect during and after the procedure.
- Provide emotional support to relieve anxiety and apprehension.
- Encourage patient to come for follow-up after 2 weeks and to report any untoward symptoms, e.g. heavy bleeding, pain or fever immediately.
- Discuss with patient the various contraceptive measures especially barrier contraceptives, i.e. condoms for prevention of infections and use of emergency contraceptive devices.
- Provide emotional support to the woman who is grieving for the loss of her pregnancy. Give time and opportunities in order to express her emotions. If required she may be referred to a counselor for further assistance.

PELVIC INFLAMMATORY DISEASE

Definition

Pelvic inflammatory disease refers to an infectious condition of the pelvic cavity that involves the upper genital tract such as endometrium (endometritis), fallopian tubes (salpingitis), ovaries (oophoritis), and pelvic peritoneum (peritonitis or tuboovarian abscess).

Etiology and Risk Factors

- *Neisseria gonorrhea* and *Chlamydia trachomatis* are the most common organisms.
- Other organisms such as anaerobes, streptococci, mycoplasma and gram-negative rods may also cause infections.
- Organisms gain entrance during unprotected sex or after pelvic surgery or termination of pregnancy or child birth.
- Multiple sex partners, presence of intrauterine contraceptive devices and vaginal douches may increase the risk of infection.

Pathophysiology

- Organisms enter through vagina, pass through cervical cannal, colonize the endocervix and move upward into the uterus.
- Organisms reach fallopian tubes, ovaries and into the pelvis to cause inflammation of these structures.
- In bacterial infections that occur after childbirth or abortion organisms reach the parametrium directly through the uterine or cervical lymphatics and blood vessels and usually results in unilateral infection.
- In gonococcal and chlamydial infections, organisms multiply rapidly in the uterine environment and proceed to the falloplan tubes resulting into acute bilateral salpingitis. Pus and debris drain from infected fallopian tubes in the peritoneal cavity resulting in pelvic peritonitis or a tuboovarian abscess.
- Infection may also spread from pelvic cavity itself such as *E. coli* from ruptured bowel and cause pelvic peritonitis.
- Rarely organisms such as tuberculosis reach reproductive organs such as fallopian tubes, ovaries, uterus and pelvic peritoneum through blood stream from the lungs to cause infection.

Clinical Manifestations

- Lower abdominal pain starts gradually and is constant, severe aching pain on both sides of the abdomen or pelvis, increases while walking, voiding, defecation, during intercourse and menses.
- Anorexia, nausea, vomiting, malaise, fever, chills and tachycardia.
- Heavy, purulent, odorous cervical or vaginal discharge.
- Spotting after intercourse.
- Intense lower abdominal tenderness on palpation or movement of the cervix.

Complications

1. Septic shock due to release of endotoxins from the infecting organisms to general circulation.
2. Fitz-Hugh-Curtis syndrome due to spread of infection to liver causing perihepatitis. (patient has acute right upper quadrant pain but normal liver function test results).
3. Pelvic or generalized peritonitis from leaking of tuboovarian mass.
4. Embolism from thrombophlebitis of pelvic veins.
5. Ectopic pregnancy from adhesions and strictures developing in fallopian tubes.
6. Infertility.
7. Chronic pelvic pain

Diagnostic Studies

a. History of acute lower genital tract infection, sexual habits and contraceptive use (IUD).
b. Bimanual pelvic examination detects intense lower abdominal tenderness on palpation and positive cervical motion tenderness.
c. Cultures obtained from abnormal vaginal or cervical discharge reveals gonor-

rhea, chlamydia or any other offending organism.

d. Test for pregnancy to rule out ectopic pregnancy.
e. Colposcopy visualizes the status of pelvic organs.
f. Ultrasonography may identify an abscess.

Medical Management

- **Out-patient treatment for mild cases**:
  1. Broad-spectrum antibiotic therapy.
  2. Rest.
  3. Plenty of oral fluids.
  4. Examination and treatment of sexual partner.
  5. Advise to avoid sexual activity ; douching; or other activities that increases the infectious process.
  6. Follow-up after 48 to 72 hours.
- **In-patient treatment for acutely ill**:
  1. Bed rest in semi-Fowler position to promote drainage of the pelvic cavity and to prevent abscess formation high in the abdominal cavity.
  2. Parenteral antibiotics.
  3. IV fluids to prevent dehydration.
  4. Analgesics to relieve pain.
  5. Sitz bath to increase circulation and decrease pain.
  6. Corticosteroids may be given to reduce inflammation and for faster recovery.
  7. Draining of abscess by laparoscopy or laparotomy if abscess fails to resolve with antibiotic therapy.
  8. Hysterectomy if severe infection or severe chronic pelvic pain.

NURSING MANAGEMENT

Assessment

Subjective data

Lower abdominall pain, pelvic pain, low back pain, pain during menses and dyspareunia. Abnormal vaginal bleeding or discharge, irregular menses. Urinary frequency, urgency. Malaise, nausea, vomiting, chills and fever. Past history of pelvic inflammatory disease, gonorrhea and Chlamydia infections, infertility, multiple sexual partners, unprotected sex, and recent abortion or any pelvic surgery.

Objective data

Heavy, purulent and odorous vaginal discharge, lower abdominal tenderness during bimanual examination and presence of mass on lower abdominal palpation.

Nursing Diagnoses

1. Lower abdominal pain related to infection of pelvic organs as evidenced by patient's verbal complaints.
2. Risk for infection transmission.
3. Low self-esteem related to the PID secondary to sexually transmitted infections.
4. Ineffective health maintenance due to knowledge deficit regarding the disease process, its prevention and treatment as evidenced by recurrence of infections and inaccurate statements about health maintenance.

GOALS

1. Relief of lower abdominal pain
2. Prevention of infection transmission
3. Improved self-esteem
4. Effective health maintenance.

Nursing Intervention

Relief of lower abdominal pain

- Assess pain, its location, character, onset, and duration. Monitor intensity of pain by a pain scale.

- Administer antibiotics, pain medications as advised by the physician.
- Encourage patient to have plenty of fluids to prevent dehydration. Administer IV fluids if the patient is very sick to drink enough fluids.
- Provide sitz bath at least thrice a day to increase circulation, promote, healing and decrease pain.
- Provide bed rest in Fowler position to promote drainage of the pelvic cavity and to prevent abscess formation high in the abdomen.

Prevention of infection transmission

- Discuss with patient about different factors causing the infection and ways to prevent recurrence.
- Advise patient that treatment of her sexual partner is essential to prevent recurrence.
- Teach patient safe disposal of perineal pads and meticulous hand washing.

Improved self-esteem

- Assess patient's psychological status.
- Establish open communication with the patient to establish rapport.
- Plan and provide time for the expression of feelings and concerns of the patient.
- Provide support to the patient and partner.

Effective health maintenance

- Assess patient's knowledge regarding the cause of disease, treatment and prevention.
- Explain patient that it is very important to undergo treatment of both the sexual partner together.
- Teach patient to use condom during coitus to prevent infection.

ENDOMETRIOSIS

Definition

The presence of functioning endometrial tissue in sites outside the endometrial cavity is called endometriosis.

Sites of Ectopic Endometrium

Abdominal—Ovary, pouch of Douglas, uterosacral ligament, broad ligament, rectovaginal septum, rectum and pelvic nodes, gut, appendix, ureters and urinary bladder.

Extra abdominal—Abdominal scar of hysterectomy, cesarean section, tubectomy and myomectomy, umbilicus, episiotomy scar, vagina and cervix.

Remote sites—Pleura, lungs and deep tissues of arms and thighs.

Incidence

- Incidence of endometriosis is increasing.
- It occurs in 10% of women of reproductive age group.
- Incidence is high (30–40%) among the infertile women.

Etiology

- Cause remains unclear but the following theories regarding its cause have been proposed:

Retrograde menstruation theory

During menstruation retrograde flow of menstrual blood passes through the fallopian tubes into the pelvis. Viable endometrial fragments present in menstrual blood get implanted in the peritoneal surface of different pelvic organs. Chronic irritation of the pelvic peritoneum by the menstrual blood may cause metaplasia that result in endometriosis.

Vascular and lymphatic dissemination theory

Metastasis or spread of endometrial tissue occurs through the vascular and lymphatic system to sites outside the uterus. This explains occurrence of endometriosis in remote sites.

Genetic susceptibility theory

Endometrial or decidual tissues when implanted in new sites start to grow in susceptible individual. Incidence of endometriosis is 6 to 7 times more in first degree relatives which suggest genetic factors may be involved in its causation.

Pathophysiology

- Endometrial tissue in the ectopic site responds to ovarian hormonal stimulation.
- During menstruation this ectopic tissue bleeds in areas having no outlet.
- Trapped menstrual blood undergoes various changes such as inflammation, nodule formation, scarring and adhesions at these extrauterine sites. The inflammatory lesions are typically small with blue/brown/gray powder or blue black appearance indicating concealed bleeding.
- Repeated cyclic bleedings due to hormonal stimulation of the endometrial tissue give rise to extensive scarring and adhesions that cause the peritoneal surface and organs to become fixed to one another resulting in pain and infertility.
- With normal ovarian regression associated with menopause these endometrial tissues undergo atrophy. They also regress during pregnancy.

Clinical Manifestations

Manifestations depend more on the ectopic site than to the extent of the disease. 25% of women may remain asymptomatic. Symptomatic women may show wide range of manifestations. Most common manifestations are:

- Secondary dysmenorrhea—There is progressively increasing secondary dysmenorrhea. Pain starts a few days prior to menstruation, gets worse during menstruation and continues even after cessation of period. Site of pain is deep-seated and on the back or rectum.
- Abnormal menstruation such as menorrhagia, epimenorrhagia or polymenorrhea.
- Infertility.
- Dyspareunia.
- Chronic pelvic pain located in several areas. Pain aggravates during periods.
- Abdominal pain of varying degrees during periods may be experienced by some patients. Acute pain may occur due to rupture of chocolate cyst (when the condition occurs in the ovary).
- Frequency, dysuria or even hematuria may occur if the lesion is in bladder.
- Dyschezia (painful defecation), diarrhea, rectal bleeding or even melena may occur if the lesion is in sigmoid colon and rectum.
- On palpation a mass may be felt in lower abdomen. Mass is tender and fixed.
- Pelvic tenderness, nodules in the pouch of Douglas, fixed retroverted uterus, etc. may be found during bimanual pelvic examination.

Diagnosis

1. Pelvic examination finding is suggestive of endometriosis.

2. Laparoscopic examination or laparotomy confirms the diagnosis.

Medical Management

Management depends on age of the woman, number of children, or desire for children, severity of symptoms and extent and location of the disease.

Conservative therapy (when symptoms are mild)

- 'Watch and wait'.
- Mild analgesics, e.g. NSAIDs for pain relief.

Drug therapy

Drug therapy is carried out when symptoms are severe and the woman wants to conceive. Drugs induce pseudo pregnancy or pseudo menopause by inhibiting estrogen production by the ovary, so that the ectopic endometrial tissue shrinks. The drugs given are:

1. Combined oral contraceptives (estrogen and progestogen) for continuous 9 months to suppress ovulation and to produce pseudo pregnancy.
2. Danazol (a synthetic androgen) inhibits anterior pituitary to release gonadotrophin. It produces pseudo menopause (ovarian suppression) with atrophy of endometrial tissue.
3. Gonadotropin-releasing hormone (GnRH) agonists such as cause hypoestrogenic state resulting in amenorrhea.

Surgical therapy

Surgical therapy is the only cure for the disease. Surgery may be:

Conservative—Conservative surgical therapy is carried out for women who wish to become pregnant and are young. The procedure involves removal of implants that are blocking the fallopian tubes, excision of adhesions from the tubes, ovaries and pelvic structures by laparoscopic laser surgery or by laparotomy.

Definitive surgery—Definitive surgery carried out when all other interventions fail and the woman does not want to preserve her, fertility. Uterus, fallopian tubes, ovaries and as many implants as possible are removed.

NURSING MANAGEMENT

Assessment

Subjective data

Secondary dysmenorrhea, lower abdominal pain or backache, painful bowel movements, bleeding per rectum, diarrhea, melena, dyspareunia, menstrual irregularities such as menorrhagia, polymenorrhea, premenstrual symptoms, infertility, frequency, and hematuria, dysuria, chronic fatigue and history of use of analgesics.

Objective data

Anxious look, distress due to pain, abdominal mass on palpation, mass tender and fixed. Pelvic tenderness, nodules in the pouch of Douglas, fixed retroverted uterus and unilateral or bilateral adnexal mass of varying sizes on bimanual pelvic examination. Bluish spots in the posterior fornix seen during speculum examination.

Nursing Diagnoses

1. Chronic lower abdominal pain related to inflammation, scarring and adhesions of ectopic endometrium as evidenced by patient's complaints and distressed look.
2. Anxiety and depression related to possible infertility, perceived loss of femi-

ninity as evidenced by frequent crying, weeping, verbalization of perceived loss of femininity and inability to conceive.

GOALS

1. Relief of pain
2. Avoidance of infertility.

Nursing Interventions

Relief of pain

- Teach patient the nature of the disease and reassure that it is not a life-threatening condition so that she accepts a more conservative and gradual treatment approach.
- Teach patient to understand the medicines that have been prescribed to her. Teach patient the side effects of pain medications, e.g. NSAIDs and the precautions to be taken while taking these drugs.
- Teach patient to practice different non-pharmacologic methods of pain relief when pain is not severe.
- Explain patient about the side effects of hormonal drugs such as weight gain, acne, hot flashes and hirsutism during treatment with danazol, hot flashes, vaginal dryness, osteoporosis, and emotional lability with GnRH agonists are common.

Avoidance of infertility

- Assess patient's and her partner's psychological responses regarding the possibility of infertility.
- Provide emotional support that with timely intervention pregnancy is possible.
- Help patient in decision-making regarding in vitro fertilization or adoption if pregnancy is not at all possible.

BENIGN TUMORS OF THE FEMALE REPRODUCTIVE SYSTEM

Uterine Fibroids

Definition

Uterine fibroids or leiomyomas are benign tumors of smooth muscle and fibrous connective tissue.

Incidence

- It is the most common benign tumor of the female genital tract.
- 20% of women at the age of 30 years have fibroid, but most are asymptomatic.
- Incidence is 2 to 3 times more in African-American women than white women.
- It occurs more commonly in nulliparous or those having one child infertility.
- Common in women approaching menopause, highest prevalence is 35 to 45 years of age.

Etiology

- Cause of tumor development is unknown.
- Growth of tumor is believed to be related to estrogen stimulation which is evident by:
  - Increased growth during pregnancy.
  - They do not occur before menarche.
  - Following menopause growth ceases, atrophies and there is no new growth at all.

Pathophysiology

- Fibroid arises from the single smooth muscle cell of the myometrium.
- Growth is due to the proliferation of the smooth muscle cells.
- Proliferation of the muscle cells is due

to the influence of ovarian hormones as evident by the fact that fibroids grow slowly during the reproductive years and regress after menopause.

Classification

According to the location fibroids are classified

Subserosal—It is found on the outer surface under the serous layer of the uterus. Tends to become pedunculated, multiple and large, backache, constipation and bladder problems are common with it.

Intramural—It is found in the uterine wall surrounded by myometrium. Common features are large abdomen, dysmenorrhea, and metrorrhagia.

Submucosal—It is located under the endometrium, involving the endometrial cavity. It may become pedunculated. Associated with prolonged vaginal bleeding with cramps.

Cervical—Tumor occur in the cervix. It may obstruct cervical canal.

Wandering or parasitic—Pedunculated tumor that breaks off and attaches to other tissues such as omentum.

Intraligamentary—It is found on the pelvic ligaments.

Clinical manifestations

- Majority remain asymptomatic.
- Symptoms depend upon the size of the tumor, its location and number of tumors.
- Most common symptoms are:
  - Abnormal uterine bleeding (hypermenorrhea).
  - Pain, dysmenorrhea, dyspareunia.
  - Lower abdominal, bladder and rectal discomfort due to pelvic pressure.
  - General enlargement of the abdomen when tumor is large.
  - Miscarriage or infertility may also be the only presenting symptoms.
  - Urinary frequency or retention of urine may also occur due to pelvic pressure.
  - Vaginal discharge which is foul smelling, water-tinged or blood-tinged

Diagnosis

1. History of presenting features.
2. Abdominal and pelvic examination findings.
3. Ultrasonography shows abnormal uterine size and shape.
4. Test for pregnancy and cancer to be performed to rule out these conditions before initiation of therapy.

Medical management

Treatment depends on presenting symptoms; age of the patient; desire to preserve fertility and location and size of the tumor.

Minimum symptoms

- Keep under surveillance under a physician.
- Instruct woman to avoid using aspirin.
- GnRH analogs (leuprolid) may be given to shrink the size of the tumor.

Severe symptoms

- Heavy persistent bleeding or rapidly growing tumor requires surgery.

Surgical procedure

Myomectomy—It is the removal of the tumor without removing the uterus. Performed in women who want to preserve their fertility. Carried out by laparotomy. Laparoscopic myomectomy may also be performed.

Uterine artery embolization—In this procedure, small plastic or gelatin beads is injected into the uterine artery and carried to the fibroid branches to stop the blood supply to fibroid.

Cryosurgery—This procedure involves removal of fibroid by freezing of its tissue.

ExAblate 2000 system—The procedure uses magnetic resonance imaging (MRI) guided focused ultrasound to target and destroy uterine fibroids.

Hysterectomy—It is the removal of the uterus along with the fibroids. This is the preferred method when mother completes her family. Other methods which preserve the uterus do not rule out recurrence.

NURSING MANAGEMENT

- Nursing management of woman undergoing hysterectomy is discussed later.
- Nursing management of woman undergoing myomectomy is like laparotomy.
- Postoperative teaching after myomectomy regarding self-care include:
  - Explanation regarding the type of operation she has undergone and the possibility of pregnancy.
  - To attend regular gynecological follow-up.
  - To avoid coitus until physician permits.
  - Eat a well-balanced diet and take adequate rest.
  - Avoid heavy lifting for about 6 weeks and other activities such as aerobic exercise, prolonged standing to prevent pelvic congestion.
  - Report any vaginal bleeding or any abnormal discharge to the physician.
  - When coitus is resumed to use birth control measures until her physician permits her suitable for pregnancy.

BENIGN OVARIAN TUMORS

Benign ovarian tumors are of different types. Primarily they are either solid tumors or cysts.

Types

Most commonly occurring ovarian tumors

1. Mucinous cyst adenoma
2. Serous cyst adenoma
3. Brenner tumor
4. Dermoid cyst.

Mucinous cyst adenoma

- Arises from the totipotent surface epithelium of the ovary.
- 20% to 25% of all ovarian tumors are mucinous cyst adenoma.
- If left untreated may attain a huge size.
- They are the largest ovarian tumors.
- Wall of the tumor is smooth, lobulated, whitish or bluish white color. In some places wall is thin and translucent.
- Tumors may be bilateral in some patients.
- Chance of malignancy is 10%.

Serous cyst adenoma

- Arises from the totipotent surface epithelium of the ovary.
- About 40% of all ovarian tumors are serous cyst adenoma.
- Occur bilaterally in 40% cases.
- Chance of malignancy is about 40%.
- Wall of the cyst is smooth, shiny and grayish white with papillary projections.
- Cut section shows multilobulated.
- The content fluid is clear, rich in serum albumin and globulin.

Brenner tumor

- 1% to 2% of all ovarian tumors is Brenner tumor.
- 8% to 10% of them are bilateral.
- It occurs in women above the age of 40.
- Most of them are solid tumors and less than 2 cm in diameter.

- It arises from squamous metaplasia of surface epithelium.
- They look like fibroma on naked eye.
- The tumors secrete estrogen resulting in abnormal vaginal bleeding.

Dermoid cyst

- Dermoid cyst arises from the germ cells arrested after the first meiotic division and contains any type of body tissue such as hair or teeth.
- 15% to 20% of all ovarian tumors are dermoid tumor.
- It may occur bilaterally.
- Dermoid cyst is of moderate size.
- Capsule is tense and smooth.
- Cut section shows primarily sebaceous material with hair.
- Most common tissue element of the cyst is ectodermal but there may be endodermal or mesodermal tissues also.
- Beside dermal components bone, cartilage, neural tissue, thyroid and salivary gland tissues are often present.

Clinical Features of Ovarian Tumors

Ovarian tumors are mostly asymptomatic, detected accidentally by a physician during routine abdominal examination or during pelvic examination. Common symptoms are:

- Heaviness in the lower abdomen.
- A gradually increasing mass in lower abdomen.
- Dull aching pain in lower abdomen. Pain is severe when cyst twists on its pedicle.
- Untreated tumor may be so big that it may fill whole abdomen.
- Nausea, indigestion, constipation and urinary frequency may occur due to pressure of tumor on the abdomen.
- Menstrual pattern usually remain unaffected.
- Menorrhagia, postmenopausal bleeding or precocious puberty may occur in some hormone producing tumors.
- General condition of the patient usually remains unaffected but with huge mucinous cyst adenoma patient may be cachetic.
- Pitting edema on legs due to pressure of huge tumor on the great veins.
- Per abdomen bulging of the lower abdomen is seen. Mass may be located centrally or in one side. Visible veins under the skin are seen.
- Pelvic examination reveals a mass or an enlarged ovary.

Diagnostic Studies

1. Ultrasonography identifies the tumor.
2. Transvaginal sonography with color Doppler determines tumor volume, cyst wall, and vascularity and distinguishes between benign and malignant tumors.
3. Straight X-ray abdomen may show shadow of bones or teeth if dermoid cyst. An outline of soft tissue shadow may also be seen.
4. Examination under anesthesia is done in virgins.
5. Laparoscopy differentiates painful cystic mass with ectopic pregnancy.
6. Laparotomy is performed when other diagnostic methods fail.
7. Cytology rules out malignancy if ascites or pleural effusion.

Management

Once an ovarian tumor is diagnosed, surgery should be performed immediately.

Surgical procedures

Ovarian cystectomy—It is the removal of the tumor leaving behind healthy ovarian tissue. This procedure is performed in young patients.

Ovariotomy (salpingo-oophorectomy)—It is performed when a large tumor has destroyed almost all ovarian tissue.

Total hysterectomy with bilateral salpingo-oophorectomy—It is performed in women who have completed family and around 40 years of age.

NURSING MANAGEMENT

Nursing management of patients with ovarian tumor undergoing surgery is like nursing management of patients undergoing laparotomy.

PELVIC ORGAN PROLAPSE

Definition

Pelvic organ prolapse involves descent of the vaginal wall and or the uterus. The other organs that descend with pelvic organ prolapse are the urethra, bladder, bowel and rectum.

Incidence

The condition is very common amongst menopausal women.

Etiology and Risk Factors

1. Decreased level of circulating estrogen after menopause causes the supporting structures of the pelvic floor to lose their elasticity and ability to support the pelvic organs.
2. Multiparity.
3. Childbirth trauma.
4. Obesity.
5. Chronic cough.
6. Straining during defecation.
7. Congenital weakness of the supporting structures.

Clinical Types

1. Vaginal prolapse—It occur independently without uterine descent.
2. Uterine prolapse—It is usually associated with vaginal prolapse.

Vaginal prolapse

Cystocele—It is formed by laxity and descent of the upper two-thirds of the anterior vaginal wall and there is herniation of the urinary bladder through the laxed anterior wall.

Urethrocele—It is formed by laxity and descent of the lower-third of the vaginal wall. The urethra herniates through laxed anterior vaginal wall. It may occur independently or along with cystocele and is known as cystourethrocele.

Rectocele—It is formed by laxity of the middle-third of the posterior vaginal wall and the rectovaginal septum, allowing herniation of the rectum through the lax area.

Uterine prolapse

Uterovaginal prolapse—It is the prolapse of the uterus, cervix and upper vagina. Cystocele occurs first which causes traction effect leading to uterovaginal prolapse.

Congenital uterine prolapse—It is the herniation of the uterus along with upper vagina due to congenital weakness of the supporting structures. It is found in nulliparous women and is termed as nulliparous prolapse.

Degrees of uterine prolapse

First degree—The uterus descends down from its normal anatomical position to half way between the ischeal spine and the hymenal ring, i.e. the external os still remains inside the vagina.

Second degree—The uterus descends to the hymenal ring. External os protrudes outside the vaginal introitus but the uterine body is still inside the vagina.

Third degree/complete/procidentia—The uterine body descends to lie outside the introitus. Prolapse of the uterus occurs along with eversion of the entire vagina.

Pathophysiology

- Vaginal mucosa becomes stretched. When exposed to air gets dry, thickened and pigmented due to keratinization.
- The mass lying outside the introitus initially gets keratinized and ultimately infected and ulcerated. There is diminished circulation due to constriction of the prolapsed mass through the vaginal opening and narrowing of the uterine vessels due to the stretching effect.
- Herniation of the bladder results in sharp angulation of the urethra, causing incomplete emptying of the bladder. Incomplete emptying ultimately gives rise to infection and hypertrophy of bladder wall.

Clinical Manifestations

Variable manifestations are noticed irrespective of the progress of the prolapse. Usual manifestations are:

- Feeling of something coming down from vagina especially during standing or walking. Discomfort during walking. Symptoms increase after cough or lifting heavy objects.
- Backache or dragging pain in the pelvis.
- Dyspareunia.
- Urinary symptoms (when cystocele is present):
  - Difficulty in passing urine.
  - Frequent urge to pass urine may be due to incomplete emptying of the bladder and possible infections of urinary bladder.
  - Stress incontinence.
  - Retention may occur rarely.
- Bowel symptoms (when rectocele is present)
  - Difficulty in passing stool.
  - Unable to empty rectum completely (the woman has to push the stool out by putting her fingers in the vagina).
  - Fecal incontinence.
- Excessive white or blood stained discharge per vagina due to associated vaginitis or decubitus ulcer.

Diagnosis

- A detail history to evaluate the etiology of prolapse.
- Thorough pelvic examination by inspection and palpation of vagina, rectum, in both standing and lying down positions.

Management

Preventive management

1. Adequate antenatal and intranatal care. Delivery to be performed by skilled professionals.
2. Encouraging early ambulation after delivery and postnatal exercises (pelvic floor exercises) in postnatal period.
3. Teaching women to avoid strenuous activities, chronic cough, constipation and heavy lifting.
4. Encourage spacing between childbirths and avoid too many pregnancies by contraceptive practices.

Conservative management

Conservative treatment is prescribed for women who have mild symptoms; who are absolutely unfit for surgery and who are pregnant.

1. Improvement of general conditions such as avoiding strenuous activities, heavy weight lifting; treatment of chronic cough and constipation.
2. Estrogen replacement therapy in postmenopausal women.
3. Pelvic floor exercises to strengthen pelvic muscles (Kegel exercises).
4. Use of pessary, a device that is placed in vagina to help support the uterus.

Surgical management

Surgery is the only curative treatment for prolapse. Different types of operations that are carried out are:

1. Anterior colporrhaphy to correct cystocele.
2. Perineorrhaphy or colpoperineorrhaphy to correct prolapse of posterior vaginal wall.
3. Pelvic floor Repair (PFR) to correct both anterior and posterior vaginal wall prolapse and relaxed perineum.
4. Fothergill's or Manchester operation to correct uterine prolapse along with cystocele and rectocele, when preservation of the uterus is desired. The procedure involves—(a) Dilatation and curettage of cervix, (b) amputation of cervix, (c) plication of Mackenrodt's ligament in front of cervix, (d) anterior colporrhaphy, (e) colpoperineorrhaphy.
5. Vaginal hysterectomy with pelvic floor repair (Ward Mayo's operation) performed in menopausal and perimenopausal women with uterovaginal prolapse.
6. Cervicopexy or sling operation (Purandare's operation) performed in congenital or nulliparous prolapse without cystocele. The procedure involves pulling up cervix mechanically through abdominal route and stitching of strips of rectus sheath from both sides to the anterior surface of the cervix by silk.

Complications of Vaginal Repair Operations

1. Hemorrhage
2. Injury to bladder and rectum
3. Retention of urine
4. Sepsis
5. Dyspareunia
6. Recurrence of prolapse, vault prolapse
7. Vesico vaginal fistula
8. Recto vaginal fistula
9. Pelvic abscess
10. Thrombophlebitis
11. Pulmonary embolism.

NURSING MANAGEMENT OF SURGICAL PATIENT

Preoperative Care

- Prepare patient psychologically by explaining the nature and extent of the surgery, what the patient will expect after surgery, and effect of surgery on future reproductive and sexual functions.
- Shave perineum the evening before surgery.
- Cathartic and enema to be given as ordered.
- Usual routine preparation for general anesthesia to be carried out.

Postoperative Care

- Prevent postoperative wound infection by giving perineal care with aseptic technique twice a day and after each urination and defecation.
- Postoperatively indwelling catheter remains in situ for at least 3 to 4 days to prevent strain on the sutures. Provide catheter care twice a day to prevent ascending infection.
- Administer analgesic as ordered to give relief from postoperative pain. Ice pack may be given locally to lessen initial discomfort, later sitz bath may be

given to increase circulation and thus promote healing and provide comfort.
- Provide low residue diet and administer stool softener if the patient has undergone posterior colporrhaphy.
- During discharge, advise patient to prevent constipation by taking laxatives as ordered, avoid heavy lifting, prolonged standing, sitting or walking and avoid intercourse until physician permits.
- Reassure patient that loss of vaginal sensation is temporary.

Nursing Management of Medical Patient

- Teach patient perineal floor exercises (alternately tightening and relaxing rectal and vaginal muscles as if to hold back a bowel movement or a stream of urine for a few seconds). Encourage patient to perform the exercises frequently during the day.
- Teach patient pessary care (to remove daily and to reinsert it after cleaning with mild soap and water).
- To apply estrogen cream at vagina twice a day at bed time.
- Encourage patient to come for follow-up after 15 days for reevaluation of vaginal mucosa.

MALIGNANT TUMORS OF THE FEMALE REPRODUCTIVE SYSTEM

Cervical Cancer

Incidence

- Incidence of invasive cervical cancer is steadily decreasing in the developed world whereas that of in situ cervical cancer is increasing. Reason being the regular screening program of women with Papanicoalou test (Pap smear test).
- In developing countries, where facilities for screening of women by Pap smear test is not readily available or inadequate, incidence of invasive cancer among women is very common.
- In India cancer cervix is the second most common cancer in women, followed by breast.

Etiology and risk factors

Exact cause is unknown but the following factors are believed to cause the disease:
- Chronic irritation or repeated injuries to the cervix.
- Sexual exposure to human papilloma virus.
- Multiple sexual partners or a partner who has had multiple sexual partners.
- Early age of first intercourse.
- Smoking tobacco.
- Low socioeconomic status.
- Untreated chronic cervicitis.
- Sexually transmitted diseases.
- Woman having a sexual partner with history of penile or prostate cancer.

Pathophysiology

- Repeated injuries and exposure of carcinogenic factors to the cervix cause dysplasia (early premalignant changes) and ultimately to invasive cancer. Progression of normal cervical cells to dysplasia and then to invasive cancer takes place very slowly may be over a period of 5 to 10 years.
- Most cervical cancers (85%–90%) are squamous cell carcinoma that begins at the squamocolumnar junction near the external end of cervix. About 10% to 15% of cervical cancers are adenocarcinoma. Adenocarcinoma develops from the endocervical canal and generally involves the endocervical glands.
- Cervical carcinoma spreads first by direct extension to the vaginal mucosa, the body of the uterus, parametrium,

pelvic wall, bladder and bowel. Regional metastasis occurs mainly through lymphatics to the pelvic lymph nodes. Bloodborne metastasis takes place in late stage by veins to lungs, liver or bone.

Clinical features

In precancerous stage or in early stage of the disease patient usually remains asymptomatic. An abnormal Pap smear result is suspicious and demands need for further assessment. Symptoms when appear are commonly:

- Vaginal bleeding especially after coitus. Initially it may be spotting; later bleeding is heavy and irregular. Metrorrhagia, postmenopausal bleeding and polymenorrhea may be present.
- Vaginal discharge normally thin and watery becomes dark and foul smelling as the disease advances.
- Frequency of micturition, dysuria, hematuria or true incontinence may occur due to pressure on bladder or fistula formation.
- Diarrhea, rectal pain, bleeding per rectum or even rectovaginal fistula may occur if rectum is involved.
- Frequent attacks of pyelonephritis due to obstruction of the ureter by the tumor.
- Pelvic pain of varying degree is usually a late manifestation.
- Cachexia, anemia, edema legs develop in late stage due to progressive obstruction of lymphatics and veins by the growing tumor.
- On speculum examination ulcerative or fungating growth is seen that bleeds easily to touch.

Complications

1. Hemorrhage.
2. Pyelitis, pyelonephritis and hydronephrosis.
3. Pyometra if the lesion is endocervical.
4. Vesicovaginal fistula.
5. Rectovaginal fistula.

Diagnostic tests

1. Pap smear test is the primary diagnostic tool for cervical cancer. Abnormal finding requires further examination and testing.
2. Thinprep is a newer liquid-based technique for Pap test, which enhances the possibility of accurate finding in Pap smear test.
3. Biopsy followed by cytological test confirms the diagnosis of cancer. Various biopsy techniques are used:
   - Punch biopsy—It is done with a punch biopsy forceps in out patient department.
   - Cone biopsy—It is the excision of a cone shaped section of the cervix, may be used both for diagnosis and treatment. The excision or conization may be performed by— (i) Cryotherapy (freezing), (ii) Laser vaporization and (iii) Loop electrocautery excision procedure (LEEP).
4. Other tests—CT scan, MRI, intravenous urography, cystography and barium X-ray may be performed for staging of the disease (Table 10.1).

Management

Preventive

- Primary prevention.
  - Identifying high risk woman.
  - Encourage use of condom during sexual activity.
  - Human papilloma virus (HPV) vaccine to all women before sexual exposure.

Table 10.1: Staging of cervical cancer

Preinvasive	
Stage 0	Carcinoma in situ
Invasive	
Stage I	Carcinoma confined to cervix
Stage II	Carcinoma extends beyond the cervix
Stage III	Carcinoma extends to one or both pelvic walls
Stage IV	Carcinoma extends beyond the true pelvis

Medical Surgical Nursing Lewis, et al.

- Secondary prevention
  - Regular screening of all sexually active women.
  - Down staging screening- suggested by WHO as an alternative to regular cytological screening by Pap smear. The procedure involves inspection of the cervix for abnormality by speculum examination. Reddish, red or white areas of patch, growth or ulcer on the surface of the cervix that bleeds to touch are considered to be abnormal. The women with abnormal findings to be referred to a center where diagnosis and treatment of premalignant and malignant lesions are done.

Curative management

- Modalities employed for the treatment of carcinoma cervix are:
  - Primary surgery
  - Primary radiotherapy
  - Chemotherapy
  - Combination therapy.
- Selection of the treatment modality depends on:
  - Stage of the disease (Table 10.1 for staging of cervical cancer).
  - Age and general condition of the patient.
  - Treatment facilities available.
  - Patient's choice of treatment regimen.

Primary surgery

Cervical conization—Performed for non invasive (in situ) cancer. Removal of a small cone of tissue is done either by a sharp scalpel, cryotherapy or laser therapy.

Radical hysterectomy—Removal of the uterus, fallopian tubes, ovaries, upper-half of the vagina, parametrium (most of cardinal and uterosacral ligaments), and the draining primary cervical lymph nodes.

Pelvic exenteration—Performed rarely in a few selected cases of stage IV disease without metastasis to outside the pelvis. It involves radical hysterectomy, removal of urinary bladder, and rectum with a permanent colostomy and an ileal bladder.

Primary radiotherapy: Radiotherapy may be a treatment of choice in all stages of carcinoma cervix. It may be given as teletherapy or brachytherapy.

- **Teletherapy**—In this therapy external beam radiation for 5 days a week given for a period of 4 to 6 weeks followed by 1 or 2 treatments of brachytherapy.
- **Brachytherapy**—in this method small radioactive sources packed in needles or tubes are placed in the cervical tissue (interstitial) or in the uterine cavity (intracavitary) for a period of 1 to 3 days.

Complications of radiotherapy

1. Intestinal and urinary strictures
2. Fistula formation
3. Vaginal fibrosis and stenosis
4. Radiation menopause.

Chemotherapy: Cisplatin-based combination chemotherapy (cisplatin, ifosfamide, paclitaxel or vinorelbine) have been used in advanced cancer. 3 cycles of chemotherapy followed by surgery or radiotherapy have shown improved survival rates.

Combination therapy: In the combination therapy either the surgery or the radiotherapy precedes or follows the other.

a. Surgery followed by radiotherapy, such as in case of positive lymph nodes detected during or after surgery.
b. Radiotherapy followed by surgery, e.g. bulky tumor first treated by radiotherapy to shrink its size to facilitate operative removal afterwards.

OVARIAN CANCER

Ovary is a common site of primary as well as metastatic lesions from other cancers.

Incidence

- It is the 4th leading cause of cancer deaths in women.
- It is more prevalent in USA and Scandinavian countries and less in Asian countries including India.
- Occurs mostly between the age of 55 and 65.

Etiology and Risk Factors

Etiology is unknown. Risk factors include—

- Family history of ovarian cancer. BRCA 1 and BRCA 2 gene mutations have been observed in 80% to 95% of cases of all familial ovarian cancers.
- Family history of breast or colon cancer.
- Personal history of breast or colon and hereditary nonpolyposis colorectal cancer.
- Increasing age.
- Nulliparity.
- High fat diet.
- Mumps before puberty.
- Early menarche, late menopause (increased number of ovulatory cycles lead to increased exposure to estrogen).
- Hormone replacement therapy, use of infertility drugs.

Risk of ovarian cancer decreases with

- Use of oral contraceptives for more than 5 years.
- Breast feeding.
- Multiple pregnancies.
- Early age at first birth.

(These factors reduce the number of ovulatory cycles and thus reduce the exposure to estrogen).

Pathophysiology

- 90% of ovarian cancers are epithelial carcinoma that arise from the surface epithelial cells.
- 10% are germ cell tumors.
- Ovarian cancer tends to grow and spread silently. Symptoms occur when tumor causes pelvic pressure on nearby organs.
- Direct spread occurs by shedding malignant cells, which usually implant on fallopian tubes, uterus, other ovary, bladder, bowel and omentum.
- Distant metastasis takes place when the pelvic blood vessels are involved. Usual route of metastasis is by drainage through the retroperitoneal lymph nodes and iliac and inguinal lymph nodes.

Clinical Manifestations

In early stage nonspecific symptoms of short duration appear, e.g.

- Feeling of vague abdominal discomfort and abdominal distention.
- Indigestion, flatulence, bloating after meals, feeling of fullness, loss of appetite and change of bowel habits.

In later stage more pronounced symptoms appear, e.g.

- Abdominal swelling.
- Persistent dull abdominal pain or pelvic pain.
- Sudden loss of body weight, cachexia, pallor.
- Respiratory distress due to ascites or pleural effusion.
- Menstrual irregularities.
- Jaundice may be present, liver enlarged, mass may be felt on hypogastrium.
- Enlarged left supraclavicular lymph nodes.
- Edema leg or vulva.

Diagnostic Studies

No screening test exists for ovarian cancer. Bimanual pelvic examination if performed yearly may detect ovarian mass at an early stage.

Palpable pelvic mass of any size in a postmenopausal woman is highly suspicious of ovarian cancer.

Screening procedure for high-risk women includes yearly pelvic examination, ultrasound, and test for tumor marker CA-125.

1. CA-125—It is elevated in 80% of women with epithelial ovarian cancer. It is used for monitoring of the course of the disease. It may be elevated in other benign conditions, e.g. endometriosis or fibroids.
2. Abdominal or transvaginal ultrasound detects ovarian mass.
3. Exploratomy laparotomy may establish the diagnosis and stage of the disease.
4. Cytologic examination of fluid collected by abdominal paracentesis or cul-de-sac aspiration confirms malignancy.
5. Histological examination of excised ovarian tumor confirms the diagnosis, identifies the type and grade of malignancy.
6. Other tests, e.g. X-ray chest, barium enema, CT scan, MRI, PET scan, etc. may be done to identify the extent of spread.

Medical Management

Preventive treatment

1. Identification of high-risk women based on family and personal history and genetic screening for BRCA 1 and BRCA 2.
2. Combined oral contraceptives to high-risk women.
3. Prophylactic oophorectomy along with hysterectomy in high-risk women.

Curative treatment

Treatment of ovarian cancer depends on the stage of the disease.

Treatment option is surgery/chemotherapy/radiotherapy /combined therapy.

Surgery

- **Early stage disease**:
  1. Unilateral oophorectomy (removal of the diseased ovary) in young women.
  2. Hysterectomy and bilateral salpingo oophorectomy in elderly women. Procedure involves removal of both the ovaries, uterus along with the fallopian tubes.
- **Advanced stage disease**:
  - Exploratory laparotomy followed by cytoreductive or debulking surgery. The procedure involves total

abdominal hysterectomy, bilateral salpingo oophorectomy, complete omentectomy and resection of any metastatic tumor.

Chemotherapy

1. Chemotherapy with paclitaxel and carboplatin is used as adjuvant therapy after surgery to improve the survival rate in stage I disease that is poorly differentiated. Drugs are given for 5 to 6 cycles at 3 to 4 weekly interval.
2. In advanced disease primary chemotherapy with carboplatin and paclitaxel is used before cytoreductive surgery.
3. Intraperitoneal chemotherapy with paclitaxel and carboplatin is used for minimal or microscopic residual disease.
4. Altretamine (hexalen) or gemcitabine (genzar) with carboplatin is used to treat recurrent ovarian cancer.

Radiotherapy

1. Intraperitoneal radioisotopes may be instilled into the peritoneal cavity for early stage disease.
2. External abdominal and pelvic radiation may be given in stage II disease after tumor reducing surgery.

Combined therapy

1. In early stage disease combined therapy in the form of radiotherapy or chemotherapy aften surgery is performed.
2. Surgical debulking in conjunction with chemotherapy for advanced disease.

NURSING MANAGEMENT OF PATIENTS WITH CANCERS OF THE FEMALE REPRODUCTIVE SYSTEM

Nursing management of patients with cancers of the female reproductive system includes those related to the patient's treatment plan, e.g. surgery, chemotherapy or radiotherapy.

Overall objectives of care are:

1. Active participation of patients in treatment decision.
2. Relief from pain and other presenting problems.
3. Early detection and management of problems arising due to treatment regimen.
4. Helping patient to maintain a quality lifestyle as long as possible.

NURSING INTERVENTIONS OF PATIENTS UNDERGOING SURGERY

Preoperative Care

- Assess potential varied emotional reactions of the patient such as fear due to the diagnosis of cancer, anxiety due to prospect of surgery on her future reproductive and sexual functions, loss of femininity, change in bowel and bladder pattern (in case of pelvic exenteration operation) or feelings of relief due to the prospect of having no menstrual periods or becoming pregnant.
- Explain patient the expectations after surgery on prospective reproductive and sexual functions or bladder and bowel functions as appropriate in simple languages and with the aid of diagrams. Include partner in the discussion.
- Spend time to listen to the concerns of the patient and provide emotional support.
- Explain and provide usual preoperative care to the patient:
  - Carry out usual abdominal or perineal skin preparation.
  - Administer enema and/or vaginal douche if ordered.
  - Introduce an indwelling catheter, which is commonly ordered or empty the bladder before sending to the operating room.

- Provide elastic compression stockings to prevent thromboembolic phenomena.

Postoperative Care

- Assess abdominal dressings or perineal pad (in vaginal hysterectomy) for any sign of bleeding during the first 8 hours after surgery (moderate amount of serosanguinous drainage on the perineal pad is normal after vaginal hysterectomy). Monitor vital signs for tachycardia and hypotension that indicate hemorrhage.
- Assess and monitor urinary drainage from indwelling catheter, which is commonly used for 1 to 2 days postoperatively to maintain constant drainage of the bladder and prevent strain on the sutures. Report any complaint of backache or decreased urine output that may arise due to accidental ligation of a ureter during such operation. Provide catheter care to prevent urinary infection.
- Assess patient for abdominal distention caused due to the effect of anesthesia and sudden release of pressure on the intestines after removal of a large tumor. Withheld food and fluids orally till nauseated and return of bowel sounds. Pass a flatus tube if abdominal distention. Provide abdominal binder that gives relief until the distention subsides. Encourage early ambulation to aid passage of flatus and relieve distention.
- Place the patient on Fowler position to facilitate drainage. Change position every 2 hours, avoid high Fowler position, and avoid pillows under knees to minimize stasis and pooling of blood. Encourage leg exercises, early ambulation to promote circulation and prevent deep vein thrombosis.
- Assess emotional reactions of patient postoperatively since some women experience grief over loss of uterus and ability to bear children. Provide time and allow the woman to express her feelings and concerns so that appropriate care and support may be provided.
- Start hormone replacement therapy as ordered, if, both the ovaries are removed and the woman experiences surgical menopause due to sudden withdrawal of ovarian hormone.
- Teach patient to resume activities gradually. She should avoid heavy lifting for 2 months and avoid activities that may increase pelvic congestion such as dancing and walking swiftly and avoid sexual intercourse until healing is complete.
- Patient undergoing pelvic exenteration has a radical hysterectomy, an abdominal perineal resection and an ileostomy or a colostomy. She will have an urinary or fecal diversion in the abdominal wall, a reconstructed vagina and the onset of menopausal symptoms. Provide understanding and support to the patient and family member during the long rehabilitative process. Patient need to verbalize her concerns regarding her altered body structures.

  (Nursing management of ileostomy or colostomy is discussed in separate section)

NURSING MANAGEMENT OF PATIENT UNDERGOING RADIATION THERAPY

1. Prepare the patient for radiotherapy by explaining the procedure of therapy, the expectation during the therapy and possible side effects she may experience and how to manage those.

2. Explain patient that for brachytherapy:
   - A specially prepared applicator is inserted into the endometrial cavity and vagina and later loaded with predetermined amounts of radioactive materials.
   - The patient will remain isolated in a specially prepared room for 24 to 72 hours depending upon the dose of radiation.
   - She has to remain still in the bed as much as possible in order to prevent dislodgement of the applicator. An indwelling catheter will be inserted and a low residue diet will be given to prevent bowel movement and thus prevent dislodgement of the applicator.
   - Visitors will be restricted and if at all needed will be allowed for a very short period. Nurses will remain near bedside for minimum period of time that may be needed for giving proper care and attention to the patient.
   - She may experience abdominal fullness, cramping, backache and urge to void, which are normal due to therapy and may be relieved by medications such as analgesics, sedatives or muscle relaxants.
3. Assist the physician to place the applicator in the vagina of the patient, which is done under anesthesia in the operating room.
4. After the applicator is placed, transfer patient to the treatment room, place patient on bed in supine position and elevate head to 15°.
5. Instruct patient to move from side to side gently if at all needed, practice deep breathing and coughing and flex the feet to promote circulation and thus prevent hazards of prolonged rest. Apply elastic compression stockings to prevent thromboembolic phenomena.
6. Assess and monitor patient's body temperature, urinary drainage, nausea, vomiting if any and placement of the applicators.
7. After the prescribed period of treatment, help the physician to remove the applicator.
8. Encourage patient for gradual ambulation, take a shower bath but avoid tub bath to prevent infection (the cervix still remains dilated).
9. Offer diet as tolerated.

HYSTERECTOMY

Definition

Hysterectomy is the surgical removal of the uterus.

Types

1. Subtotal (supracervical) hysterectomy is the removal of the uterus and leaving the cervix in situ.
2. Total hysterectomy is the removal of both uterus and cervix.
3. Hysterectomy with bilateral salpingo-oophorectomy (panhysterectomy) is the removal of the entire uterus along with fallopian tubes and ovaries.
4. Radical hysterectomy involves removal of the uterus, tubes, ovaries of both the sides, upper one-third of vagina, adjacent parametrium and the draining lymph nodes of the cervix (performed in malignant conditions).

Indications

- Certain types of reproductive system cancers (uterine, cervical, ovarian, endometrium) or tumors, including uterine fibroids that do not respond to more conservative treatment options.
- Severe and intractable endometriosis (growth of the uterine lining outside

the uterine cavity) and/or adenomyosis (a form of endometriosis, where the uterine lining has grown into and sometimes through the uterine wall musculature).
- Chronic pelvic pain that has not been cured with medical treatment.
- Postpartum to remove either a severe case of placenta praevia (a placenta that has either formed over or inside the birth canal) or placenta percreta (a placenta that has grown into and through the wall of the uterus to attach itself to other organs), as well as a last resort in case of excessive obstetrical hemorrhage.
- Several forms of vaginal prolapse.

Conditions when hysterectomy may be done other than the disease of reproductive organs—
- Prophylaxis against certain reproductive system cancers, especially if there is a strong family history of reproductive system cancers (especially breast cancer in conjunction with BRCA1 or BRCA2 mutation).
- Part of overall gender transition for transmen.

Techniques

Hysterectomy can be performed in different ways—
1. Abdominal hysterectomy is performed by abdominal incision.
2. Vaginal hysterectomy is performing the hysterectomy through the vaginal canal.
3. Laparoscopic assisted vaginal hysterectomy (LAVH) is performed with additional instruments inserted through a small hole, frequently close to the naval.
4. Total laparoscopic hysterectomy (TLH) is performed solely through the laparoscopes in the abdomen, starting at the top of the uterus. The entire uterus is disconnected from its attachments using long thin instruments through the ports. Then all tissue to be removed is passed through the small abdominal incisions.
5. 'Robotic hysterectomy' is a variant of laparoscopic surgery using special remotely controlled instruments that allow the surgeon finer control as well as three-dimensional magnified vision.

Advantages and disadvantages of different techniques

Abdominal hysterectomy
- Requires longer recovery time and longer hospital stay.
- Potential for infections.
- Possible to explore the abdominal cavity and perform complicated operations.

Vaginal hysterectomy
- Shorter healing time and shorter stay in hospital than abdominal hysterectomy.
- Less complications.
- Exploration of the abdominal cavity not possible.

Laparoscopic assisted vaginal hysterectomy (LAVH)
- Allows better exploration and slightly more complicated surgeries than the vaginal procedure.
- The technique begins with laparoscopy but completes with final removal of the uterus through vaginal canal.
- Requires longer operation time
- More costly.

Total laparoscopic hysterectomy
- It is more advanced than LAVH.
- Does not require double- set up, laparoscopic and vaginal.
- Requires longer operation time.
- More costly.

- Healing time is less.
- Blood loss is minimum.

Complications

- Injury to adjacent structures such as bladder, ureter, or intestine.
- Hemorrhage.
- Shock.
- Urinary complications like retention, anuria (due to accidental ligation of the ureters) and incontinence.
- Infection leading to cystitis, abdominal wound infection, pneumonia, phlebitis, peritonitis, etc.
- Deep vein thrombosis.
- Vault prolapse.
- Incisional hernia.

NURSING MANAGEMENT

Assessment Preoperative

Subjective data

Routine preoperative history and history about the disease.

Objective data

Complete physical examination, pelvic examination, findings of different laboratory tests and special investigation.

Anxiety, sleeplessness, repeated questioning, crying and weeping as a result of psychosocial responses to perceived loss of femininity and ability to conceive or fear of cancer.

Postoperative Assessment

Subjective data

Pain and discomfort, difficulty in voiding.

Objective data

General condition, level of consciousness, pulse, respiration, body temperature, blood pressure, capillary refill, breath sounds, bowel sounds, dressings on wound for bleeding or perineal pad for bleeding, drainage from the urinary catheter, pain severity, emotional response like crying, weeping or relaxed.

Nursing Diagnoses

1. Anxiety related to the (diagnosis of cancer), fear of pain, perceived loss of femininity and child bearing potential as evidenced by repeated questioning, anxious look, sleeplessness.
2. Disturbed body image related to altered fertility and fears about sexual relationship with partner as evidenced by verbalization of perceived loss of femininity, inability to conceive, depression, crying and weeping.
3. Acute pain related to the surgery as evidenced by verbalization of pain and discomfort.
4. Deficient knowledge about the perioperative aspects of hysterectomy and postoperative self-care as evidenced by inaccurate statements, repeated questioning.
5. Risk for postoperative complications such as hemorrhage, deep vein thrombosis, urinary problems.

GOALS

1. Relieving anxiety.
2. Improving body image.
3. Relieving pain.
4. Providing knowledge about perioperative care and postoperative self-care.
5. Monitoring and managing potential complications.

Nursing Interventions

Relieving anxiety

- Explain in simple language the disease process of the patient and need for undergoing this operation.

- Orient patient with operation theater and introduce her to the theater nurse if possible.
- If possible, orient the patient with other patients who are recovering from same operations.
- Explain patient that nurses would be available whenever she is examined by a doctor or sent for any investigation in order to minimize her embarrassment during exposure of genitalia in the preoperative period.
- Provide explanation of all preoperative routine procedures and postoperative outcomes and expectations (menopausal syndrome, risk and benefits of hormone replacement therapy, inability to bear children) to the patient in advance.
- Provide time to listen to the concerns of the patient.

Improving body image

- Assess patient's varied emotional reactions towards hysterectomy.
- Explore her concerns such as inability to bear more children, religious beliefs, fears about prognosis and the effects of surgery on sexual relationships.
- Discuss with patient along with significant family members the need of undergoing the surgery and its possible effects on her physical and psychological well-being.
- Reassure patient that majority of women are able to lead a normal sexual life after the surgery as hysterectomy leaves the vagina intact.

Relieving pain

- Assess pain in the incision site with the help of a pain scale.
- Assess discomfort associated with abdominal distention, insertion of nasogastric tube, in situ intravenous drip and urinary catheter.
- Explain patient that postoperative pain and discomfort are very common and will persist for short periods of time.
- Administer analgesics as prescribed. Administer SOS analgesics before pain becomes severe.
- Aspirate gastric content at periodical interval to prevent abdominal distention in a patient with abdominal hysterectomy till peristalsis returns. Apply heat to the abdomen followed by introduction of a flatus tube if abdominal distention.
- Encourage patient turning side to side, leg exercises, deep breathing and early ambulation as these facilitate early return of normal peristalsis.
- Schedule timings of analgesic administration with periods of postoperative exercises and ambulation.

Providing knowledge about perioperative care and postoperative self-care

- Assess patient' knowledge about preoperative routine and postoperative expectation.
- Inform patient beforehand about all the preoperative routine preparations with rational such as need for preoperative skin preparation, early morning enema and fasting, etc.
- Teach patient postoperative self-care such as: adequate rest, adequate diet and fluid intake, regular bowel and bladder functions and personal and perineal hygiene.
- Teach patient to resume activities gradually. Instruct patient not to sit for a long-time, lifting, straining, driving, as these increase pelvic congestion.
- Teach patient to maintain abstinence until her physician permits.
- Encourage patient to report to physician if persistent pain, excessive vaginal bleeding, foul odor in vaginal

discharge, redness and pain in legs and elevated temperature.

Monitoring and managing potential complications

Hemorrhage

- Monitor amount of bleeding postoperatively by observing and counting the perineal pads if vaginal hysterectomy and drainage from the dressings if abdominal operation.
- Monitor vital signs, oxygen saturation and blood pressure as they are the indicators of postoperative shock and bleeding.
- Teach patient activity restrictions after discharge till healing occurs as mentioned above.

Deep vein thrombosis

- Provide an elastic compression dressing before sending the patient for operation to minimize the risk of development of deep vein thrombosis which arises due to position during operation, postoperative edema and immobility.
- Encourage patient to turn in bed and perform leg and feet exercises frequently.
- Encourage and assist in early ambulation.
- Teach patient to avoid sitting for a longtime, keeping pillows under the knees, sitting at crossed legs and inactivity.
- Assess pain, redness, edema and warmth in legs for the development of deep vein thrombosis.

Bladder dysfunction

- Monitor urinary output and assess lower abdomen for distention of bladder after removal of urinary catheter when the patient is ambulated.
- Assist patient in going to the toilet, applying heat to lower abdomen or pouring warm water over perineum if the patient experiences difficulty in micturition.
- Reassure patient that this difficulty is temporary and you will provide all necessary help in resolving the situation.

BENIGN PROSTATIC HYPERPLASIA (BPH)

Definition

Benign prostatic hyperplasia is an enlargement of the prostate gland sufficient to obstruct the urethral outlet resulting from an increase in the number of epithelial cells and stromal tissue.

Incidence

It occurs in 50% of men over 50 years of age and in 90% of men over the age of 80 years.

Etiology and Risk Factors

Exact cause of BPH is not understood.

Possible cause is changes in endocrine system with aging

- Imbalance between the level of dihydrotestosterone (DHT) and 5 alpha reductase (the enzyme that converts testosterone to DHT in the prostate gland).
- Defect in the local substances that causes apoptosis (programed cell death).
- Imbalances of local growth hormone.
- Local inflammation.

Risk factors for BPH

- Family history.
- Obesity (particularly increased abdominal girth).
- Diet high in saturated fatty acids.

- Frequent use of alpha adrenergic agonists commonly found in over the counter cold medication or diet pills increases the severity of lower urinary tract symptoms associated with BPH.
- Diet high in lycopene (found in cooked tomatoes), yellow and green vegetables appear to be protective for BPH.
- Physical activity found to decrease the risk, possibly by reducing obesity.

Pathophysiology

- Benign hyperplasia of prostate develops in the inner part of the prostate, i.e. the glandular or stromal cells near the urethra.
- Hyperplasia enlarges the prostate and the enlarged prostate narrows the lumen of the section of the urethra passing through it and also encroaches upon the bladder neck producing symptoms of obstruction.
- Further growth of prostate and exacerbation of urethral obstruction leads ultimately to detrusor muscle's inability to evacuate bladder by micturition resulting into urinary retention.
- Back pressure of retained urine gradually dilates the ureters and kidneys causing hydro ureter and hydronephrosis respectively.
- Retained urine also serves as medium for growth of organism and gives rise to urinary tract infections.

Clinical Manifestations

Manifestations of BPH may be classified as storage and voiding.

1. Storage symptoms include urinary frequency, urgency (compelling need to void that cannot be deferred), urgency incontinence, feelings of incomplete voiding and voiding at night (nocturia).
2. Voiding symptoms include decrease in the volume and force of urinary stream, hesitancy (needing to wait for the stream to begin), intermittency (when the stream starts and stops intermittently during voiding), straining to void, and dribbling at the end of urination. Pain and dysuria are usually not present.

Complications

BPH is a progressive disease, specially if left untreated and may give rise to following complications:

1. Urinary tract infection and potential sepsis from the stasis of bacteria in the bladder.
2. Bladder calculi from the crystallization of salts in the residual urine.
3. Acute urinary retention.
4. Chronic urinary retention when residual urine volume gradually increases and the bladder distends.
5. Renal failure or obstructive nephropathy due to hydronephrosis resulting from chronic urinary retention and pyelonephritis.
6. Bladder damage.

Diagnostic Studies

1. Digital rectal examination reveals presence of symmetrically enlarged, firm and smooth prostate gland.
2. Urinalysis and culture determines presence of inflammation and infection.
3. Blood urea nitrogen and serum creatinine estimation are done to rule out renal insufficiency.
4. Prostate specific antigen level in blood is estimated to rule out malignancy.
5. Complete blood studies and coagulation profile are performed as hemorrhage is a potential problem of prostate surgery.

6. Uroflowmetry assesses volume of urine flow expelled from bladder per second and indicates the degree of obstruction.
7. Transrectal ultrasound detects size of the enlargement, amount of residual urine and condition of the urinary bladder.
8. Transrectal prostatic biopsy may be done to rule out cancer.

Medical Management

Goals

- To restore bladder drainage
- To relieve the patient's symptoms
- To prevent or treat complications.

Management depends on degree of obstruction and condition of the patient and not on the size of the prostate.

Watchful waiting

For patients with mild symptoms of obstruction watchful waiting or wait and watch approach is used. Teachings for lifestyle modification are given, e.g. restricting fluid intake from evening; limiting spicy or acidic foods, artificial sweeteners, caffeinated beverages and alcohol; avoiding over the counter decongestant and anticholinergic medications and following a timely voiding schedule. Patients are clinically monitored periodically for increase in sign and symptoms of obstruction for further management.

Drug therapy

It is used when patient is having mild to moderate symptoms.

a. Alpha-adrenergic receptor blockers promote smooth muscle relaxation in the prostate gland and bladder neck that facilitates urinary flow through the urethra. Alfuzosin (Uroxatral), doxazosin (Cardura), tamsulosin (Urimax) and terazosin (Hytrin) are used.
b. 5 alpha-reductase inhibitors reduce size of the prostate gland. Finasteride (proscar, fincar) blocks the enzyme 5 alpha-reductase that converts testosterone to dihydroxytestosterone, the important intraprostatic androgen. Suppression of androgens cause regression of hyperplasic tissue and thus decreases the size of the prostate.

Herbal therapy

Saw palmetto extract from serenoa repens has been found to be effective in certain individuals.

Invasive therapy

It is indicated in patients with:

- Sufficient discomfort due to decrease in urine flow.
- Persistent residual urine.
- Acute urinary retention.
- Hydronephrosis.

A. Intermittent catheterization or insertion of indwelling catheter gives immediate relief in acute urinary retention. Patients with poor surgical risk may be taught self-catheterization by clean technique.
B. Transurethral resection of prostate (TURP) is carried out by inserting a resectoscope through the urethra. Through the resectoscope cystoscope is inserted. by using a movable loop through the resectoscope prostate tissue is excised and cauterized. Bladder is irrigated by introducing irrigating fluid through the resectoscope to remove the resected tissue and debris.
C. Transurethral incision of the prostate is a surgical procedure whereby incisions are made in the prostatic tissue to enlarge the lumen of the prostatic urethra. This is a surgical option for

men with moderate to severe symptoms with a small prostate and also for men with poor surgical risk. The procedure is done under local anesthesia.

D. Open prostatectomy is done in patients with large prostate. By making external incision the prostate gland is excised. The incision may be done by three possible approaches:
   i. Suprapubic prostatectomy—in this procedure through a lower abdominal incision, an incision is made into the bladder and the enlarged prostatic tissue is enucleated by blunt dissection. Postoperatively both suprapubic and urethral catheters are inserted to drain bladder.
   ii. Retropubic prostatectomy—In this procedure through a low abdominal incision without entering the bladder the prostate gland is visualized and dissected.
   iii. Perineal prostatectomy—This procedure involves making an incision in the perineum between anus and scrotum to view the prostate for dissection. It is a less commonly performed operation due to potential for infection.

Minimally invasive therapy

It is an alternative to 'watchful waiting' and surgical therapy. These procedures may be carried out as an out patient procedure.

i. Transurethral microwave thermotherapy (TUMT)—a transurethral probe inserted through the urethra to deliver microwaves directly to prostate to raise the temperature of the prostate tissue to about 113°F or 45°C. The heat destroys hyperplasic tissue and thus relieves obstruction.
ii. Transurethral needle ablation (TUNA)—In this procedure low-wave radiofrequency is used to heat the prostate tissue that is in direct contact of the needle inserted through the urethra. This procedure provides greater precision in destroying and removing the target tissue than TUMT.
iii. Transurethral electro vaporization of the prostate (TUVP)—Under visual or ultrasound guidance laser beam is delivered transurethrally by a fiber instrument to cut, coagulate and vaporize prostatic tissue. The affected prostatic tissue gradually sloughs in the urinary stream.
iv. Intraprostatic urethral stent may be inserted into the prostatic urethra to relieve symptoms in patients who are very poor operative risks.

Complications after Surgery

Complications depend upon the type of surgical procedures.

1. Hemorrhage.
2. Infection.
3. Persistent obstruction (usually associated with minimally invasive therapies).
4. Accidental displacement of the catheter.
5. Stenosis of the urethra or bladder neck.
6. Epididymitis.
7. Urinary incontinence.
8. Erectile dysfunction.
9. Retrograde ejaculation.

NURSING MANAGEMENT OF THE MEDICAL PATIENT

Nursing Assessment

Subjective data

Decreased urinary stream, hesitancy in starting urination, dribbling after urination, urgency, frequency, incontinence, nocturia, hematuria, dysuria, low abdominal discomfort, acute pain in lower abdomen, sensation of incomplete voiding, sexual dysfunction, medication for BPH, over the counter medication or prescribed drugs for other conditions, herbal drugs and voluntary control of water intake.

Objective data

Distended bladder on palpation, smooth firm elastic enlarged prostate on digital rectal examination, enlarged prostate and residual urine on ultrasound, decreased flow of urine on uroflowmetry, presence of WBC, RBC, bacteria in urine examination, increased serum creatinine and blood urea nitrogen levels if kidney involvement.

Nursing Diagnoses

1. Ineffective therapeutic regimen management related to lack of knowledge about the condition, its manifestations and treatment options as manifested by frequent questioning, repeated attendance in outpatient department.
2. Acute pain related to impaired urinary elimination secondary to increasing urethral obstruction as evidenced by patient's complain of pain, inability to void and distended bladder.
3. Risk for infection related to urinary stasis and insertion of catheters.

GOALS

1. Understanding of the disease and treatment procedures.
2. Restoration of urinary drainage.
3. Prevention and treatment of urinary tract infection.

Nursing Interventions

Understanding of the disease and treatment procedures

- Assess knowledge of the patient regarding the disease and its treatment option.
- Explain patient in simple language with diagram about BPH.
- Teach patient adequate fluid intake at daytime and less in the evening in order to lessen bladder irritation and chances of infection due to stasis.
- Teach to avoid excessive intake of tea, coffee and alcohol as these increase the symptoms of BPH due to its diuretic effect.
- Explain patient the medical regimen as prescribed in detail, e.g.
  - 5-alpha-reductase inhibitors reduce the size of the prostate gland, and alpha adrenergic receptor blockers promote smooth muscle relaxation in the prostate and facilitates urinary flow through urethra.
  - 5-alpha-reductase inhibitors should be taken on a continuous basis for best therapeutic results and it may require 3 to 6 months to be effective, so the patient should have patience.
  - The side effects of 5-alpha-reductase inhibitors are decreased libido, decreased volume of ejaculate and erectile dysfunction.
  - The side effects of alpha-adrenergic blockers are orthostatic hypotension, dizziness, retrograde ejaculation and nasal congestion. These drugs should be taken at bedtime in order to reduce the hazards of orthostatic hypotension.
- Teach patient to inform all health care providers of their BPH, since several medications, e.g. calcium channel blockers, certain antidepressants and antipsychotics may affect bladder function and increase the risk of acute urinary retention.
- Teach patient to avoid medications

containing alpha-adrenergic agonists, e.g. cold medicines and diet pills as they may cause acute urinary retention and over the counter medications, e.g. diphenhydramine (benadryl).

Restoration of urinary drainage

- Advise patient to void every 2 to 3 hours and when first feeling the urge in order to reduce the chance of acute retention.
- Encourage patient to maintain normal fluid intake to avoid dehydration or fluid overload.
- Assist physician in inserting an urinary catheter if acute obstruction.
- Observe patient for hourly urine output, shock, hematuria caused by postobstructive diuresis.
- Clean the urinary meatus with soap and water several times a day to prevent infection.
- If indicated teach patient intermittent self-catheterization.

Prevention and treatment of urinary tract infection

- Assess patient's symptoms, e.g. burning during voiding, dysuria, and lower abdominal pain indicating urinary tract infection.
- Send urine specimen to laboratory for microscopic examination and culture as indicated.
- Administer antibiotics as ordered.
- Encourage patient to drink enough fluid at daytime and void every 2 to 3 hours when first feeling the urge to prevent stasis and thus increase infection.
- Maintain strict aseptic technique during insertion of catheters.
- Clean urinary meatus and the catheter with aseptic technique to prevent ascending infection.

NURSING MANAGEMENT OF THE PATIENT UNDERGOING PROSTATE SURGERY

Assessment

Subjective data

Please see assessment of the medical Patient. In addition, prescribed medications, over the counter medications, any herbal drugs or vitamin supplementations, e.g. vitamin E having anticoagulant effect, patient's statement about postoperative expectation regarding voiding and sexual functioning, pain after surgery, bladder spasms, urinary incontinence.

Objective data

Bladder distention, drainage through catheter, anxious and apprehensive look, hemorrhage, bleeding or leaking from suprapubic drain, patency of urinary catheter, amount and color of drainage, amount of urine.

Nursing Diagnoses

1. Risk for injury related to presence of urinary catheters, suprapubic drains, irrigation and hemorrhage.
2. Acute pain related to surgery and bladder spasms as manifested by patient's verbal complaints and facial expression.
3. Ineffective therapeutic regimen management related to lack of knowledge about postoperative follow-up care and activity restriction as manifested by frequent questioning and inaccurate statements.

Goals

1. Prevention of injury: Hemorrhage, obstruction or dislodgement of catheters, infection and incontinence.

2. Control of pain.
3. Understanding of follow-up care and activity restrictions.

Nursing Interventions

Prevention of injury

- Monitor patient for bleeding through the catheter, pulse and blood pressure for shock. Maintain pressure through the balloon of indwelling catheter and pulling the catheter out to provide traction.
- Inform physician if severe bleeding.
- Monitor urinary catheter for patency, drainage, kinks and dislodgement.
- Take care so that the tubing is connected to the catheter securely and there is no kink in the tubing.
- Maintain irrigation through the catheter to prevent blockage by debris and blood clots.
- Do not force irrigating fluid through the catheter. If there is no return of irrigating fluid, inform physician.
- Teach patient how to get in and out of bed with the catheter and tubes so that there is no pull on the catheter and no accidental dislodgement. In case of accidental dislodgement inform the surgeon promptly. Secure catheter tubing with bed linen with a clamp to prevent pull on catheter.
- Observe color of drainage for presence of frank blood and blood clots.
- Assess patient for local or systemic signs of infection.
- Maintain closed irrigation system to prevent infection.
- Maintain strict aseptic technique and cleanliness while handling the catheter and suprapubic drainage system.
- Keep skin around the catheter and drainage site clean, dry and protected. Change dressings around the suprapubic catheter whenever soiled.
- Explain patient that temporary retention or incontinence may occur after removal of catheter and will take some time to resolve. Counsel patient for use of devices, e.g. absorbent pads that may be needed temporarily.
- Teach patient pelvic muscle exercises, e.g. Kegel's exercises that help to regain continence.

Control of pain

- Assess intensity, quality and duration of pain.
- If incisional pain administer analgesic as ordered.
- Teach patient nonpharmacologic measures of pain control, e.g. relaxation, deep breathing or music to enhance the effect of pain relieving drugs.
- If bladder spasms observe drainage for blockage.
- Administer antispasmodic medications, e.g. belladona and opium suppositories or propantheline bromide (probanthine), etc. as prescribed to control bladder spasms.
- Administer stool softener with antispasmodics to prevent constipation and straining at stool and thus lessen the chance of bleeding.
- Observe drowziness and acute confusion in older patients after administration of antispasmodics.

Understanding of follow up care and activity restrictions

- Teach patient with the help of written materials about post discharge maintenance schedule planned for the patient.
- Demonstrate catheter and wound management if the patient is discharged with the catheter.
- Discuss lifestyle changes that may be

required to prevent complications, e.g. avoiding heavy lifting, strenuous activity, prolonged sitting, riding stairs, sexual activity, driving or riding prolonged automobile ride for at least 2 weeks or until permitted by the physician to prevent increases in intraabdominal pressure and the possibility of bleeding.
- Teach patient measures to prevent constipation and straining during defecation by diets rich in soluble fibers and stool softeners to prevent bleeding from the operative site.
- Teach patient to avoid alcohol, caffeine and smoking as these irritate bladder mucosa. Coughing during smoking also places strain in surgical site.
- Teach patient pelvic muscle exercises to regain continence. Refer patient to a physical therapist if required.
- Counsel patient along with his partner regarding alteration in sexual activity. Refer patient to a sexual counselors if required.

PROSTATE CANCER

Definition

Prostate cancer is a form of cancer that develops in the prostate, a gland in the male reproductive system.

Incidence

- Incidence of prostate cancer varies widely across the world.
- Incidence is less in South and East Asia than in Europe and USA.
- In USA, it is the secondmost diagnosed cancer and second leading cause of cancer death in men.
- In India, the incidence of prostate cancer is rising.

Etiology

The etiology of prostate cancer is not yet understood. The following risk factors are noted:

Heredity

Men who have first degree family members with prostate cancer have double the risk compared to men without prostate cancer in the family. Risk appears to be greater for men having an affected brother than for men having an affected father. Several genes have been implicated for prostate cancer, e.g. BRCA1, BRCA2, hereditary prostate cancer gene 1 and the androgen receptor, and the vitamin D receptor.

Age

It is uncommon in men below 45 years of age but common in older age. Majority (more than 75%) occur in men over the age of 65 years. Average age at the time of diagnosis is 70 years.

Race

The incidence of prostate cancer is more in African American than any other ethnic group. African American men are found to have more aggressive tumors at the time of diagnosis and also have a higher mortality rates from prostate cancer.

Dietary factors

Diets composed of red meat and dairy products rich in saturated animal fats; deficient in vitamin D are believed to increase the risk, whereas diets high in green and yellow vegetables or lycopene (carotenoids found in cooked tomatoes) believed to decrease the risk. Green tea may prevent or decrease the progression of prostate cancer. Supplements of selenium and zinc may lower the risk.

Environmental and occupational factors

Living in urban areas may increase the risk and occupational exposure to fertilizers, textile and rubber industries and work with batteries containing cadmium may be associated with higher risk.

Testosterone and dihydrotestosterone level

It plays an important part in the development and progression of prostate cancer. Male pattern baldness (high testosterone level) is associated with increased risk. Absence of functioning testes is associated with absence of BPH and prostate cancer.

Medications

Statin drugs used to treat hyperlipidemia have been proved to increase survival following brachytherapy for localized cancer and beta-blockers and long-term use of alpha-blockers may prevent prostate cancer.

Obesity

Lack of exercise and hypertension may increase the risk of prostate cancer.

Pathophysiology

- Prostate cancer is an androgen dependent adenocarcinoma (more than 90%).
- It occurs mostly in the outer aspect or peripheral zone of the gland unlike BPH which occurs in the transitional zone of the gland.
- It is usually a slow-growing tumor but aggressive forms are also noted. It is clinically noted when local extension or distant metastasis impairs the functioning of urinary tract or other organ systems.
- Spread of prostate cancer takes place by 3 routes, e.g. 1) direct extension to seminal vesicles, urethral mucosa, bladder wall and external sphincter; 2) lymphatic system to the regional lymph nodes; and 3) blood stream to the pelvic bones, lower lumbar spine, head of femur, lungs and liver.
- Extent of spread is measured by staging system. In stage I and II the tumor is localized within the prostatic capsule and in stage III and IV the tumor extends beyond prostatic capsule and are classified as advanced stage prostate cancer. These stages are usually associated with metastasis to lymph nodes and distant organs.
- Gleason score of 2 to 10 is given to prostate cancer to determine its grade (the degree of differentiation) where 10 is considered as the most undifferentiated cancer.

Clinical Manifestations

- In the early stage patient usually remain asymptomatic.
- In later stage sign and symptoms of urinary obstruction (similar to BPH) occurs, e.g. hesitancy, dribbling, frequency, urgency, nocturia, dysuria, hematuria, blood in the ejaculation, decreased urinary stream, retention and inability to urinate and painful ejaculation.
- Backache, pain in legs, perineal and rectal discomfort, weakness in legs urinary and fecal incontinence, anemia, weakness, weight loss, and pleural effusion indicates metastasis. Often any of these symptoms may be the first indication of prostate cancer.

Diagnostic Studies

1. History of urinary obstruction.
2. Digital rectal examination may reveal

a nodule within the substance of the gland or as hardening in the early stage. Advanced stage cancer is felt as stony hard, nodular, asymmetric, and fixed.

3. Blood test for prostate-specific antigen (PSA)—Elevated level of PSA (normal level is 0–4 ng/mL or 0–4 mcg/L) indicates prostate pathology but not necessarily prostate cancer. When prostate cancer exists PSA level is used to determine the success of prostate cancer treatment and prognosis, as higher the PSA level the greater the tumor mass.
4. Blood test for prostatic acid phosphatase (PAP)—Elevated level of PAP indicates prostate cancer and its extracapsular spread. Elevated level of serum alkaline phosphatase indicates bone metastasis.
5. Biopsy taken by TRUS (transrectal ultrasound biopsy) and histological examination of the prostate tissue confirms the diagnosis of prostate cancer.
6. Bone scan, CT scan and MRI using an endorectal probe are done to determine the location and extent of the spread of the cancer.

Screening for Early Detection

After the age of 50 years (45 years for high risk men) men should undergo yearly digital rectal examination and blood test for PSA. But result of PSA is not conclusive, as high PSA result is often detected in conditions of prostate other than cancer.

Urine Test for the presence of the protein Engrailed-2 (EN2) is found to be more reliable and accurate than existing tests.

Management

Strategies of management of prostate cancer depend on:

- Stage of the disease, grade and PSA level
- Age and general health of the patient
- Patient's views about potential treatments and their possible side effects.

Conservative management

Active surveillance

- Active surveillance (previously known as watchful waiting) is carried out for a slow growing or self-limited tumor in men age 70 years or older.
- It involves monitoring the tumor over time for signs of growth or appearance of symptoms with the intention of cure if there is any sign of cancer progression.
- Monitoring is done by serial PSA, physical examination of the prostate and/or repeated biopsies.
- Goal is to avoid overtreatment and at the same time serious, permanent side effects of treatment for a slow-growing or self-limited tumor that would never cause any problems for the patient.
- The approach may cause anxiety for the patient who wrongly believe that all cancers are deadly.
- 50% to 75% of patients with a slow growing prostate cancer may best be treated by this method.

Aggressive management

- Surgical therapy
  - Radical prostatectomy.
  - It is the treatment of choice when the disease is localized in the prostate; patient is under 70 years of age and is in good health.
  - It is the most effective treatment for long-term survival.
  - The entire prostate gland, seminal vesicles, part of the bladder neck along with retroperitoneal lymph node is removed.
  - The operation may be performed

by retropubic (more common) or perineal approach.
  - In retropubic approach a low midline incision is given to access prostate gland and to dissect the lymph nodes. After operation the patient has a large indwelling balloon catheter via urethra for about 2 weeks and a drain in surgical site usually for 3 to 4 days.
  - In perineal approach the incision is made in between the scrotum and anus. In this approach there is high incidence of infection. Lymph nodes also cannot be removed in this approach.
  - Laparoscopic approach to radical prostatectomy with robotic assistance is used in some centers. This approach is technically advanced, causes less bleeding, less pain and faster recovery than traditional approach.
  - Complications after a radical prostatectomy are erectile dysfunction, urinary incontinence, hemorrhage, urinary retention, infection, wound dehiscence, deep vein thrombosis and pulmonary emboli.
- Cryosurgery
  - It is a surgical procedure that destroys cancer cells by freezing the tissue.
  - It may be used as initial treatment and as a second line treatment after failure of radiation therapy.
  - A transrectal ultrasound probe is used to visualize the prostate gland. Liquid nitrogen is then instilled via a probe to destroy prostate tissue by freezing. The procedure does not require abdominal incision and may require 2 hours time under general or spinal anesthesia.
  - Complications include damage to the urethra, urethrorectal fistula (rare), or a urethrocutaneous fistula, tissue sloughing, erectile dysfunction, urinary incontinence, prostatitis and hemorrhage.

Radiation therapy

- Radiation therapy is commonly done for patients over 70 years of age, who are poor surgical risk or who want to avoid surgery.
- It may be given as only treatment option or may be combined with surgery.
- Both the forms of therapy, e.g. teletherapy and brachytherapy are used in the treatment of cancer.
- Teletherapy or external beam radiotherapy is given to treat disease confined in the prostate gland and/ or surrounding tissue, i.e. stage I, II and III. Patients receive 6 to 7 weeks of radiation, 5 days a week on an outpatient basis.
- Brachytherapy involves implantation of interstitial radioactive seeds under anesthesia into the prostate gland allowing higher doses of radiation to the prostate while sparing the surrounding tissue.
- It is a onetime outpatient procedure and is carried out for stage I and II disease.

Drug therapy

- Hormone therapy—Prostate cancer growth largely depends on the level of circulating androgens. Various hormones, e.g. luteinizing hormone-releasing hormone, androgen receptor blockers, estrogen are given to decrease the level of circulating androgen or its production. Orchiectomy or removal of both the testes is another method of reducing level of androgens. Hormone therapy may be used before surgery or radiation therapy to reduce tumor mass or may be used inpatients with advanced disease.

Disadvantage of hormone therapy is that almost all tumors gradually become hormone resistant.

- Chemotherapy—Chemotherapy is not very successful in the treatment of prostate cancer. Chemotherapeutic agents singly or in combination may be used for palliation of hormone resistant tumor. Drugs commonly used include cyclophosphamide, mitoxantrone, doxorubicin, idarubicin, epirubicin and estramustine. A recently found drug docetaxel when given in combination with prednisone, estramustine or mitoxantrone has found to improve survival rates in patients with hormone resistant cancer.

NURSING MANAGEMENT OF PATIENT UNDERGOING RADICAL PROSTATECTOMY

Assessment

Subjective data

Hesitancy in starting urination, decreased urinary stream, urgency frequency, dribbling after urination, retention, hematuria, dysuria, low back pain, bone pain, pain at the incision site, anorexia, weight loss, increasing fatigue, malaise, high fat diet and positive family history of prostate cancer.

Objective data

Older adult male, anxious look, anemia, distended bladder on palpation, hard irregular nodular prostate on digital rectal examination, elevated PSA, elevated prostatic acid phosphatase level, large irregular and nodular prostate on ultrasonography, positive findings of histopathology after biopsy and decreased hemoglobin level, amount of drainage, urine output, tachycardia and low blood pressure.

Nursing Diagnoses

1. Anxiety related to the impending surgical procedure and its uncertain effect on life, lifestyle and sexual functioning.
2. Acute pain related to surgery, bladder spasms and bone metastasis if any.
3. Risk for injury related to presence of indwelling catheters and drainage tube, hemorrhage and deep vein thrombosis.

GOALS

1. Understanding about the effect of surgery on future lifestyle and functioning.
2. Relief of pain.
3. Prevention of injury and complication.

Nursing Intervention

Understanding about the effect of surgery on future lifestyle and functioning

- Explain patient with the help of diagrams the surgical procedures planned for him by the physician. Reiterate information given by the physician in simple language. Explain patient the postoperative limitation with regard to urinary continence and sexual functioning.
- Teach patient with the help of written materials about postdischarge maintenance schedule planned for the patient.

Relief of pain

- Assess patient's pain with help of pain scale
- Administer prescribed analgesics, e.g. nonsteroidal antiinflammatory drugs, oral morphine along with nonpharmacologic interventions, e.g. relaxation, music, deep breathing for optimum pain relief.

- Administer antispasmodics, e.g. belladonna and opium suppositories to control bladder spasms.
- Encourage patient to change position, early ambulation that promote muscular relaxation and lessen pain.

Prevention of injury and complication

- Observe drainage tube and urinary catheter for patency, amount of drainage and urine respectively and hemorrhage.
- Take care so that there is no pull or compression on the tubings.
- Maintain strict aseptic technique during changing of drainage dressing and catheter care.
- Demonstrate catheter and wound management if the patient is discharged with the catheter.
- Apply antithrombotic stockings to prevent deep vein thrombosis.
- Teach patient to apply abdominal binder to enhance venous and lymphatic drainage and thus promote circulation.
- Encourage patient leg exercises and pelvic muscle exercises (Kegel's exercise) in order to prevent deep vein thrombosis and achieve continence. Refer patient to a physical therapist.
- Discuss lifestyle changes that may be required to prevent complications, e.g. avoiding heavy lifting, strenuous activity, prolonged sitting, riding stairs, sexual activity, driving or riding prolonged automobile ride for at least 2 weeks or until permitted by the physician to prevent increases in intraabdominal pressure and the possibility of bleeding.
- Teach patient measures to prevent constipation and straining during defecation by diets rich in soluble fibers and stool softeners to prevent bleeding from the operative site.
- Teach patient to avoid alcohol, caffeine and smoking as these irritate bladder mucosa. Coughing during smoking also places strain in surgical site.

11

Nursing Management of Patients with Disorders of Breast

ASSESSMENT OF BREAST DISORDERS

Subjective Data

Obtain a complete health history focusing on symptoms of breast disorders:

Demographic history

Age and race.

History of present illness

Pain in breast (mastalgia), swelling, redness, nipple discharge, skin changes over breast, breast pain or tenderness during menstruation, lumps or masses and location and duration of symptoms.

Personal history

Smoking, use of alcohol and practice of breast self-examination.

Psychosocial history

Occupation, marital status, financial conditions and availability of support people.

History of existing diseases

Diabetes, hypertension, obesity, menstrual disorders, hypothyroidism and infertility.

Medication history

Prescription and over the counter drugs, herbs, oral contraceptives, treatments for infertility, hormonal therapy and vitamins.

Menstrual history

Age at menarche, menstrual cycle—Frequency, regularity and flow. Any complaints regarding menstruation. Date of last menstrual period.

Obstetrical history

History of each pregnancy, childbirth and lactation. Age during first pregnancy.

Dietary history

Dietary habits, consumption of high fat and high calorie diet.

Objective Data

Physical examination and clinical examination of breast.

- Inspection of breasts for size, symmetry; skin over breasts for color, venous pattern, thickening and edema.
- Palpation of breast for mass, its location, size, shape, consistency and mobility.

- Palpation of axillary and clavicular area for enlarged lymph nodes.

Diagnostic Studies

- Mammography is a breast imaging procedure in which internal structure of the breast is visualized using X-rays. Mammography can detect tumors and cysts at early stage that cannot be felt by palpation.
- Digital mammography is a newer technique in which X-ray images are digitally coded into a computer. This allows more accurate and clear image than usual conventional mammography.
- Galactography is a mammography after introduction of radiopaque dye into the duct in the areola through a canula. Performed when abnormality in the duct is suspected, e.g. bloody nipple discharge.
- Ultrasound differentiates benign tumor from malignant tumor.
- Magnetic resonance imaging is highly sensitive, nonspecific diagnostic tool for women at high risk for breast cancer.
- Histologic examination of biopsied tissue confirms the type of tumor or cysts. Various methods of biopsy technique are available, e.g. fine needle biopsy, core needle biopsy, excisional biopsy and incisional biopsy.
- Stereotactic core biopsy and ultrasound guided core biopsy are reliable method of obtaining tissue specimen from an abnormal lesion found in mammogram.

BENIGN CONDITIONS OF BREAST

Mastalgia

Definition

Mastalgia refers to pain in breast.

Incidence

It is a common breast related complaint in women.

70% of women experience it sometimes during their lifetime.

Types and characteristics

1. Cyclic mastalgia
   - Pain in breasts coincides with menstrual cycle.
   - It is the most common type.
   - Pain is due to hormonal sensitivity.
   - Woman describes pain as diffuse breast tenderness or heaviness.
   - Symptoms may last for 2 to 3 days or most of the month and decrease after menopause.
2. Noncyclic mastalgia
   - The condition has no relationship to the menstrual cycle.
   - Pain may be due to trauma, fat necrosis or ductal ectasia.
   - Woman may complain constant or intermittent pain throughout the month.
   - Pain may continue for several years and even after menopause.
   - Woman describes pain as burning, aching or soreness in the breast.

Diagnostic studies

1. Mammography is performed to rule out cancer.

Medical and nursing management

1. Restriction of dietary fat, salt and caffeine.
2. Supplementation of vitamin E, A and B complex, and gamma-linolenic acid may provide some relief.
3. Oral contraceptives or danazol may be prescribed in severe cases.
4. Wearing supportive bra continuously.

Fibrocystic Changes

Definition

Fibrocystic changes in the breast is a benign condition characterized by development of excess fibrous tissue, hyperplasia of the epithelial lining of the mammary ducts, proliferation of mammary ducts and cyst formation.

Etiology and risk factor

- Condition is believed to occur due to excessive responsiveness of breast tissue and stroma to circulating estrogen and progesterone.
- Condition is more common in women between 35 to 50 years of age.
- It is common in women with premenstrual abnormalities, nulliparous women, women with early menarche and late menopause, women with history of spontaneous abortion, and women who do not use oral contraceptives.

Clinical manifestations

- One or more palpable mass that are round, clearly defined and movable.
- Discomfort, pain or tenderness.
- Size and tenderness increase before menstruation.
- Discharge from nipple is milky, watery milky, yellow or green.

Diagnostic studies

1. Mammography may be able to differentiate between cystic mass and solid mass.
2. Ultrasonography better distinguishes between cystic mass and solid mass.
3. Biopsy and cytological studies to rule out malignancy.

Medical management

- Dietary modifications, e.g. low-salt diet, restriction of coffee and chocolate, supplementation of vitamin E.
- Danazol to decrease follicle-stimulating hormone and leutinizing hormone that ultimately reduce estrogen production resulting in decreased nodularity and pain.
- Analgesic to relieve pain.
- Advice to wear good supporting bra and stress reduction.
- Aspiration of cyst or surgical biopsy (in case of recurrence) followed by cytological examination.

Nursing management

- Teach patient to take the prescribed medications regularly.
- Teach woman that fibrocystic changes may recur before menopause and symptoms will increase before menstruation.
- Reassure woman that fibrocystic changes do not turn into cancer but she should perform regular breast self-examination carefully as it is very difficult to find new growth or mass in a breast with fibrocystic changes.
- Teach patient to attend regular follow-up visits as prescribed throughout her life.

Fibroadenoma

Definition

Fibroadenomas are benign tumors developed in the breast.

Incidence

It is a common cause of breast mass in younger women between the ages 15 to 25 years.

The condition is more common in African American women.

Etiology

It may be caused by increased estrogen sensitivity in a localized area of the breast.

Clinical manifestation

- It appears as small, painless, mobile mass with round, and clear margin.
- Mass is solid, firm and rubbery in consistency.
- Usually single but multiple bilateral masses are also reported.
- Slow-growing tumor and growth ceases when the size reaches 2 to 3 cm.

Diagnostic studies

1. Mammography and ultrasound detects the lesion.
2. Histological examination after biopsy confirms the condition.

Medical management

1. Surgical excision of the fibroadenoma.
2. Cryoablation—Under ultrasound guidance a cryoprobe is inserted. Extremely cold gas is piped into the tumor. The frozen tumor dies and gradually shrinks.

Nursing management

- Reassure woman that fibroadenomas are benign tumors.
- Encourage for regular self-breast examination and follow-up care.

Nipple Discharge

Cause

- Idiopathic.
- Galactorrhea or inappropriate lactation due to drugs, endocrine problems and neurological disorders.
- Benign or malignant diseases, e.g. cystic disease, intraductal papilloma, ductal ectasia (dilation of one or more larger ducts of the breast and filling with secretions) and malignancies.

Manifestations

Secretions may be milky, serous, grossly bloody, and brown or green.

Diagnosis

Microscopic examination of slides prepared with discharge detects the cause.

Management

- Treatment depends on the cause of nipple discharge.
- Reassure patient that all nipple discharges are not due to malignancy.

Intraductal Papilloma

Definition

Intraductal papilloma is a benign, wartlike growth found in the mammary ducts, usually near the nipple.

Manifestations

- Occurs in women of 40 to 60 years of age.
- Usually associated with serous or serosanguinous nipple discharge or mass or both.
- A single duct or multiple ducts may be involved. Multiple papillomas increase breast cancer risk.

Treatment

Surgery to excise the papilloma, involved duct or duct system.

Ductal Ectasia

Definition

Ductal ectasia is a benign disorder of the breast involving the ducts in the subareolar zone. It is a condition in which one or more of the larger ducts of the breast is dilated and filled with thick secretions.

Manifestations

- The condition usually occurs in perimenopausal or postmenopausal women.
- Appearance of nipple discharge that may be sticky and multicolored is the primary symptom.
- Painless in the beginning but burning, itching and pain appear as the condition progresses.
- Signs of inflammation, swelling in the areolar area, palpable dilated duct and nipple retraction may be found on examination.

Management

1. Warm compress and antibiotics if inflammation and abscess formation.
2. Surgical excision of the involved ducts.
3. Reassure patient that it is not a malignant disease.

Mastitis

Definition

Mastitis is an inflammatory condition of the breast tissue.

Types

1. Lactation mastitis occurs most commonly in the lactating women within 2 to 4 weeks after childbirth.
2. Nonlactation mastitis is a rare condition, occurs in women in late adolescence or middle age.

Etiology

- Bacteria, most commonly staphylococcus organisms.
- Organisms gain entry through a cracked nipple from patient's hands, oral or eye infections of a breast-fed infant or by blood-borne organisms.

Manifestations

- Dull to severe pain in the infected region.
- Erythema in the affected region.
- Tenderness on palpation.
- Purulent discharge from the nipple may appear.
- Fever.
- Abscess may form if the inflammation does not resolve after several days of antibiotic therapy.

Management

1. Antibiotics.
2. Local cold compress to relieve discomfort.
3. Teach patient:
   - To continue breast feeding if no purulent discharge or abscess formation.
   - To feed the baby with the help of nipple shield or by hand express milk till pain subsides.
   - To maintain proper personal hygiene specially hand washing.
   - To wear a supporting bra.
   - To take adequate rest, fluid and diet.
   - To inform physician for further follow-up care and evaluation if the condition is not relieved by above measures.
4. Ultrasound-guided drainage of the abscess or surgical incision and drainage if abscess formation followed by culture and sensitivity of the drainage.
5. Antibiotics according to the result of sensitivity test.
6. Teach woman to express milk manually and discard it until the abscess is resolved.

BREAST CANCER

Definition

Breast cancer (malignant breast neoplasm) is a type of cancer originating from breast tissue, most commonly from the inner lining of milk ducts or the lobules that supply the ducts with milk.

Incidence

- Breast cancer is the most common cancer among women worldwide.
- According to estimates, in the 2004 alone breast cancer caused 519,000 deaths worldwide. It is the fifth most common cause of cancer deaths worldwide.
- Incidence increases with age. It mostly occurs in women over the age of 50 and the risk is specially high for women over age 60.
- It may occur in both men and women. Men to women ratio are 1:100.
- Globally, the incidence of breast cancer is the highest among American women.

Classification

Classification of breast cancer like all other cancers helps the physician and the family to choose treatment options and to determine the prognosis. Breast cancers are classified according to the following factors:

Histopathology

It describes the tissue of origin of cancer and its invasiveness.

- Ductal carcinomas arise form the epithelial lining of the ducts.
- Lobular carcinomas arise from the epithelial lining of the lobules.
- Carcinoma in situ is growth of low grade cancerous or precancerous cells within a particular tissue compartment, e.g. the mammary duct without invasion of the surrounding tissue.
- Invasive carcinoma does not confine itself to the initial tissue compartment.

Grade

Grading compares the difference in appearance of breast cancer cells to that of normal breast tissue cells (degrees of differentiation).

- Low grade tumor comprises of well-differentiated cells.
- Intermediate grade tumor consists of moderately differentiated cells.
- Cells of high grade tumors are poorly differentiated. High grade tumor has poor prognosis.

Stage

Using TNM system breast cancer stage is determined where T is the size of the tumor, N is cancer spread to the lymph nodes and M means whether the cancer has metastasized. According to this system:

- Stage 0 is a precancerous condition, either ductal carcinoma in situ (DCIS) or lobular carcinoma in situ (LCIS).
- Stages 1 to 3 are within the breast and regional lymph nodes.
- Stage 4 is metastatic cancer that has a poor prognosis.

Receptor status

Breast cancer cells have receptors on their surface and in their cytoplasm and nucleus. Chemical messengers such as hormones bind to receptors and bring changes in their structure and cause death. Breast cancer may be classified according to the presence or absence of three important receptors:

- Estrogen receptor (good prognosis)
- Progesteron receptor
- HER2 receptor (worse prognosis).

Etiology and Risk Factors

Exact cause is not yet understood but the following factors are thought to relate to the cause of breast cancer:

- Female gender.
- Increasing age.
- Race—White and African American women have higher incidence than Hispanic and Asian.
- Personal history of breast cancer—A woman who had breast cancer in one breast has an increased risk of getting a second breast cancer.
- Family history—A woman's risk of breast cancer is higher if her first degree relative had the history of breast cancer.
- Genetic mutations (BRCA 1 and BRCA 2) are responsible for inherited breast cancer cases.
- Lack of childbearing or breastfeeding.
- Higher hormonal levels.
- Early menarche.
- Late menopause.
- Nulliparity.
- First child after 30 years of age.
- Hormone therapy.
- Economic status—Higher incidence is noted among higher income group.
- Dietary iodine deficiency, a high fat diet, alcohol intake.
- Weight gain and obesity after menopause.
- Benign breast disease with atypical hyperplasia and lobular carcinoma in situ increase the risk.
- Environmental factors, e.g. smoking, exposure to radiation during adolescence or early adulthood and shift work.

Pathophysiology

- Breast cancers begin at the epithelial lining of the lobule or of the ducts with a genetic alteration in a single cell and takes time to divide and double in size. A carcinoma may double in size 30 times to become 1 cm or larger and clinically palpable.
- Regional spread of the cancer occurs most commonly to the axillary lymph nodes via lymphatic channels. Other sites of regional spread are internal mammary, and supraclavicular nodes.
- Distant metastasis may affect any organ but most common sites are bone, lungs, brain, liver, pleura and adrenals.
- Majority of breast cancers are adenocarcinoma and located in the upper outer quadrant of the breast.

Clinical Manifestations

- Presence of a lump that is painless, nontender, hard, irregular and nonmobile.
- Lump in axillary lymph nodes may also indicate breast cancer.
- Changes in breast size and shape.
- Unilateral nipple discharge that may be clear or bloody.
- Nipple retraction.
- Skin over breast appears orange peel texture (peau d'orange).
- Infiltration, induration and dimpling of overlying skin occur in advanced cases.
- Mammogram detects earliest sign of breast cancer that is not yet palpable.
- Nonspecific symptoms, e.g. unexplained weight loss, fevers or chills, bone and joint pains, jaundice or neurological symptoms may also appear in metastatic breast cancer depending upon the site of metastasis.

Complications

- Most common complications are—
  1. Local or regional recurrence of breast cancer that may appear near the mastectomy site and internal mammary lymph nodes, or axillary lymph nodes.
  2. Metastasis to distant organs, e.g. bone, lung, brain and liver.

Diagnostic Studies

1. Mammography indicates early sign of cancer even when the tumor is not clinically palpable.

2. Histological analysis of breast tumor tissue obtained by various biopsy techniques confirms the diagnosis of cancer. Various biopsy techniques are:
   a. Fine needle aspiration biopsy
   b. Core needle biopsy
   c. Excisional biopsy.
3. Axillary lymph node biopsy and cytology to detect the status of axillary nodes.
4. Lymphatic mapping and sentinel lymph node dissection done to find out the status of lymph nodes that drain first from the tumor site.
5. Estrogen progesterone receptor status of the tumor indicates prognosis of breast cancer. Receptor positive tumors are usually well-differentiated, have less chance of metastasis and treatable with hormones.
6. Blood test for HER-2 receptors also indicates prognosis. Over expression of HER-2 indicates poor prognosis
7. Ultrasonography, CT scan, bone scan and MRI may be required to evaluate staging of the disease.

Screening

Breast cancer screening refers to testing otherwise—healthy women for breast cancer in order to diagnose the disease early.

The screening methods include

- Self breast examination starting from age 25.
- Clinical examination at least every 3 years for women at 20s and 30s and annually for women at 40s.
- Mammography every year recommended from age 40 and for high-risk women should begin at age 25.
- Genetic screening may be performed for high-risk women.
- Ultrasound.
- Magnetic resonance imaging may be performed in women with BRCA 1 and BRCA 2 mutation.

Prevention

- In general women can reduce their risk of breast cancer development by:
  - Maintaining a healthy body weight.
  - Being physically active and performing regular exercise.
  - Drinking less alcohol, avoiding smoking.
  - Breast feeding their children.
- Breast cancer if developed may be detected at an early stage by taking part in regular screening programs.
- Chemoprevention aims at preventing the disease before it starts. Tamoxifen and raloxifene prescribed to the postmenopausal women have been found to reduce the incidence of invasive breast cancer.
- Prophylactic bilateral mastectomy may be considered in women with strong family history and BRCA 1 and BRCA 2 mutation.

Medical Management

Various management modalities are available for treatment of breast cancer. Selection of the appropriate strategy depends on the size, stage, rate of growth and other characteristics of the tumor.

Surgical therapy

1. Breast conservation surgery with radiation therapy involves removal of the entire tumor along with a margin of normal tissue. Axillary node dissection or sentinel node dissection may also be performed. Following surgery radiation therapy is given to entire breast.
2. Modified radical mastectomy includes removal of the breast and axillary lymph nodes on the same side but preservation

of the pectoralis muscle. It is selected over breast conservation surgery when the tumor is too large to excise and good cosmetic result is not possible. Patient may also choose the option as she may undergo breast reconstruction surgery along with this procedure or after postoperative recovery.

3. Axillary lymph node dissection (ALND) and sentinel lymph node dissection (SLND). Axillary lymph node dissection involves removal of 12 to 20 axillary lymph nodes and used to be the standard practice in all invasive breast cancer. Recently sentinel lymph node dissection has replaced axillary node dissection in women with early stage cancer with negative sentinel lymph nodes. ALND has many complications while SLND has fewer complications but success rate is same.

Complications of surgery

- Lymphedema
- Postmastectomy pain syndrome
- Hematoma or seroma formation
- Infection
- Cellulitis.

Radiation therapy

- Radiation therapy is used in the treatment of breast cancer as:
  - Primary treatment to prevent local recurrence after breast conservation surgery.
  - Primary treatment in women with poor surgical risk.
  - Adjuvant treatment after mastectomy to prevent local and nodal recurrences.
  - Palliative treatment to relieve pain caused by metastases or local recurrence.
- Radiation therapy may be given as external beam radiotherapy or teletherapy or as high dose internal radiation or brachytherapy.
  - In teletherapy the region of the tumor bed and regional lymph nodes are irradiated daily over a 5 to 6 weeks period using an external beam of radiation.
  - High dose brachytherapy involves implantation of multiple catheters in the breast and then delivering a radioactive seed in each catheter to treat the tumor area or tumor bed after operation.
  - High dose brachytherapy requires only 5 days to treat compared to 5 to 6 weeks of traditional radiotherapy.
  - Radiation can also be given during operation as intraoprative radiation therapy.

Side effects of radiation therapy

- Fatigue.
- Mild to moderate erythema at the site of radiation.
- Breast edema.
- Skin breakdown at axilla or under the breast towards the site of treatment is a rare complication.

Nursing management of patient undergoing radiation therapy

- Explain patient that fatigue during the period of radiation treatment is normal.
- Teach patient to take care of skin over breast to prevent side effect of radiation, e.g. daily bathing without rubbing; avoid using deodorant, lotion, etc. without the advice of physician; keeping the area dry; avoid tight clothing, exposure to sun, exposure to excessive hot or cold climate.

Chemotherapy/medication

Chemotherapy is the use of cytotoxic drugs to destroy cancer cells. Chemotherapy or other types of medications are used in the treatment of breast cancer.

Indication

- Before operation to reduce the size of tumor in order to perform a less extensive surgery—called neoadjuvant therapy.
- After surgery in stage II or III cancer to prevent recurrence—called adjuvant therapy

Drug regimen

Three main groups of drugs used are:

1. Hormone blocking therapy
2. Chemotherapy
3. Monoclonal antibodies.

Hormone blocking therapy

- Some breast cancers require estrogen for their growth and are identified by the presence of estrogen receptors (ER+) and progesterone receptors (PR+) on their surface.
- ER+ cancers may be treated with tamoxifen that block the receptors or by an aromatase inhibitor, e.g. anastrozole or letrozole that block the production of estrogen. Aromatase inhibitors are only suitable for postmenopausal women.

Chemotherapy

- Chemotherapy or use of cytotoxic drugs is used for stage 2 to 4 diseases and particularly useful for estrogen negative tumors.
- Chemotherapeutic drugs are given in combination usually for 3 to 6 months.
- Some of the common combinations used in breast cancer are—(1) cyclophosphamide and doxorubicin (Adriamycin) known as AC; (2) cyclophosphamide, doxorubicin and taxane (paclitaxel or docetaxel) known as CAT; (3) cyclophosphamide, methotrexate, 5 fluorouracil (5FU) known as CMF.

Monoclonal antibodies

- Trastuzumab (Herceptin), a monoclonal antibody to HER-2 is effective in patients with metastatic breast cancers whose tumor overexpresses HER-2.
- The antibody attaches to the antigen; it is taken up by the cells and ultimately kills them.
- It can be used alone or in combination with chemotherapy in any stage of the disease following surgery.
- The drug has been found to improve the 5 year disease free survival of stage 1-3 HER-2 breast cancers.
- The drug is expensive.
- About 2% of patients treated with this drug have been found to develop significant heart damage.
- Studies are going on with other monoclonal antibodies.

NURSING MANAGEMENT OF PATIENT UNDERGOING LUMPECTOMY AND MASTECTOMY (PREOPERATIVE CARE)

Nursing Assessment

Subjective data

Change in breast contour, size and symmetry, palpable mass found on self-breast examination, clear or milky or bloody discharge from one breast, history of breast cancer in the first degree relative, early menarche and late menopause, nulliparity or first pregnancy after the age of 30, use of hormones such as oral contraceptives or hormone replacement therapy after menopause, history of previous cancer, exposure to radiation, alcohol use, etc.

Objective data

Hard, irregular, nonmovable breast lump, nipple inversion or retraction, orange peel skin on breast, dimpling, erythema, palpable axillary or supraclavicular lymph nodes, obese, stressed and anxious.

Possible findings

Positive findings in mammography or ultrasonography, positive results in fine needle or surgical biopsy.

Nursing Diagnoses

1. Fear and anxiety related to the diagnosis of cancer, treatment and potential body image changes as evidenced by crying, insomnia and repeated questioning about prognosis.
2. Decisional conflict regarding treatment options related to knowledge deficit as evidenced by repeated questioning and verbalizing inaccurate statements.

Goals

1. Relief of fear and anxiety
2. Active participation in the decision making process related to treatment options.

Nursing Intervention

Relief of fear and anxiety

- Explain patient that various treatment options are available for the treatment of breast cancer.
- Reassure patient that diagnosis of cancer is not always frightening and one may lead a normal life for many years after treatment if detected early.
- Explain and reinforce information given by the physician regarding the treatment option planned for the patient.
- Explain patient what to expect before, during and after surgery, e.g. admission the day before surgery and discharge the day after surgery if patient is having breast conservation surgery. Patient with mastectomy may remain in hospital little longer if they have immediate breast reconstruction surgery.
- Explain patient that surgical drains will be placed at the incision site and also at the axilla, if axillary lymph node dissection is done.
- Explain patient that prior instructions will be provided to her before discharge about the care of drain, pain relief measures and postoperative arm exercises.
- Introduce the patient with the social workers, psychiatrist, support group and breast cancer survivors as and when required.
- Maintain open communication and reassure patient that clarification of any doubts will be available whenever needed.

Active participation in the decision making process related to treatment options

- Explain patient and significant family member about treatment options.
- Explain the merits and demerits of each option for example breast conservation surgery requires 6 to 7 weeks of radiotherapy and the patient has to attend radiotherapy 5 days a week for 6 to 7 weeks and spend extra money for this additional treatment options.
- Help the patient to choose option that would be realistic and practical for her.
- Once the patient has taken a decision support her so that she realizes that the decision is best suited for her.

Postoperative Care

Nursing assessment

Subjective data: Pain at the incision site, verbalization of concern of change in body image.

Objective data: Grief and depression, tachycardia, operative wound, drain, amount and character of drainage, movement of hand at the operative site.

Nursing diagnoses

1. Pain and discomfort related to surgical procedure as evidenced by patient's verbal complain.
2. Disturbed body image related to perceived effects of mastectomy or lumpectomy as evidenced by verbalization of loss of femininity and refusal to see the incision.
3. Self-care deficit related to limitation of movement of upper extremity on the surgical side.
4. Ineffective therapeutic regimen management related to lack of knowledge regarding disease process and postoperative care as evidenced by frequent questions regarding disease and treatment, after care and prognosis.
5. Risk for injury related to increased risk of infection and lymphedema secondary to axillary node dissection.

Goals

1. Controlling pain and discomfort.
2. Promoting positive body image.
3. Increasing participation in self-care activities.
4. Acquiring knowledge regarding therapeutic regimen.
5. Absence of infection and lymphedema.

Nursing Interventions

Controlling pain and discomfort

- Perform a comprehensive assessment of pain, its location, severity, quality, onset and duration of pain, and factors that increase or decrease pain.
- Administer analgesics as prescribed regularly in order to reduce pain.
- Teach patient nonpharmacologic measures, e.g. distraction, listening music, relaxation, etc. to use along with analgesic or in place of it.
- Teach patient to report onset of pain before it becomes severe so that pain control measures are initiated timely.

Promoting positive body image

- Assess psychological reaction of the patient if she has a mastectomy.
- Assist patient to discuss changes caused by surgery in order to ventilate her grief.
- Introduce patient to other persons who have had mastectomy and leading a normal life at present in order to instill hope for recovery and a normal future.
- Teach patient that various measures, e.g. prosthesis, or breast reconstruction are available in order to improve appearance.
- Refer patient to support group, psychologist or social worker as and when required.

Increasing participation in self-care activities

- Teach patient to participate in self-care activities with the hand on the operative site from the first postoperative day.
- Administer analgesic liberally to control pain which will enhance self-care activity and use of the arm on affected side.

Acquiring knowledge regarding therapeutic regimen

- Teach patient and a significant relative if required how to care for the incision site, drainage tube, signs of inflammation at the insertion site, obstruction or dislodgement of the tube(avoid any pull on the drainage tube), emptying the drainage bottle, recording amount of drainage, etc.
- Take a return demonstration before discharge to ensure whether patient or significant family member is self-sufficient in own care or patient's care.
- Teach patient when to come for follow-up or to report any significant untoward changes in patient's condition, e.g. changes in surgical site or any changes in breast or chest wall.
- Teach patient regular self-breast examination and attending regular follow-up visits for periodical mammogram for early identification of recurrence in the same breast or other breast.

Absence of infection and lymphedema

- Assess signs of infection, e.g. elevated temperature, chills, redness, swelling, tenderness, foul smelling discharge at the incision site for evidence of infection.
- Administer prophylactic antibiotics as prescribed to prevent infection.
- If infection develops send swabs from the infected incision site for culture and sensitivity and administer antibiotics accordingly.
- Teach patient to maintain personal hygiene, cleanliness of clothes and beddings, good diet to prevent infection.
- Take special care to control blood sugar in diabetic patient and in patient with immune disorder.
- Assess patient's arm on the operative site for transient edema and later on for lymphedema, e.g. heaviness, localized pain for early detection and necessary intervention.
- Reassure patient that transient edema is normal and it is not lymphedema.
- Elevate arm after operation with a pillow so that the elbow is at the level of the heart and the forearm is just above the elbow to promote lymphatic drainage.
- Instruct patient to squeeze hand gently after the opeartion and start practicing postmastectomy exercises several times from the first postoperative day to promote development of collateral lymphatic channels and thus prevent lymphedema as well as joint stiffness and contracture.
- Instruct patient to avoid keeping hand in dependent position for increased venous return and allow proper healing.
- Teach patient to avoid injury and infection on the hand at the operative site.
- Do not use the hand on the operative side for injections, venipuncture and blood pressure measurement.
- If lymphedema develops advise patient to wear elastic sleeve or use of pneumatic compression and massage by a physiotherapist for good venous return.

12

Oncological Nursing: Nursing Management of Patients with Cancer

ONCOLOGICAL NURSING

Definition of Terms

Oncology

It refers to the medical specialty that deals with the diagnosis, treatment and study of cancer.

Oncologist

It is a physician who specializes in cancer treatment.

Tumor

The term tumor refers to lump, mass or swelling.

Neoplasm

It refers to an abnormal mass of tissue that serves no useful purpose but may harm the host. Neoplasm may be benign or malignant.

Benign neoplasm: It is usually a harmless growth of well-differentiated cells that resembles normal cells of the tissue from which it originated; usually encapsulated and does not invade other tissues; grows usually slowly; does not metastasize; usually gives rise to localized symptoms. It may be harmful or even fatal if located near a vital organ e.g. brain or near a major vessel or tube obstructing circulation or drainage.

Malignant neoplasm: Malignant neoplasm or cancer is a harmful mass of undifferentiated cells that does not resemble normal cells of the tissue from which it originated, capable of invading and destroying tissues, vascular and lymphatic channels; metastasizes to distant organs; grows usually faster than the benign tumor. It causes generalized effects, e.g. anemia, weight loss, etc. and extensive tissue damage as the cancer outgrows its blood supply or grows on the blood flow of the area. If the growth cannot be controlled death is imminent.

Incidence of Cancer

- Cancer is a major health problem affecting people worldwide.
- Worldwide about 10 million people are diagnosed with cancer and 6 million die with it each year.
- It occurs in people of all age group but incidence is more (76%) in people over 55 years of age and is considered a disease of old age.

- Incidence is higher in men than women, in industrialized nations and industrial sectors and in more developed countries.
- It is the second leading cause of death in USA and UK.
- In India 2 to 2.5 million cases of cancers exist at any given point of time.
- 7 to 9 lakh new cases detected each year and half of these die each year. Iit is one of the 10 leading causes of death.
- Four more frequent cancers in males in India are mouth or oropharynx, esophagus, stomach, lower respiratory tract, e.g. trachea, bronchus, and lungs.
- In women more frequent cancers in India are breast, cervix, mouth/oropharynx and esophagus.

Oncological Nursing

Cancer is a disease which has profound impact on physical, psychological, and social well-being of individual patients, and their families.

The disease causes great deal of sufferings and is a leading cause of death.

Despite improvements in cure rates many uncertainties concerning the nature, causes, methods of prevention, and cure lead to various myths and fears about the disease.

Nurses educated in oncological nursing are in a key position to educate the public to remove fears and apprehension and promote a realistic attitude and behavior about cancer.

Goals of Cancer Nursing

1. To assist individual to understand, reduce, or eliminate their risk of development of cancer.
2. To encourage patient and family to comply with cancer detection and cancer treatment regimens.
3. To support the patient and family experiencing a wide range of physical, emotional, social and spiritual crisis.

PATHOPHYSIOLOGY OF MALIGNANT PROCESS

Cancer is a group of diseases characterized by uncontrolled and unregulated growth of abnormal cells originating from multiple causes.

Any cell of the body which escapes normal regulatory mechanisms of proliferation and differentiation may turn into cancer. In other words, defective cellular proliferation and defective cellular differentiation result in development of cancer.

Defective Cellular Proliferation

Normal cell proliferation originates in stem cells (a population of predetermined differentiated cells) and begins when cell enters cell cycle. A mature cell continues to function until it dies. An intracellular mechanism activates cell proliferation when some cells die or there is a physiological need for more cells. Normally rate of cell proliferation equals rate of cell degeneration or death in order to maintain a dynamic equilibrium. Malignant cells respond differently than normal cells to the intracellular mechanism that regulates dynamic equilibrium and proliferates indiscriminately and haphazardly. Another control mechanism that exists in normal cell proliferation is contact inhibition. Normal cells respect their territories surrounding them and do not enter a territory that is not their own. Malignant cells have no regard for contact inhibition and thus do not respect cellular boundaries and continue to proliferate beyond their boundaries in between normal cells.

Defective Cellular Differentiation

Genetically identical cells in the embryo ultimately develop into various structures and assume various specialized functions. This process of development is known as cellular differentiation. The growth and function of a specific cell line is the result of expression of protooncogenes (that promote growth) and suppression of tumor suppressor genes. Transformation of a normal cell to a malignant cell may occur at any point in the process of differentiation through genetic mutation that alters the expression of protooncogenes and activate them to function as oncogenes or tumor-inducing genes and cells assume appearance and characteristics of previous undifferentiated cells.

Development of Cancer

The process of transformation of normal cells into malignant cells is called carcinogenesis. Carcinogenesis is not a rapid process but an orderly three-step cellular process occurring over a period of time:

Initiation

It is the first step of carcinogenesis occurs when a carcinogen damages DNA and results in mutation in the cell's genetic structure. The altered cell has the potential for developing into a group of identical altered cells but do not develop cancer as they have not the ability to self-replicate and grow, instead many of them undergo apoptosis (genetically programed cellular death).

Promotion

It occurs with additional insults to the initiated cells by promoting agents (co-carcinogens) and result in reversible proliferation of the altered cells. The activity of the promoting substances is reversible. But repeated exposures to promoting agents result in an increase in the altered cell population and possibility of further genetic mutations and malignant conversion. A varying period of time from years to decades elapses between the initial genetic alteration and the clinical evidence of cancer. This period of time called latent period comprises of both initiation and promotion phases.

Progression

It is the final stage of carcinogenesis. In this stage there is increased growth of malignant cells to a mass of clinically evident tumor and increased invasiveness and spread of the cancer to a distant site or metastasis.

Etiology

Definite causes of cancer are yet to be discovered but epidemiological studies have identified several factors known as carcinogenic factors that may be implicated in the development of cancer.

Carcinogenic factors may be intrinsic or extrinsic.

Intrinsic factors

Heredity and familial susceptibility: Genetic factors believed to play a role in cancer development. Abnormal chromosomal patterns have been detected in certain cancers, e.g. Burkitt's lymphoma, chronic myelogenous leukemia, meningiomas, acute leukemias, retinoblastomas, Wilms tumor, etc. High incidence of leukemia has been noted in children with Down syndrome and Bloom syndrome. Many cancers have been found to display a familial predisposition, e.g. breast, ovarian, endometrium, colorectal, prostate, stomach and lung cancers. BRCA1, and BRCA2 have been identified in certain percentage of women with breast cancer.

Hormones: Tumor growth are believed to be promoted by excessive production of body's own hormone or by administration of exogenous hormones. Prolonged effect of estrogen in women with early menarche, late menopause and nulliparity is associated with increased incidence of breast cancer. Oral contraceptives and prolonged estrogen replacement therapy are associated with increased incidence of hepatocellular, endometrial and breast cancers.

Immunity: Impaired immune system is believed to be associated with cancer. Increased incidence of Kaposis sarcoma is found in patients with AIDS. Persons receiving immunosuppressive drugs (organ transplant recipients) are at increased risk of developing cancer. Persons treated with chemotherapeutic drugs like alkylating agents for Hodgkin's disease is found to develop secondary malignancies.

Age: Incidence of cancer rises with increased age. It may be due to prolonged exposure to carcinogen or decreased resistance to the effect of carcinogen that normally occurs with aging.

Preexisting disease: Tissue subjected to constant irritation or disease process are prone to develop cancer, e.g. ulcerative colitis may develop into colorectal cancer; pernicious anemia may turn into gastrointestinal cancer.

Stress: Stress is found to alter the growth of certain tumors. Traumatic life events experienced by patients, whose cancer were well controlled have been found to exaggerate the illness and even death.

Extrinsic factors

Physical agents: Excessive exposure to ultraviolet rays of sun specially in fair-skinned, blue or green-eyed people increases the risk of skin cancer.

Exposure to ionizing radiation is associated with several types of cancers. Increased incidence of leukemia, lymphoma, thyroid cancer and other cancers are noted in survivors of atomic bomb explosion in Hiroshima and Nagasaki. Increased incidence of bone cancer occurs in persons exposed to radiation in certain occupations, e.g. uranium miners and radiation technologists. A higher incidence of childhood cancers occurs in children exposed to radiation in fetal life.

Chronic irritation or inflammation increases the risk of cancers, e.g. oral cancers from defective teeth and ill-fitting dentures, esophageal cancer from gastrointestinal reflux disease.

Chemical agents: Tobacco smoke or tobacco use in any form is believed to be the singlemost carcinogen and accounts for 22% of cancer mortality per year worldwide. It is strongly associated with cancers of the lung, head and neck (esophagus, larynx, tongue, lip, mouth, and pharynx), urinary bladder and kidneys, uterine cervix, breast, pancreas and colon.

Other chemicals, which are suspected to be carcinogens are aromatic amines and aniline dyes, soot and tars, pesticides, arsenic, asbestos, benzene, betel nut and lime, polyvinyl chloride, cadmium and chromium compounds, wood dust and certain drugs, e.g. alkylating agents and immunosuppressive agents.

Bacteria and viruses: *Helicobacter pylori* has been associated with an increased incidence of gastric cancer. Epstein-Barr virus is suspected to cause Burkitt's lymphoma, some types of non-Hodgkin's lymphoma and Hodgkin's disease. Herpes simplex virus, cytomegalovirus and human papilloma virus are associated with cancer of the cervix. Hepatitis B virus cause liver cancer and human immunodeficiency virus is associated with Kaposi's sarcoma.

Dietary factors: Dietary factors are believed to be related to one-third of all environmental cancers. Dietary substances can be proactive or protective, carcinogenic or co-carcinogenic. Risk of cancer increases with long-term ingestion carcinogenic or cocarcinogenic substances, e.g. fats and oils, alcohol, salt cured or smoked meat and fish, nitrate or nitric acid containing foods, high caloric diet. Cancer risk is believed to be less with diets containing high fiber (whole grain cereals), certain vegetables (cabbage, broccoli, cauliflower, and sprouts), carotenoids (carrots, tomatoes, spinach, dark green and yellow vegetables) and probably vitamins C and E and zinc and selenium. Obesity is associated with breast and endometrial cancers and it may also increase the risk of cancers of the colon, kidney and gallbladder.

Manifestations of Cancer

- Manifestations of cancer occur due to the direct or indirect effect of cancer, on the location, size, type of tumor and on the extent of metastasis.

Manifestations arising from direct effects of the tumor

- Dysphagia, constipation duc to obstruction in esophagus and rectum.
- Gangrene or ischemia due to compression of major blood vessels.
- Pain or paralysis due to pressure on regional nerve.
- Loss of organ functions due to reduction of normal tissue and invasion of cancerous tissue.
- Hemorrhage due to erosion of local blood vessels.
- Ulceration or necrosis as tumor reduces local blood supply.
- Increased susceptibility to infection due to malnutrition, ongoing cancer treatments or metastatic invasion of bone marrow resulting in decreased hematopoiesis.
- Metabolic imbalances such as disturbances in glucose metabolism in pancreatic cancer; hypercalcemia in cancers of breast, bone, lung and kidney.

Manifestations arising from indirect tumor effects or paraneoplastic effects

- Skin changes
- Peripheral neuropathy and myopathy
- Degeneration
- Anemia
- Generalized endocrine disturbances
- Cancer cachexia.

Classification of Cancer

Cancers are classified according to the following ways.

Anatomic site

It is the classification of cancer based on the anatomic site, e.g. breast, lung, stomach and according to the tissue of origin, e.g. carcinomas originate from embryonal ectoderm, i.e. skin and glands and endoderm, i.e. mucous membrane lining of the respiratory tract, gastrointestinal tract, and genitourinary tract; sarcomas develop from embryonal mesoderm, i.e. connective tissue, bone, muscle and fat; and lymphomas and leukemias originate from the hematopoietic system.

Histologic classification

Histologic classification of cancer is based on the degree of differentiation of the cells of the tissue from which the cancer is originated. Histologic classification classifies cancer in the following four grades:

Grade I: Cells of the cancer are well-differentiated. Appearance of cancer cells differ slightly from that of normal cells.

Grade II: Cells are moderately differentiated. Appearance of cancer cells is more abnormal.

Grade III: Cells are poorly differentiated. Appearance of cancer cells is very abnormal.

Grade IV: Cells are undifferentiated. Cells are immature and primitive and do not have any resemblance to the original cells from which they have originated.

Well-differentiated cancers have better prognosis than undifferentiated cancers.

Extent of the disease

Classifying cancers according to the extent and its spread is called staging. Clinical staging system (described by American Joint Committee on Cancer) determines the anatomic extent of the cancer by the following stages:

- Stage 0: Cancer in situ.
- Stage I: The tumor is limited to the tissue of origin, localized growth.
- Stage II: Localized growth of the tumor.
- Stage III: Extensive local growth and regional spread.
- Stage IV: Cancer spreads to distant organs—metastasis.

TNM classification

This system is the modification of the clinical staging of cancer. According to this system the extent of the disease is determined by 3 parameters: tumor size and invasiveness (T), involvement of the disease in regional lymph nodes (N), and metastasis to distant organ (M). Clinical staging or TNM staging is not applied for leukemias as they are not solid tumors.

Primary tumor (T)

- T_0 No evidence of tumor.
- T_{is} Carcinoma in situ.
- T_{1-4} Tumor size and involvement in ascending order.
- T_X Tumor cannot be measured or found.

Regional lymph nodes (N)

- N_0 No regional node involvement.
- N_{1-4} Involvement of regional nodes in ascending order.
- N_x Lymph node involvement cannot be assessed.

Distant metastases (M)

- M_0 No evidence of distant metastasis.
- M_{1-4} Degrees of metastatic involvement along with distant nodes.
- M_x Metastasis cannot be determined.

PREVENTION AND SCREENING OF CANCER

Nowadays much emphasis is being given to the primary prevention (reducing the risk of cancer in healthy people) and secondary prevention (detection and screening to achieve early diagnosis and prompt treatment to control the cancer process).

Nurses are in a key position to disseminate the knowledge among common people in order to remove the fear and myths about cancer that prevent early detection.

By observing the following 10 healthy-life style patterns people may reduce the risk of cancers as well as other health problems.

1. Avoid exposure to known carcinogens:
   - Do not smoke; do not smoke in front of others.
   - Avoid excessive exposure to the sun. Tan slowly, avoid sun burn, and use sun filter preparations. Take special care if you are fair-skinned or burn easily.
   - Follow health and safety instructions especially in a working environment that is associated with production,

handling or use of any substance that may cause cancer.
2. Eat balanced diet. Eat fresh fruits, vegetables and high fiber diets. Cut down on fatty foods. Moderate your consumption on alcoholic drinks.
3. Participate in a regular exercise program. Avoid being overweight.
4. Take adequate consistent rest.
5. Eliminate, reduce or change the perception of stressors and enhance ability to cope.
6. Participate in regular health examination.
7. Learn and practice self examination. Testicular self examination for male members and breast self examination for women.
8. Participate in regular cancer screening program on a regular basis to detect cancer at an early stage, e.g. regular pap smear testing for cancer cervix, mammogram for breast cancer, digital rectal examination and prostate specific antigen blood test for prostate cancer.
9. Know the 7 warning signs of cancer 'CAUTION':
   C— Change in bladder and bowel habits.
   A— A sore that does not heal.
   U— Unusual bleeding or discharge.
   T— Thickening or lump in breast or anywhere in the body.
   I— Indigestion or difficulty in swallowing.
   O— Obvious change in wart or mole.
   N— Nagging cough or hoarseness.
10. Seek medical care whenever unusual symptoms appear.

Diagnosis of Cancer

- Health history to find out the risk factors, e.g. personal or family history of cancer, exposure to known or occupational carcinogen, presence of chronic inflammatory diseases, ingestion of hormones or cancer chemotherapeutic drugs, dietary habits, and lifestyle.
- Complete and thorough physical examination specially of respiratory system; gastrointestinal system including colon, rectum and liver; the lymphatic system, the breasts, testes and prostate in male and cervix, uterus and ovaries in female, musculoskeletal system and neurologic system.
- Diagnostic studies are performed according to the suspected site of cancer. The various studies and procedures that are performed include:
  - Cytology of cervical smear or Pap test and bronchial washings.
  - Biopsy (obtaining tissue from the suspicious area surgically) followed by histologic examination is the only definitive method of diagnosing cancer. Biopsy procedure may be—(1) Needle or aspiration biopsy, (2) Incisional biopsy, (3) excisional biopsy and (4) by endoscopic procedure.
- Chest X-ray.
- Blood test for complete blood count and blood chemistry.
- Liver function studies.
- Blood test for tumor markers, e.g. PSA, CEA, CA-125, AFP and genetic markers, e.g. BRCA-1 and BRCA-2.
- Bone marrow examination.
- Radiologic studies, e.g. mammography, ultrasound.
- CT scan, PET (positron emission tomography) and MRI.
- Radioisotope scan e.g. thyroid scan, bone scan.
- Endoscopic procedures, e.g. gastroscopy, colonoscopy, sigmoidoscopy.

MANAGEMENT OF CANCER

Goals

Treatment options offered to cancer patients for each specific type of cancer are:

Cure

When cure is the goal, treatment options are offered for complete eradication of malignant disease.

Control

When cure is not possible, treatment options are offered to slow disease process and to prolong life.

Palliation

When either cure or control is not possible, treatment is offered to alleviate distressing symptoms of cancer and to maintain a satisfactory quality of life.

Treatment modalities

Multiple modalities of treatment either singly or in combination are offered to the cancer patients. The main modalities of treatment of cancer are—(1) Surgery (2) radiation therapy, (3) chemotherapy, and (4) biologic and targeted therapy. Factors that determine the selection of treatment modalities are:

1. Type of cancer (cell type), size, location and systemic spread of cancer.
2. Physical condition, presence of associated diseases, psychosocial status, and personal likings of the patient.

Surgery

Surgical removal of the entire tumor is the ideal and most frequently used method of cancer treatment. Surgery plays a major role in the diagnosis, staging and treatment of cancer. It may also be used for rehabilitation, and palliation in patients with cancer and less frequently used for prevention.

Diagnostic surgery

Cancer is diagnosed by identifying malignant cells from tumor tissue under microscope. A variety of surgical procedures, called biopsy are used to obtain tissue for microscopic examination.

Excisional biopsy

- It is performed in small size tumor (2–3 cm) and which is easily accessible, e.g. skin, breast, upper respiratory tract.
- Removes entire tumor plus surrounding tissue.
- Helps pathologist in staging and grading.
- Decrease likelihood of recurrence by residual microscopic cells.
- It may be performed by endoscopy.

Incisional or subtotal biopsy

- It is performed when tumor is too large to remove.
- A part of the tumor is excised
- Excised part should contain representative sample in order to make a diagnosis.
- It may also be performed through endoscopy.

Fine needle aspiration biopsy

- Involves withdrawing tumor cells from the tumor with a needle and syringe.
- It is performed for easily accessible masses, e.g. breast, lung, thyroid liver, etc.
- It is a fast, relatively inexpensive and easy to perform procedure.
- Patient experiences slight discomfort.
- Scanning may be performed to guide the needle.

Core needle biopsy: It is similar to fine needle aspiration biopsy except a specially designed larger size needle is used to obtain a small core of tissue.

Nursing management

- Patient undergoing diagnostic procedure for cancer is anxious and afraid.
- Nurse should act as a liaison between doctor and patient and reiterate the explanation about the procedure to be performed.
- Give time to patient to ask questions and think what has been explained.

Surgery as primary treatment

Goals

- To remove the entire tumor and any involved surrounding tissue and regional lymph nodes.
- To remove the tumor as much as possible when the tumor cannot be removed completely (debulking or cytoprotective procedure).

Approaches of surgery

Local excision

- Performed when mass is small.
- Entire mass and surrounding margin is removed.

Wide or radical excision

- Involves removal of primary tumor, lymph nodes.
- Adjacent involved structures and high-risk normal tissue.
- This procedure may result in disfigurement and altered functioning.
- Performed when chances of cure or control are good.

Video-assisted endoscopic surgery

- Video-assisted endoscopic surgeries nowadays are replacing conventional surgeries.
- Requires short incision and short recovery time.

Salvage surgery: It involves use of extensive surgical approach to treat the local recurrence of the cancer after a less extensive approach had been used. Viz. mastectomy to treat local recurrence of breast cancer after initial treatment of lumpectomy and radiotherapy.

Electrosurgery: Instead of using traditional surgical blades or scalpels to excise cancerous tissue, electric current is used to destroy tumor tissue.

Cryosurgery: In cryosurgery liquid nitrogen is used to freeze tissue and thus cause cell destruction.

Chemosurgery: In chemosurgery chemotherapeutic drugs are administered topically while the tumor tissue is excised layer by layer surgically.

Laser surgery: Laser (light amplification by stimulated emission of radiation) is directed in precise location and depth of cancerous tumor to vaporize cancer cells and thus their destruction.

Stereotactic radiosurgery: In stereotactic radiosurgery a single, highly precise high dose radiation is administered in some types of cancers of brain, head and neck. This precise and high dose radiation is highly effective in destroying the cancerous tissue and is considered to be effective as traditional surgery.

Prophylactic surgery

- Surgical intervention is used to remove nonvital organs or tissues that are likely to develop cancer.
- Performed in persons with certain underlying conditions that increase their risk of cancer development. Viz. preventing colorectal cancer in a person with familial adenomatous polyposis by a prophylactic total colectomy and a prophylactic mastectomy in a woman who has genetic mutations of BRCA 1 or

BRCA2 and has a strong family history of early onset breast cancer.
- Preoperative counseling and teaching is required before deciding on this type of surgery.

Palliative surgery

- Performed when cure or control of cancer is no longer possible.
- Surgical intervention is used to give the patient as comfortable life as possible and to promote a satisfying and productive life for as long as possible.
- Some of the surgeries performed for palliation of symptoms associated with cancer are colostomy for a patient with inoperable colorectal cancer and debulking of tumor to relieve pain and pressure.
- Patient and family must be properly informed about the purpose of surgery openly in order to avoid false hope and disappointment.

Rehabilitative or reconstructive surgery

- Rehabilitative or reconstructive surgery usually follows curative or radical surgery.
- Is performed to improve function or to obtain a more desirable cosmetic effect (since many of the curative cancer surgeries cause disfigurement and altered function).
- May be performed in one single operation during the time of primary surgery or later or by multiple operations in stages.
- Examples of rehabilitative or reconstructive surgeries are: creation of a bladder reservoir during cystectomy, tracheostomy in head and neck cancer surgery, reconstruction of breast after mastectomy, etc.
- Proper assessment of individual disabilities and needs to be done before deciding this type of surgery.

Nursing Management

Patient requires general preoperative and postoperative care and additional care specific to patient's age and impairment of organ which has been described in respective chapters.

- Points to emphasize are:
  - Thorough assessment of nutritional deficits, coagulation disorders, altered immunity, problems and complications associated with adjuvant chemotherapy or radiotherapy, e.g. infection, impaired wound healing, altered pulmonary and renal function and development of deep vein thrombosis that may affect postoperative outcome.
  - Assessment of patient and family for their knowledge about the surgical procedures, possible findings, postoperative expectations and limitations, changes in normal body functions and prognosis; patients and family's needs and coping mechanisms.
  - Provide education and emotional support. Encourage patient and family to take active role in decision-making regarding treatment options whenever possible.
  - Clarify information given by the physician or other health team members. Provide repeated explanations as required. Coordinate with other health care team members in order to provide accurate and consistent information.
  - Postoperatively assess patient's response to surgery, and monitor for presence of complications, e.g. infection, bleeding, thrombophlebitis wound dehiscence, organ dysfunc-

tion, fluid and electrolyte disturbances, etc.
- Relief pain and provide comfort as much as possible.
- Teach patient activity, early ambulation; wound care, prevention of infection, nutrition, medications to be taken.
- Discuss with patient and family plans for discharge, follow-up and home care, use of community resources or referral center well in advance.

RADIATION THERAPY

Definition

Radiation therapy involves treatment of malignant diseases by using ionizing radiation.

Radiation oncology is a medical speciality in which ionizing radiation is used to treat cancer or other diseases.

Ionizing radiation

- The emission and distribution of rays having very much energy level.
- A form of transferring energy.
- Capable of penetrating body tissue.
- Harmful for both normal and malignant cells when it is absorbed into tissue.

Types of Radiation

Different types of ionizing radiations are used in the treatment of cancer

1. Particulate radiation, e.g. alpha particles, electrons, protons, neutrons (less powerful).
2. Electromagnetic radiation, e.g. X-rays and gamma rays (more powerful). Ionizing radiation are either obtained from the decay of naturally occurring radioactive substances, e.g. radium, polonium, uranium and artificially produced isotopes, e.g. cobalt 60, cesium 137 or may be generated by an electric machine, e.g. linear accelerator.

Effects of Radiation

- Radiation causes ionization of atoms and molecules in living cells.
- During ionization electrons are knocked off from one atom and are taken up by another creating one negatively charged and one positively charged atom, both unstable.
- The local energy in ionizing radiation and the resultant free radicals break the chemical bonds in DNA. Damage to cellular DNA retards cell metabolism that disrupts cell's ability to reproduce and ultimately leads to cell death.
- Damage to cellular DNA may be lethal (causes irrepairable damage) or sublethal. In sublethal damage there is potential for tissue repair in between radiation doses or there is potential for accumulated damage to occur with repetitive doses.
- Radiation damages DNA of cancer cells as well as normal cells. But rapidly dividing cells are more vulnerable to radiation than slowly dividing cells. Since cancer cells are rapidly dividing and are in cell cycle, the effect of radiation is more on cancer cells than normal cells. Normal cells of certain tissues, e.g. skin, mucous membrane of gastrointestinal tract and urinary tract, gonads, bone marrow are rapidly dividing. So radiation damages these cells giving rise to untoward side effect. So the radiation oncologist while treating a cancer by radiation tries to deliver sufficient dose of radiation to the cancer cells while sparing the normal cells as much as possible.
- In addition to the effects of DNA, a complex chain of chemical reactions occur in the extracellular fluid resulting

in the formation of free radicals. Well-oxygenated tumors show greater response to ionizing radiation than poorly oxygenated tumors. Oxygen-free radicals formed during ionization interact readily with nearby molecules, causing cellular damage. A well-oxygenated tumor is therefore more sensitive to ionization radiation than the same type of tumor if it is poorly vascularized.

Radiation Dosage

Dose of radiation depends on—(1) Size of the tumor and (2) sensitivity of the target tissue to radiation.

In order to achieve cure lethal tumor dose (the dose that destroys 95% of tumor yet preserve normal tissue) is given. The total radiation dose is given over a period of several weeks (fractionated dose) to achieve maximum cell kill as well as to allow healthy tissue to repair the damage.

Methods of Radiotherapy

Radiation is delivered to the tumor sites by external or internal means.

External radiation or teletherapy

It is delivered by placing the source of radiation at a distance from the tumor. In this technique radiation beam passes through external tissues to reach the internal tumor. Different types of machines, e.g. cobalt-60 machine (emits gamma rays), a cyclotron (protons and neutrons) and a linear accelerator (X-rays) are used for this purpose.

Internal radiation or brachytherapy

Involves placing the source of radiation within the tumor (interstitial) or in close proximity of the tumor (intracavitary) in order to deliver maximum dose to the tumor while sparing the surrounding healthy tissue. Sources of radiation in brachytherapy include temporary sealed sources, e.g. cesium-137, iridium-192 and permanent sealed sources, e.g. iodine-125, gold-198. These sources are supplied in the forms of seeds or ribbons into a special catheter or metal tube that has been implanted into the tumor and is left in place for previously calculated hours to deliver the total dose of radiation.

Radiopharmaceutical therapy

It is performed by administering orally a liquid unsealed source of radioactive material such as iodine-131 for the treatment of thyroid cancer.

Radiation Protection

While a patient is receiving radiation, care should be taken in order to prevent radiation exposure to others as well as health care personnel.

During teletherapy the patient is treated in a specially constructed treatment room alone, the patient is monitored and the teletherapy machine is operated from outside. Duration of treatment is for brief period. The patient does not remain radioactive as soon as the radiation is turned off.

When patient receives brachytherapy with temporary sealed source the patient emits radioactivity as long as the temporary radioactive source is within the patient. While caring for this patient the nurse should maintain the following principles of radiation protection.

Time

Nurse should spend as little time as possible in giving direct care to the patient.

Distance

She should maintain a safe distance from the patient, the distance determined by the radiation safety officer.

Shielding

If at all she has to be in the close proximity she should use shield. She should always wear a film badge that records cumulative amount of radiation exposure, while caring for the patient, the badge should not be used by others and should not be worn other than at work.

The patient should be explained the reason for remaining isolated during treatment and the rational for maintaining time and distance by the health care personnel.

Side Effects of Radiation Therapy

- Side effects of radiation therapy are usually localized to the region being treated.
- Side effects increase when chemotherapy is also administered along with radiotherapy.
- Local reactions occur due to the damage of surrounding normal cells present in the treatment area and normal cellular death exceeds cellular regeneration.
- Rapidly proliferating tissues such as skin, epithelial lining of the gastrointestinal tract including oral cavity and bone marrow are mostly affected when these are near the treatment area.
- Certain systemic side effects may also be noted that may be due to release of certain substances from dead cancer cells.
- Most of the side effects are temporary and subside after treatment is stopped.
- Systemic side effects—Fatigue, lethargy, nausea and anorexia
- Local side effects—
  - Skin changes—Erythema, dry desquamation (shedding of skin) and wet desquamation and alopecia in the treatment field.
  - In the oral cavity—Stomatitis, dry mouth (xerostomia), decreased salivation, change or loss of taste and dental decay (radiation caries).
  - In the neck area and esophagus—Esophageal irritation, dysphagia, hoarseness, loss of voice, dry cough, pain in chest.
  - Treatment over abdomen (stomach and colon)—Anorexia, nausea, vomiting and diarrhea.
  - Treatment over pelvis—Diarrhea, occasional rectal bleeding, cystitis, altered sexual functions, e.g. impotence, sterility in men, dyspareunia due to vaginal dryness and fibrosis, loss of libido, premature menopause and sterility.
  - In the bone marrow producing sites such as pelvis, vertebral column—Anemia, leucopenia and thrombocytopenia resulting into increased risk for infection and bleeding.

CANCER CHEMOTHERAPY

Definition

Cancer chemotherapy refers to use of chemicals or drugs as a systemic treatment of cancer.

Physiological Basis of Cancer Chemotherapy

Cell cycle—The process of cell reproduction begins in the center and the entire period from a single reproduction to a second reproduction is known as the cell cycle.

There are four phases in the cell cycle: M, G1, S, G2 (Fig. 12.1).

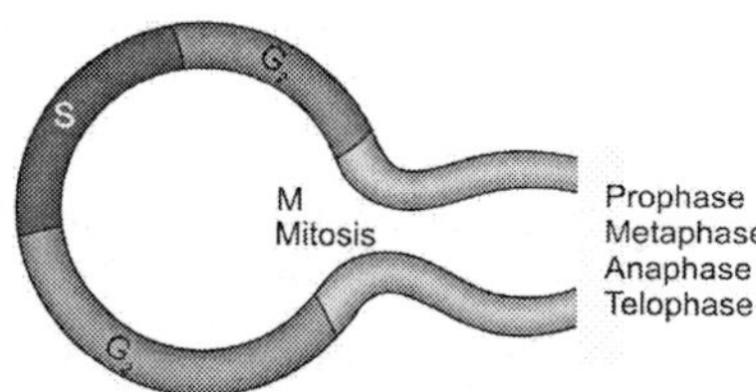

Fig. 12.1: Cell cycle

- **M phase**: It is mitosis, the brief period in the cell cycle, when actual cell division takes place. This phase is subdivided into prophase, metaphase, anaphase and telophase.
- **G_1 phase**: It is the postmitotic, presynthesis phase, when growth of cells takes place and cells begin to carry out their reproductive activity. RNA and protein synthesis takes place in this phase.
- **S phase**: It is the synthesis phase, when DNA synthesis takes place. DNA, is the important constituent of chromosomes that carries genetic characteristics to one cell to another cell. RNA and protein synthesis also continues resulting in two similar sets of chromosomes containing all the genetic materials needed for mitosis.
- **G_2 phase**: It is the premitotic phase when synthesis of DNA stops but RNA and protein synthesis continues. Preparation of cell division goes on, mitotic spindles necessary for mitosis form. This phase is followed by mitosis or M phase again.
- **Generation time**—Generation time is the time required for a cell to complete the cycle from the end of mitosis until the beginning of next mitosis. Cells of certain tissues such as bone marrow stem cells, cells of lymphatic tissue, ovary, testes, hair follicle, epithelial lining of the gastro intestinal tract have very short generation time (hours) whereas cells of pancreas, uterus, cartilage have long generation time (days/months/years).

Normal Cell and Cancer Cell Replication

Cancer cells replicate at the same rate with that of their counterparts. But normal regulatory mechanism is absent in cancer cell replication.

Effects of Drugs on Cancer Cells

Chemotherapeutic drugs destroy cells by interrupting or altering the synthesis of DNA.

Drugs are more effective when cells are either preparing for reproduction (G_1, S, G_2 phase) or during reproduction (M phase). The more rapid the mitotic rate (short generation time) the greater is the potential for response.

The drugs, which damage cells when in reproduction or are preparing for reproduction are called cell cycle phase-specific drugs.

The drugs capable of damaging cells whether or not the cells are reproducing or resting (G_0) are called cell cycle phase-nonspecific drugs.

Combination chemotherapy is based on combining both cell cycle phase—specific and cell cycle phase—nonspecific drugs at a time in order to achieve maximum number of cell kill.

Newly developing tumors tend to have a better response as they have a greater percentage of proliferating cells.

Tumors present in certain anatomical sites, e.g. brain are in the protective environment and are spared from the action of many chemotherapeutic drugs as they do not reach the tumor site. Only a few drugs such as bleomycin, nitrosoureas and temozolamide are able to cross blood brain barrier.

Effect of Drugs on Normal Cells (Side Effects or Toxic Effects)

Drugs are unable to distinguish normal and cancer cells. So drugs affect normal cells in the same way, they affect the cancer cells. Damage or destruction of normal cells specially those that are of short generation time or highly proliferating such as those in the bone marrow, hair follicle, the epithelium of the gastrointestinal tract gives rise to side effects of chemotherapy.

Cells of certain other normal tissue irrespective of short or long generation time may have specific drug affinity, giving rise to specific side effects or toxic effects such as bleomycin causes lung toxicity, Adriamycin results in cardiac toxicity and Vincristine gives rise to neurotoxicity.

The general and specific side effects of drugs are classified as acute, delayed or chronic according to their time of onset.

Acute side effects occur during or immediately after administration of drug. These may be nausea and vomiting, hypersensitivity and anaphylactic reactions, cardiac dysrhythmias and extravasation.

Delayed effects are nausea, vomiting, mucositis, diarrhea or constipation, alopecia, skin rashes, bone marrow suppression giving rise to anemia, leukopenia or thrombocytopenia and neuropathies.

Chronic toxicities result from damage to organs such as heart, lung, liver and kidneys.

Preparation and Administration of Chemotherapeutic Drugs

- Chemotherapeutic drugs should be prepared and administered by persons specially trained for this purpose.
- Specific guidelines for preparation and administration of the drugs to be followed strictly.
- The drugs may cause occupational hazards, so the nurse should take special caution to prevent exposure to the drug during its preparation and administration.
- Chemotherapeutic drugs may be administered by various routes such as oral, intravenous (most common), intramuscular, intracavitary, intrathecal, intrarterial, subcutaneous and topical.
- Difficulties that arise during intravenous administration of the drugs are venous access difficulties, infection through the venous access device and extravasations (infiltration of the drug into local tissue around the infusion site) resulting into local tissue damage. So patient should be closely monitored for early signs of extravasations.
- If extravasation is detected, stop the infusion immediately and take care of the infusion site as per established protocol of the hospital.

Classification of Chemotherapeutic Drugs

Alkylating agents

- Drugs of this class contain alkyl group in their structures. Alkyl group binds with DNA of both dividing and nondividing cells.
- H-ion of DNA is replaced with alkyl group.
- Damage in the structure of DNA prevents replication of DNA and also protein synthesis.
- These drugs are effective in killing cells of dividing and nondividing cells and thus are cell cycle nonspecific agents.
- These are cytocidal and cytostatic.
- Drugs belonging to this class are N2 mustard, cyclophosphamide (cytoxan), chlorambucil (leukeran), ifosfamide (flex), melphalan (alkeran), busulfan (myleran), dacarbazine, temazolomide, thiotepa.

Nitrosourea

- This group of drugs are a type of alkylating agents but are categorized separately as they have additional methods of action over alkylating agents.
- They damage structure of DNA of both dividing and nondividing cells and are cell cycle nonspecific.
- Drugs inhibit DNA repair, crosses blood-brain barrier by dissolving lipids.
- Most remarkable toxicity is delayed bone suppression usually after 3–4 weeks. Examples of this group of drugs are carmustine (BiCNU), lomustine (CeeNu), streptozocin.

Platinum drugs

- These drugs bind to DNA and RNA of cells, miscoding information thus inhibit DNA replication and cells die.
- These are cell cycle phase-nonspecific drugs.
- Drugs belonging to this group are Cisplatin (Platinol-AQ), carboplatin (Paraplatin), oxaliplatin (Eloxatin).

Antitumor antibiotics

- Drugs belonging to this group are heterogenous group of compounds produced by various bacterial and fungal organisms.
- These drugs change DNA structure by binding directly to DNA resulting in inhibition of RNA synthesis.
- They are cell cycle phase-nonspecific agents, bleomycin, mitomycin, adriamycin, daunorubicin, epirubicin, etc.

Antimetabolites

- Drugs of this group are chemically similar to the essential cellular components called metabolites.
- They are taken up by the cells instead of metabolites resulting in alteration or interruption of cellular enzymatic action necessary for DNA and RNA synthesis.
- Drugs primarily act during S-phase. So they are cell cycle phase-specific agents.
- Subdivision of this group of drugs are purine antagonist, pyrimidine antagonist, folic acid antagonist. (Purine and pyrimidine are building blocks of nucleic acid needed for DNA and RNA synthesis).
- Examples are mercaptopurine (purinethol), fludarabine, thioguanine, cladribine, pentostatin, capecitabine, cytarabine, fluoroiracil (5fu), floxuridine, methotrexate, pemetrexed, hydroxyurea (hydrea).

Mitotic inhibitors

- These drugs bind with microtubular protein necessary to form mitotic spindles of dividing cells, causing mitotic arrest.
- They act during G_2 phase and M phase. So they are cell cycle phase-specific agents.
- Examples are vinblastine (Velban), vincristine (Oncovin), paclitaxel, docetaxel.

Topoisomerase inhibitors

- These drugs act by inhibiting the normal enzymes topoisomerases that allow reversible breaks and repair in DNA necessary for DNA replication.
- They act during S phase. So they are cell cycle phase-specific drugs.
- Examples are etoposide, teniposide, topotecan and irinotecan.

Corticosteroids and other hormonal agents

- These agents act in various ways and their mechanism of action is not very clear.

- Believed to disrupt cell membrane and inhibit synthesis of protein; decrease circulating lymphocytes; inhibit mitosis, increase sense of well-being; depress immune system.
- These are cell cycle phase-nonspecific agents.
- Examples are cortisone, hydrocortisone, methylprednisolone, prednisone, dexamethasone.

Antiestrogens

- These agents selectively attach to estrogen receptors causing down regulation of them and inhibiting tumor growth.
- Interfere with hormone receptors and protein. They are also known as SERMs (selective estrogen receptor modulators).
- Examples are tamoxifen and raloxifene.

Nursing Management of Patients with Cancer Undergoing Chemotherapy/Radiotherapy

Objectives

1. To prepare patient about the therapy, what to expect during the therapy and the expected side effects of therapy.
2. To provide supportive care to the patient in order to minimize or manage the side effects of therapy.

Nursing Intervention for the Management of Common Side Effects of Chemotherapy/Radiotherapy

Fatigue

- Explain patient that fatigue is a common side effect of therapy and is not a sign of advancement of disease.
- Help patient identify the factors which cause more fatigue or make him feel better.
- Advise patient to avoid activities that cause more fatigue and to take help from others in carrying out activities.
- Encourage to take rest in between activities and to avoid over stressing the body when fatigue is tolerable.
- Encourage patient to maintain good nutritional and hydration status.
- Teach patient to control other side effects if any that may cause more fatigue.
- Encourage patient to take part in walking program that would keep him active and in good mood without overtaxing him.

Anorexia

- Explain patient that anorexia is a very common side effect of chemotherapy and it happens due to the release of certain substances (having appetite suppressing effect) from the damaged cells; due to the action of medicines or radiotherapy as well as anxiety associated with the diagnosis of the disease.
- Monitor patient's body weight twice a week and also the amount of food and fluids consumed daily.
- Encourage patient to take small amounts of food of high quality with high protein and calorie in frequent intervals.
- Teach family members to serve food according to patient's choice as much as possible in an attractive manner.

Nausea and vomiting

- Explain patient that nausea and vomiting is a common side effect of chemotherapy and in some cases of radiotherapy (radiation to chest or abdomen).
- Administer prophylactic antiemetic prior to chemotherapy and as and when required.

- Provide a light meal consisting of bland foods to the patient before therapy.
- Encourage patient to eat and drink when not nauseated.
- Assess fluid and electrolyte balance of patient expressing delayed nausea and vomiting (for a week after therapy).
- Maintain intake output chart.
- Administer antiemetics, antianxiety drugs and frequent small feeds of nonirritating high quality foods. Give patient ice cubes to suck.
- Teach patient diversional activities.

Mouth sore (stomatitis) and dysphagia (esophagitis)

- Explain patient that stomatitis or oral mucositis and dysphagia or esophagitis are very common side effects occurring in all patients receiving radiation therapy to head and neck area and in some patients receiving certain chemotherapeutic drugs, e.g. 5FU.
- Patient scheduled for radiotherapy of head and neck area to be referred to dental department for assessment of dental health and necessary prophylactic measure, e.g. extraction of defective tooth.
- Assess oral cavity and throat daily for the status of the mucous membrane, amount and consistency of saliva, ability to chew, masticate foods, feelings of lump in throat or dysphagia regularly when treatment starts.
- Teach patient dental care such as proper tooth brushing and flossing (if not contraindicated due to thrombocytopenia) before and after each meal and at bed time.
- Encourage patient to use normal saline and sodibicarb solution for mouth rinsing and gurgling and avoid commercial preparation (chlorhexidine) without physician's order.
- Provide bland and soft, high protein and high calorie diet at room temperature.
- Encourage patient to take small amount of foods at frequent intervals and to drink fluids with food to ease dysphagia. Include family members in assisting patient to eat. Avoid citrus fruits.
- Apply topical analgesics or systemic analgesics if ordered before meals if mouth or throat is too painful.
- Apply candid lotion or glycerin borax if ordered on the sores.

Dry mouth (xerostomia)

- Explain patient that dry mouth is a common symptom of patients receiving radiotherapy in head and neck area.
- Teach patient to rinse mouth with baking soda solution frequently that helps in secretions of saliva.
- Encourage patient to take plenty of oral fluids and drink sips of water frequently.
- Apply vaseline gel to lubricate lips.
- Provide mouth care before every meal to stimulate salivation.
- Offer soft foods that are easy to masticate and swallow. Avoid salty foods.
- Serve food in attractive manner so that the patient can see and smell to stimulate salivation.
- Give lozenges to stimulate salivation.

Diarrhea

- Explain patient that diarrhea is a common side effect of radiation to abdomen and pelvis and certain neoplastic drugs.
- Instruct patient to record the number, volume, consistency and character of stools per day as well as aggravating and relieving factors of diarrhea.
- Administer low residue diet before chemotherapy with drugs known to cause diarrhea.

- Encourage patient to avoid roughage, e.g. fresh fruits, vegetables, nuts, seeds and fried or highly seasoned foods to prevent diarrhea.
- Administer antidiarrheals, antimotility agents and antispasmodics when diarrhea is marked.
- Administer adequate fluid and electrolytes to prevent fluid and electrolytes deficit.
- Assess rectal area for skin breakdown and redness.
- Provide sitz bath with luke warm water, keep rectal area clean and dry.

Alopecia

- Explain patient that alopecia due to chemotherapy is temporary but due to radiation therapy may be permanent.
- Cut long hair before therapy.
- Teach patient to avoid excessive shampooing, and combing hair frequently.
- Suggest patient to use scarves, wigs, hats, etc. to cope with hair loss.

Skin changes due to radiation (dry to wet desquamation)

- Explain patient possible skin changes before the therapy and ways to minimize the effect.
- Teach patient to keep the treatment area clean by washing with tepid water and pat dry the area gently with soft cloth.
- Instruct patient to protect the treatment area from friction, extremes of heat or cold, constricting garments, harsh chemicals, cosmetics, lotions, creames, etc. unless prescribed by doctor.
- Keep dry skin lubricated with nonirritating lotion such as aloe vera as prescribed.
- Assess skin for wet desquamation.
- If wet desquamation, keep area clean with normal saline compresses.
- Protect the area from further damage by applying nonadhesive absorbent dressings.
- Expose area to air as often as possible.

Skin changes due to chemotherapy (hyperpigmentation, photosensitivity, acral erythema, urticaria, radiation recall skin reaction)

- Teach patient to remain alert for skin changes and report physician for severe symptoms.
- Initiate symptomatic management as advised (application of lotions, corticosteroids creams, etc.)
- Instruct patient to avoid sun exposure.

Leukopenia

- Monitor white blood cells count especially neutrophils.
- Teach patient warning signs of infection such as rise of temperature, cough, cold, sore throat, change in bowel and bladder habits, redness, swelling or discharge, etc.
- Teach patient to avoid infections by frequent hand washing; maintaining hygiene by bathing daily; eating freshly prepared cooked foods and avoiding raw foods; avoiding large crowds and people with infections.
- Administer white blood cells growth factors when leukopenia.

Thrombocytopenia

- Monitor platelet counts.
- Teach patient to remain alert for early signs of bleeding such as, bleeding from gums, hematuria, bleeding during defecation, ecchymosis, petechia, etc.
- Teach patient to prevent bleeding by preventing injury; avoiding using sharp instruments; avoiding strenuous

exercises, avoiding constipation; avoiding forceful blowing of nose; avoiding plucking eyebrows or other body hair; shaving with electric razor; avoiding skin piercing or tattooing, avoiding over the counter drugs like aspirin, etc.

Anemia

- Monitor hematocrit levels and hemoglobin percentage.
- Administer iron supplements and erythropoietin.
- Provide foods that promote red blood cells production such as meat, liver, fish, green leafy vegetables, legumes, whole grains, dried fruits, milk and milk products, eggs, nuts, citrus fruits, etc.

Cystitis

- Explain patient that cystitis may develop during treatment with cyclophosphamide and ifosphamide and with radiation therapy to the pelvis.
- Teach patient alarming signs of cystitis, e.g. frequency, urgency, dysuria, hematuria, etc. and to report to the physician.
- Encourage patient to drink at least 3 liters of fluid per day to increase urinary output.
- Instruct patient to void every 2 hourly at daytime and 4 hourly at night in order to prevent stasis of urine in bladder that may cause further irritation.
- Teach patient perineal hygiene.

Nephrotoxicity

- Monitor blood urea nitrogen, serum creatinine, and serum electrolytes levels of patients receiving chemotherapy particularly with cisplatin, methotrexate and mitomycin which are known to affect kidneys during their excretion.
- Encourage adequate hydration to flush out the drug as well as end products of cell breakdown that may lead to tumor lysis syndrome.
- Administer sodium bicarbonate to alkalinize urine and allopurinol to prevent formation of uric acid crystals responsible for kidney damage.

Reproductive dysfunctions (temporary or permanent sterility, loss of libido, dyspareunia)

- Discuss with patient and his partner about the possible effects of therapy on reproductive functions. (Effects on reproductive functions are more common when reproductive organs are within the radiation treatment field and during treatment with alkylating agents).
- Refer patient in reproductive age group to a counselor when permanent sterility is expected.
- Teach patient to use barrier contraceptives, e.g. condom during the period of treatment to prevent teratogenic effect.

BIOLOGIC AND TARGETED THERAPY

Biologic Therapy

Definition

Biologic therapy or biologic response modifier therapy refers to use of agents that modify the relationship between the host and the tumor by altering the biologic response of the host to the tumor cells.

Mode of action

Biologic response modifier agents alter host tumor response by:

1. Direct antitumor effects.

2. Restoring, modulating, augmenting host immune system mechanism.
3. Interfering with the cancer cells' ability to metastasize or differentiate.

Examples of biologic agents

1. Alpha-interferon
2. Interleukin-2
3. Levamisole
4. BCG vaccine.

Targeted Therapy

Definition

Targeted therapy is based on the recognition of the abnormality in the malignant cell and developing a treatment that targets the specific cellular receptors and pathways that are important in cancer growth. By targeting the specific cellular receptors and pathways necessary for cancer growth, these agents selectively kill cancer cells without damaging normal cells.

Agents for targeted therapy

1. Tyrosine kinase inhibitors (Tyrosine-kinase is an enzyme that activates the signaling pathways that regulate cell survival and multiplication).
   Example: Cetuximab.
2. Monoclonal antibodies—They bind to specific target cells including tumor cells. The binding inhibit the internalization of receptor-antibody complexes and signaling pathways. They may also stimulate immunologic response in the patient.
3. Antiangiogenic agents or angiogenesis inhibitors act by preventing the mechanisms and pathways necessary for development of blood vessels for continued growth of tumors and metastasis.
4. Proteasome inhibitors—Proteasomes are intracellular multienzyme complexes that degrade proteins. Proteasome inhibitors prevent degradation of proteins leading to altered cell function. Normal cells are able to recover the effects of proteasome inhibitors but cancer cells die due to proteasome inhibition.

Side effects of Biologic and Targeted Therapy

- Constitutional and flu-like symptoms, e.g. headache, fever, chills, myalgias, fatigue, malaise, weakness, photosensitivity, anorexia and nausea.
- Tachycardia and orthostatic hypotension.
- Capillary leak syndrome giving rise to pulmonary edema associated with interleukin-2 and monoclonal antibodies.
- Central nervous system disturbances such as confusion, memory loss, insomnia; cardiac dysfunction and hepatic dysfunction are associated with interferons and IL-2.
- Infusion-related problems such as fever, chills, urticaria, mucosal congestion, myalgia, nausea, diarrhea and anaphylaxis are associated with MoAB administration.
- Skin rashes such as erythema, acne-like rashes are common with human epidermal growth factor receptor inhibitors.
- Arterial thrombi, hemorrhage, hypertension, and proteinuria may occur with antiangiogenics.
- Bone marrow depression due to MoAB.

Nursing Management

- Explain patient that side effects may occur with biologic and targeted therapy and the side effects disappear when the agent is discontinued.
- Teach patient to take periods of rest in between activities and take help from

others whenever necessary, if feeling fatigue.
- Encourage patient to take nutritious diet in small amount and frequent intervals.
- Administer acetaminophen as ordered and large amount of fluids if flu-like symptoms.
- Teach patient for the occurrence of any neurological deficits, e.g. loss of memory, confusion, insomnia, etc and report to the physician. Institute protective and supportive measures, e.g. railed bed and assistance whenever necessary.

Other Supportive Therapies

Hematopoietic growth factors

- Hematopoietic growth factors are used to support cancer patients through the treatment of the disease. Families of glycoproteins produced by various cells, known as colony-stimulating factors (CSF), stimulate production, maturation, regulation and activation of cells of the hematopoietic system. The name of the colony-stimulating factor (CSF) is based on the specific hematopoietic cell it affects. Examples are:
- Granulocyte-macrophage colony-stimulating factor (GM-CSF) helps in myeloid cell recovery after bone marrow transplantation.
- Granulocyte-colony-stimulating factor (G-CSF) (neupogen) stimulates granulocyte production and is given in chemotherapy-induced neutropenia.
- Erythropoietin (epoetin) stimulates erythroid precursor cells to produce erythrocytes and is used to treat anemia associated with chronic cancer or anemia associated with chemotherapy.
- Interleukin-11 (platelet growth factor) given to treat therapy-induced thrombocytopenia.

Hematopoietic stem cell transplantation (HSCT)

- Hematopoietic stem cell transplantation is the common terminology used for conventional bone marrow transplantation (as the stem cells used to be obtained from bone marrow) and today's newly developed peripheral stem cell transplantation (stem cells obtained from peripheral blood).
- The procedure is effective in curing certain cancers and noncancerous diseases. Even when cure is not achieved the procedure may give a period of remission from the disease.

Types of hematopoietic stem cell transplantation

1. Allogenic transplant involves use of stem cells acquired from a donor who is HLA matched to the recipient (usually a family member).
2. Syngenic transplantation is use of stem cells from an identical twin and infusing them into the other. It is type of allogenic transplant.
3. In autologous transplant patient receives his own stem cells (which had been previously collected and harvested) back following myeloablative chemotherapy.

Procedures of hematopoietic stem cell transplantation

- The approach of this procedure is to eradicate tumor cells from the bone marrow by administering higher than normal dosage of chemotherapy with or without radiation therapy. Healthy stem cells, which have been previously collected and harvested either from a donor or self, are then infused, which rescues the damaged bone marrow through engraftment and subsequent normal proliferation and differentiation of the infused stem cells in the recipient.

- Hematopoietic stem cells are harvested by two different methods—(1) In the operating room under general anesthesia or spinal anesthesia multiple bone marrow aspirations either from iliac crest or sternum are done to obtain sufficient number of stem cells. (2) Peripheral stem cells are obtained from the peripheral blood with the help of a cell separator equipment that automatically separates the stem cells from the blood circulating through the machine and returns the rest of the blood components to the donor.
- The marrow (processed to strain out bone fragments) or peripherally collected stem cells are then bagged with preservative for cryopreservation until needed.
- Autologous stem cells are treated to remove undetected cancer cells by different pharmacologic, immunologic, physical or chemical agents.
- Cord blood which is HLA typed and cryopreserved may be used for allogenic transplant.
- Before infusion of the stem cells the patient with cancer is treated with chemotherapy with or without radiation for the underlying disease. Total body radiation may also be used for immunosuppression. This preinfusion preparation is known as 'conditioning regimen'.
- Stem cells infusion is administered by intravenous route either by slow bolus or like a blood transfusion.
- The infused stem cells reconstitute the bone marrow element and rescue the patient's hematopoietic system usually after 2–4 weeks time period. The time period of 2–4 weeks patient remains pancytopenic and must be protected from infectious agents and supported by blood transfusions, adequate nutrition and hydration to maintain blood cells in circulation.

Complications of hematopoietic stem cell transfusion

- Infections
- Graft-versus-host disease.

ONCOLOGICAL EMERGENCIES

Oncological emergencies are certain life-threatening conditions that can occur as a result of cancer or cancer treatments.

These emergency conditions may be grouped as:

1. Metabolic such as hypercalcemia, tumor lysis syndrome, SIADH.
2. Obstructive such as spinal cord compression, superior vena cava syndrome.
3. Infiltrative, such as cardiac tamponade, carotid artery rupture.

Hypercalcemia

Hypercalcemia, a common condition associated with cancer occurs when the serum calcium level rises more than 11 mg/dL.

Causes

- Metastatic cancer of the bone from solid tumors like lung, breast, head and neck, etc. or multiple myeloma.
- Parathyroid hormone-like substance secreted from certain cancers in the absence of bony metastasis.
- Immobility and dehydration exacerbate hypercalcemia.

Manifestations

Anorexia, nausea, vomiting, constipation, polyuria, excessive thirst, dry mucous membrane, poor skin turgor, fatigue, muscle weakness, diminished deep tendon reflexes, paralytic ileus, apathy, depression.

Collaborative care

- Maintain hydration and mobility to prevent hypercalcemia.

- Look for early signs of hypercalcemia.
- Treatment of primary disease to be continued.
- Administer fluid at least 3 liters per day.
- Administer loop diuretic.
- Biphosphonate—Zoledronate, or pamidronate when administered inhibits osteoclastic activity.

Syndrome of Inappropriate Antidiuretic Hormone Secretion (SIADH)

Syndrome of inappropriate antidiuretic hormone secretion is a condition where there is abnormal and sustained production of antidiuretic hormone (ADH) giving rise to water retention and hyponatremia.

Causes

- Cancer of lung (most common 80%) and also in other common cancers. Cancer cells in these cancers are able to manufacture, store and release ADH.
- Stress, infection, action of a few chemotherapeutic drugs, e.g. cyclophosphamide, vincristine, vinblastine and cisplatin stimulate release of ADH.

Manifestations

- Weight gain, weakness, anorexia, nausea, vomiting.
- Personality changes, seizures, coma.

Management

- Treament of underlying malignancy.
- Restriction of water intake to correct water-sodium imbalance.
- Administration of intravenous sodium chloride 3% if hyponatremia is severe.

Tumor Lysis Syndrome

Tumor lysis syndrome (TLS) is a metabolic condition characterized by rapid release of intracellular components from the damaged tumor cells in response to chemotherapy and less commonly with radiation therapy.

Etiology and pathology

- TLS occurs most commonly in cancers that are rapidly growing and are sensitive to chemotherapy.
- Released intracellular components in the blood stream are metabolized by liver into urea, concentrated uric acid production and give rise to metabolic abnormalities. Concentrated uric acid crystallizes in the renal tubule and lead to acute renal failure.

Management

- Prevent renal failure and severe electrolyte imbalance.
- Hydration therapy to increase urine production.
- Allopurinol is given to decrease uric acid production.

Spinal Cord Compression

- Spinal cord compression is a neurological emergency occurring by a malignant tumor in the epidural space of the spinal cord, which causes direct pressure on the spinal cord or compromise blood supply to the spinal cord.
- Depending on the rate of growth of the tumor, it may take only hours or days to progress spinal cord compression to irreversible neurological damage with paralysis and loss of bowel and bladder control.
- Early manifestations are intense, localized and persistent backache; vertebral tenderness, motor weakness and dysfunction.

Management

- Radiation therapy to shrink the tumor and thus reduce compression.
- Corticosteroids.
- Activity limitation and pain management.
- Surgical laminectomy (less commonly performed) for radioresistant tumor.

Superior Vena Cava Syndrome

Superior vena cava syndrome results from internal or external obstruction of the superior vena cava by a thrombus or a tumor.

Manifestations

- Facial edema, periorbital edema, distention of veins of head, neck and chest, seizures.

Management

- Radiation therapy to the site of obstruction.
- Chemotherapy if the tumor is sensitive to chemotherapy.

Cardiac Tamponade

Cardiac tamponade is a type of infiltrative emergency that results from fluid accumulation in the pericardial sac; constriction of the pericardium by tumor; or pericarditis secondary to radiation therapy to the chest.

Manifestations

- A heavy feeling over the chest, shortness of breath, tachycardia, cough, dysphagia, hiccup, hoarseness, nausea, vomiting, excessive perspiration, decreased level of consciousness, pulsus paradoxus, distant heart sounds, extreme anxiety and jugular venous distention.

Management

- Cardiocentesis.
- Oxygen therapy, intravenous infusion and vasopressor therapy.
- Surgical excision of pericardial window or an indwelling pericardial catheter.

Carotid Artery Rupture

Carotid artery rupture occurs when tumor is invaded into the wall of the carotid artery or due to erosion of arterial wall following surgery or radiation therapy. This condition commonly occurs in patients with head and neck cancers.

Manifestations

Oozing of blood or bleeding if the artery blows out.

Management

- Apply pressure to the site.
- Intravenous fluid or blood transfusion to stabilize patient for surgery.
- Ligation of carotid artery above and below rupture.
- Reduction of local tumor by appropriate therapy.

13

Nursing Management of Patients with Skin Disorders

ASSESSMENT OF PATIENT WITH SKIN DISORDERS

Subjective Data

- History of present illness (chief complaints)—Itching (pruritus), insomnia due to pruritus, rashes, dryness, lesions, ecchymosis (small hemorrhagic patches), lumps, masses, cosmetic appearance, changes in hair, nails and skin associated with any complaint and its onset and duration.
- Past health history—Previous trauma, surgery or any systemic disease with manifestations on skin, e.g. poor wound healing, jaundice (liver disease), cyanosis (lung disease), pallor (anemia), etc. allergies to certain drugs, substances and food, insect bites and stings.
- Family history—Presence of any skin problems or unusual skin, nails, and hairs in close family members, e.g. alopecia, atopic dermatitis, psoriasis, scabies, etc.
- Medications—Consumption of prescribed drugs or over the counter drugs. Administration of vitamins, hormones, antibiotics, corticosteroids and antimetabolites. Duration of use and effectiveness of these medications.
- Surgery or other treatments—Previous surgery including cosmetic surgery, biopsy, phototherapy, radiotherapy or treatment for cosmetic purposes, e.g. tanning, laser resurfacing, etc.
- Personal history—Health practices related to integumentary system, hygiene, use of cosmetics, use of sun protection factors or measures (umbrella), use of any chemical during work, stress at work or home, outdoor recreational activities or exposure to extreme environment.
- Dietary habits—Regular consumption of balanced diets, vitamin or nutritional supplements, and fluid intake.

Objective Data

Examine patient in a private and comfortable room with good lighting. Have the patient wear a gown so that all skin areas are examined easily. Use proper terminology to document findings.

- Inspection of skin for general color, pigmentation, moisture or dryness, skin texture, lesions, vascularity, bruising, petechiae or purpura, rash, scar, discoloration, hypopigmentation or hyperpigmentation. Color, size, distribution, location and shape of lesions if found has to be noted. Condition of hair, the distribution and growth of hair, cleanliness, presence of lies and nits, dandruff, lesions on scalp. Nail shape, thickness, curvature and surface, presence of any grooves, ridges, and detachement from nail bed.

- Palpation of skin for temperature, turgor and mobility, moisture and texture, pain or tenderness, masses or lumps. Hair oiliness, texture, integrity and smoothness of scalp. Nail for firmness, pain or tenderness, rapid blanching response.

Diagnostic Studies

Skin problems are usually diagnosed by a careful history and examination of the individual lesion. Additional diagnostic tests are required to establish a definitive diagnosis when the above measures fail.

1. Skin biopsy may be obtained by various techniques, e.g. punch, excisional, incisional and shave. Obtained specimen is examined under microscope to diagnose cancer or any other abnormality.
2. Skin culture and sensitivity identifies bacterial, viral and fungal organisms responsible for the disorders. Materials for culture are obtained either by scraping or swab of skin or from pustules, bullae, or abscesses.
3. Immunofluorescent studies are performed to detect certain abnormal antibodies present in some immune skin disorders. Antibodies are made fluorescent by attaching them to a dye. Direct immunofluoroscence test is performed on skin and indirect immunofluoroscence test detects antibodies in patient's serum.
4. Potassium hydroxide test is performed to detect fungal infection. Material for examination obtained by scraping is placed on a slide and 10% to 20% potassium hydroxide added and examined under microscope.
5. Tzanck test is performed to examine cells from blistering skin conditions such as herpes zoster, herpes simplex, varicella, and all forms of pemphigus. Secretions from suspected lesions are applied on a glass slide, stained and examined under microscope.
6. Mineral oil slides are prepared by placing samples from a lesion by scraping with a scalpel blade moistened with oil so that the scraped skin adheres to the blade. The material then transferred to a slide and examined under microscope. Test is performed to diagnose infestations, e.g. scabies.
7. Wood's lamp examination (black light) is performed to differentiate epidermal from dermal lesion and hypopigmented and hyperpigmented lesion from normal skin. Test is done in a darkroom with a special lamp that produces long-wave ultraviolet rays, which result in a characteristic dark purple fluorescence.
8. Patch test is used to determine whether patient is allergic to any testing material. Some amount of potentially allergenic material is applied under occlusion to skin on back. Development of itching, redness, elevation, papules blisters, etc. indicate positive reaction.

SKIN LESIONS

Common Terminologies to Describe Skin Lesions

Primary skin lesions

Primary skin lesions are original lesions arising from previously normal skin.

Macule—Flat nonpalpable skin color change, less than 1 cm area with circumscribed border (flat moles, petechia).

Patch—Flat nonpalpable skin color change, more than 1 cm in area and may have irregular border (vitiligo, ecchymosis).

Papule—Elevated solid lesion of less than 1 cm varying in color (warts or elevated nevi).

Plaque—Raised flat lesion formed by merging several papules (Psoriasis).

Nodule—Raised, palpable solid mass extending deeper into the dermis than a papule (lipoma, poorly absorbed injection).

Tumor—A large nodule is called a tumor.

Wheal—Elevated skin lesion with irregular and transient borders due to edema (urticaria, insect bites).

Vesicle (blister)—Elevated, sharply defined, palpable lesion containing serous fluid usually less than 1 cm in size (chicken-pox or herpes simplex).

Bulla—Large elevated fluid-filled lesion usually more than 1 cm in size (large burn blister).

Cyst—Elevated thick-walled lesion containing fluid or semisolid mass in the dermis or subcutaneous tissue.

Pustule—Pus-filled elevated lesion less than 1 cm in size (acne, furuncles, impetigo).

Secondary skin lesions

Secondary skin lesions are those primary lesions that undergo natural progression or physical change, e.g. scratching, irritation or secondary infection.

Erosion—A moist demarcated depressed area formed by loss of partial or full thickness epidermis (ruptured chickenpox, scratch marks).

Ulcer—Irregularly-shaped, exudative, depressed lesion in which all of epidermis and part of dermis is lost (pressure ulcer).

Fissure—Deep linear crack in the epidermis extending to dermis (chapped lips, athlete's foot).

Scale—Dried fragments (flakes) of sloughed epidermis, irregular in shape and size of varying colors and thickness adhering to skin (dandruff, dry skin, psoriasis).

Scar—Skin mark left after healing of a wound or lesion formed by replacement of dead tissue by scar tissue.

Crust—Dried residue of blood serum or pus on skin surface. Large adherent crust is called a scab.

Keloid—Elevated, irregularly shaped progressively enlarging scar due to excessive formation of collagen during postsurgical healing.

Lichenification—Epidermal thickening resulting in elevated accentuated skin markings due to repeated rubbing, irritation or scratching.

INFECTIOUS DISORDERS OF SKIN

Bacterial Infections

Impetigo

- Impetigo is the superficial infections of the skin caused by *Staphylococcus aureus and group A Beta-hemolytic streptococcus.*
- Commonly occurs in children in low socioeconomic background with poor personal hygiene, chronic health problems and malnutrition.
- Appears as small red macules, which turn into vesicles that rupture and covered with a honey-colored crust surrounded by erythema; usually appears

on face as primary infection; highly contagious and may spread to other parts of the body or to other members of the family by direct contact or with common linen and laundry (Fig. 13.1).

- Systemic antibiotics, e.g. oral penicillin, benzathine penicillin IM, and erythromycin (in penicillin allergic patients) is given to treat impetigo, control streptococcal infection and prevent the risk of development of glomerulonephritis. Topical antibiotic therapy after warm saline soaks and soap and water removal of crusts may be given if the lesion is localized and evidence of streptococcal infection not found.
- Nursing measures include teaching control of infection transmission to other parts of the body and to other members by maintaining personal hygiene, use of separate laundry for patient's linens, meticulous hand washing and separate washing of patient's utensils.

Folliculitis

- Folliculitis is the infection of hair follicles caused by bacteria, usually *Staphylococcus* or fungus.
- Small, superficial pustule at hair follicle with minimum erythema appear commonly in beard area of face in men and in legs of women, scalp. Pustules are tender; crust develops (Fig. 13.2).
- Localized folliculitis is treated with gentle washing, warm compresses and topical antibiotics. Healing takes place without scarring.

Furuncles and furunculosis

- A furuncle is an acute inflammation arising in one or more hair follicles by infection with staphylococci and spreading into the surrounding dermis. It is a deep form of folliculitis. Furunculosis refers to recurrent or multiple lesions.
- May occur anywhere in the body but common in areas with excessive perspiration, pressure, friction such as axillae, back of the neck, buttocks, breasts, perineum and thighs.
- Lesion begins as a small red, raised painful pimple around hair follicle. Gradually infection progresses to surrounding skin and subcutaneous fatty tissue, gives rise to pain, tenderness and surrounding cellulitis. Characteristic pointing (head) of a boil follows in a few days. Drains pus and necrotic debris on rupture of the head (Fig. 13.3).

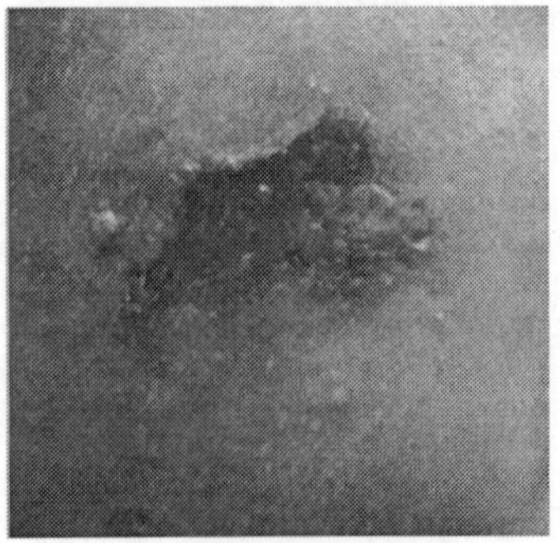

Fig. 13.1: Impetigo

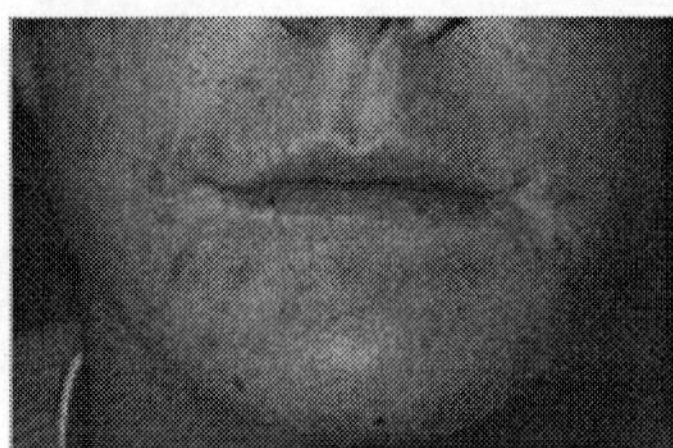

Fig. 13.2: Folliculitis

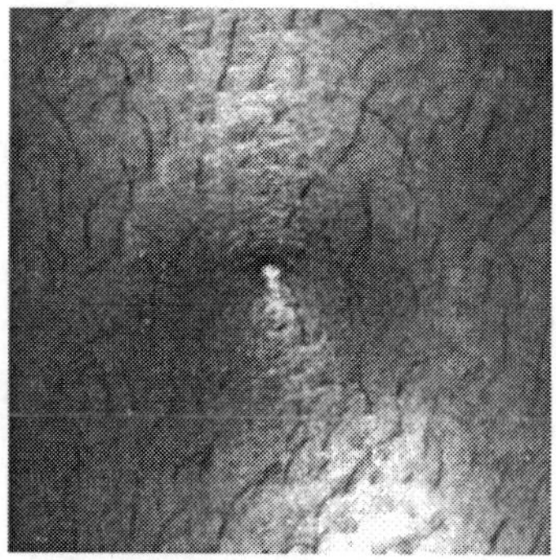

Fig. 13.3: Furuncle

- Furuncle is treated by frequent warm compresses, meticulous cleanliness of the involved skin, incision and drainage when head develops. Systemic antibiotics may be required if recurrent furuncle. Predisposing factors if any such as diabetes must be treated and meticulous personal hygiene to be maintained.

Carbuncle

- A carbuncle is an abscess of the skin and subcutaneous tissue that represents an extension of a furuncle that has affected several follicles and is large and deep-seated.
- Caused by *Staphylococcus* organism. Appears commonly in areas where skin is thick and inelastic such as nape of neck.
- Many pustules appear in a thick erythematous area (Fig. 13.4). Painful, high fever, leukocytosis and spread to blood-stream may also occur if infection is extensive in a previously weak individual, person with diabetes, or patients receiving immunosuppressive therapy.

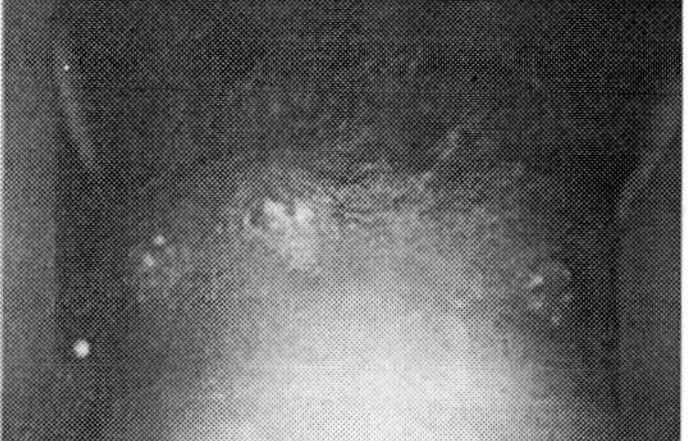

Fig. 13.4: Carbuncles

- Treatment is same as furunculosis. Systemic antibiotic therapy according to the culture and sensitivity is generally indicated. Bed rest may be advised for patient having carbuncle on buttocks to promote comfort. When the pus is localized a small incision is given to drain pus and slough.
- Nurse should provide support to the patient who are acutely ill from infection by giving bed rest, administering intravenous infusion as prescribed, implement measures to reduce fever; provide warm moist compresses several times to hasten resolution; cleaning surrounding skin gently with antibacterial soap, and applying topical antibiotics as and when advised. Care should be taken to prevent spread of infection to others by watching standard infection control measures.

Erysipelas

- Erysipelas is an acute, superficial skin infection primarily involving the dermis.
- Caused by Beta-hemolytic group A streptococci.
- Commonly appears on the face and extremities. Often recur in the same area possibly due to the lymphatic obstruction resulting from the inflammatory lesion.

- Initial lesion is small elevated and bright red, progresses peripherally to become a sharp, indurated (hard) plaque that is red hot and painful. Fever, leukocytosis, tachycardia, headache, malaise and confusion are usually present (Fig. 13.5).
- Treated with systemic antibiotics usually penicillin or according to the culture and sensitivity test of the wound specimen. Soaks may reduce edema and inflammation. Patient with complicated erysipelas may need to be hospitalized.

Cellulitis

- Cellulitis is a skin infection extending into the deeper dermis and subcutaneous tissue that results in deep, red erythema without sharp borders that spreads widely through tissue spaces.
- Caused usually by *Streptococcus pyogenes*. Other organisms may also be present. Cellulitis results as primary infection or as secondary infection. Usually occurs in older adults or in persons with lowered resistance from diabetes, malnutrition, steroid therapy, presence of ulcers or wounds, presence of edema, etc.

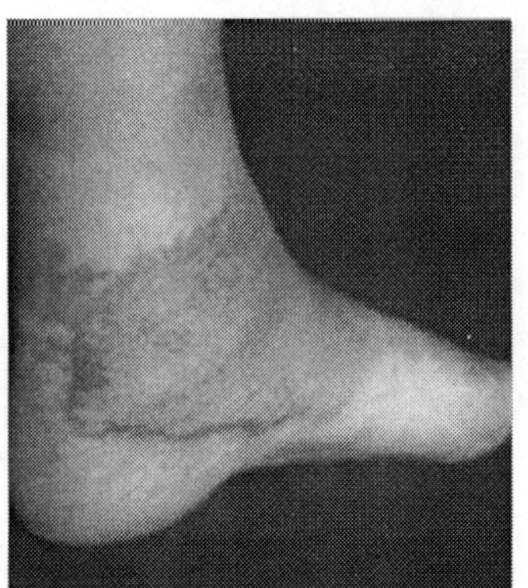

Fig. 13.5: Erysipelas

- Widespread lesion that is hot, tender, erythematous, edematous and sometimes nodular with diffuse border. Chills, malaise, fever and lymphangitis may be present. If untreated may result in sepsis, metastatic abscesses and gangrene (Fig.13.6).

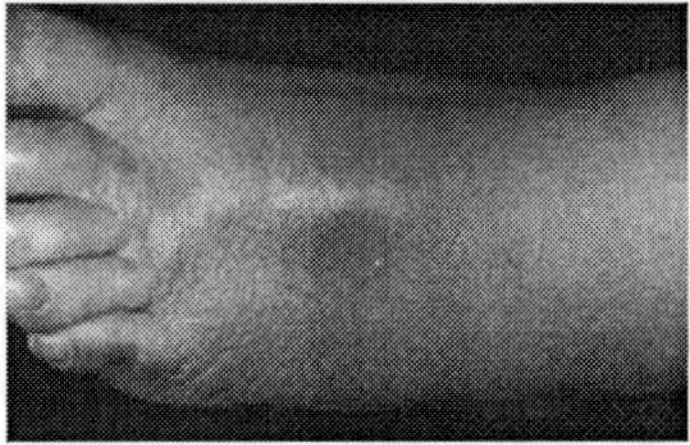

Fig. 13.6: Cellulitis

- Cellulitis is treated by application of moist heat; immobilization and elevation of affected part; systemic antibiotic therapy according to culture and sensitivity report. Hospitalization is usually indicated in severe cases.
- Nurse's responsibility is to monitor body temperature; provide optimum rest to the patient; immobilize the affected part, monitoring the condition of the affected part; administering antipyretic medications as prescribed; and teach proper handwashing technique, handling of soiled linen, clothing and dressings in order to prevent the spread of infection.

Viral Skin Infections

Herpes simplex

- Herpes simplex is a common skin infection.
- It is caused by *Herpes simplex type 1* and *Herpes simplex type 2 viruses. Herpes*

simplex type 1 causes lesion on the mouth and *Herpes simplex* type 2 causes lesion in the genital area. Both virus types may be found on both locations.

- Prevalence of type 1 virus is more common than type 2. About 85% of adults in the world are seropositive of type 1 virus, but all do not show clinical disease.
- Orolabial herpes, (herpes simplex type 1) also called fever blisters or cold sores appear as erythematous based clusters of grouped vesicles on lips. Tingling or burning with pain may occur before appearance of lesion. Increased stress and excessive exposure to sunlight may cause recurrence (Fig. 13.7).
- Genital herpes or herpes simplex type 2 causes mild to severe infections. Mild infections produce no symptoms at all. Severe primary infections with type 1 virus cause systemic flu-like symptoms. Lesions appear on vagina, penis or rectum. Lesions are symmetric grouped vesicles on an erythematous base. Lesions may continue to appear for 7 – 14 days. Regional lymphadenopathy is usually present. Recurrences are common. Burning, tingling or itching occurs before the appearance of vesicles. Vesicles rupture, causing erosions and ulcerations.

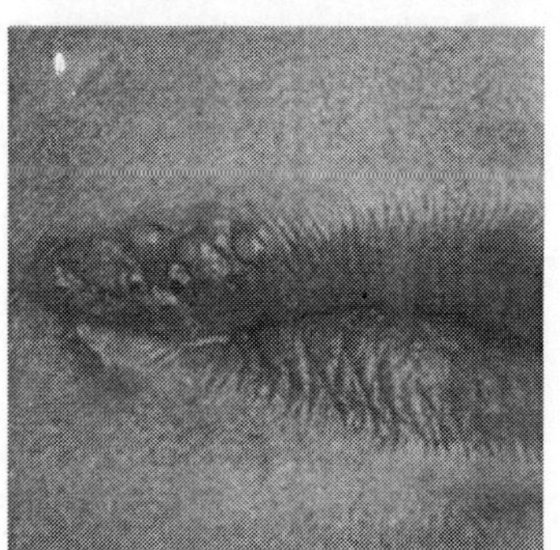

Fig. 13.7: Herpes simplex

- Herpes simplex infection is diagnosed by the appearance of characteristic lesions. In suspected cases viral cultures of swabs from vesicles or crusts may be obtained.
- Recurrent orolabial herpes is cosmetically embarrassing than a disease. Patient is advised to use sunscreen on face and lips regularly; soothing moist compresses and application of white petrolatum jelly provides comfort. Intermittent treatment with 200 mg of acyclovir 5 times a day for 5 days may be given for more severe outbreaks or in patients who have identified a trigger.
- Mild and rare appearance of genital herpes may not require any treatment. Severe form may be treated as orolabial herpes. Patients experiencing very frequent recurrences may be given suppressive therapy by oral antiviral medications.

Herpes zoster (shingles)

Definition: *Herpes zoster* is an infection caused by the varicella-zoster virus and characterized by painful vesicular eruptions along the area of distribution of the sensory nerves from one or more posterior ganglia.

Incidence

- 10% of adults get in their lifetime.
- Usually occurs in people after 50 years of age.
- Occurs in patient with weakened immunity, cancers especially leukemias, lymphomas.

Pathophysiology

- After an attack of chickenpox the varicella-zoster viruses lie dormant inside nerve cells near the brain and spinal cord.

- When immunity goes down these viruses travel by way of the peripheral nerves to the skin, where they multiply and produce a rash of small, fluid-filled blisters.

Clinical manifestations
- Eruptions comprising of patches of grouped vesicles appear on the red and swollen skin.
- Eruptions usually unilateral on trunk, face and lumbosacral areas.
- The early vesicles, which contain serum, later may become purulent, rupture and form crusts (Fig. 13.8).
- Burning pain and neuralgia over the entire region supplied by the affected nerves occur preceding outbreak. Pain becomes severe during outbreak.
- The disease may be severe and the clinical course acutely disabling if the patient is immunosuppressed.

Medical management
1. Analgesics in liberal doses during the acute phase to control pain.
2. Antiviral agents such as acyclovir, valacyclovir or famciclovir administered within 24 hours of the initial eruption halt the progress of the disease, reduce pain.
3. Wet compresses, white petrolatum on lesions may produce relief.

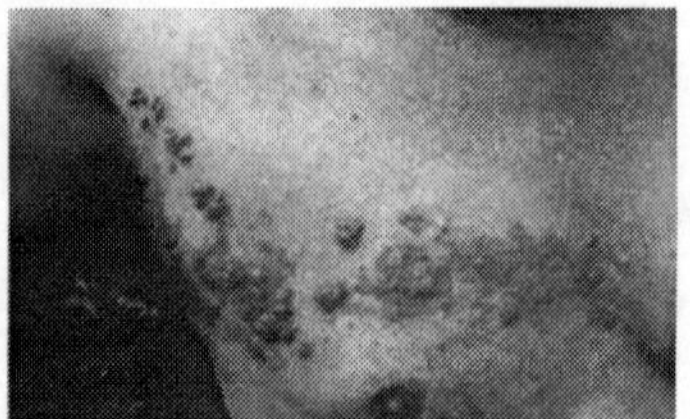

Fig. 13.8: Herpes zoster

Nursing management
- Assess patient's pain and discomfort and his response to the medications prescribed.
- Teach patient proper hand washing technique and techniques of applying medications and wet compresses to the lesions to avoid spreading the virus. If the patient is elderly and unable to care for himself, assist patient with dressings or teach a care giver to perform the dressing.
- Teach patient to take pain medications before pain becomes severe for optimum pain relief. Encourage diversional activities and relaxation techniques along with pain medication to ensure restful sleep and to alleviate discomfort.

Parasitic Skin Infestations

Pediculosis (lice infestations)

- Three varieties of lice infest humans:
  1. Pediculus humanus capities (head louse)
  2. Pediculus humanus corporis (body louse)
  3. Phthirius pubis (pubic louse).
- Lice are ectoparasites because they live on the outside of the host's body, feed on human blood and inject their digestive juices and excreta into the skin, which causes severe itching.
- Pediculosis capities is infestation of the scalp by head louse. It is more common in children and people with long hair. The female louse lays eggs (nits) close to the scalp. The eggs hatch to young lice by 10 days and reach maturity by 2 weeks.
- Head louse found commonly in the back of the head and behind ears. Nits found as silvery white oval bodies on hair. Intense itching may lead to secondary bacterial infection.

- Head louse may be transmitted by direct physical contact or indirectly by sharing combs, wigs, hats, bedding.
- Pediculosis corporis and pubis are infestations by body louse. They affect people with poor hygiene and who lives in crowded homes and are transmitted by direct physical contact and shared household linens and clothing. Pubis infestation is transmitted by sexual contact. Body louse is found on bodies in those areas where skin comes in direct contact with underclothing.
- Bites of body louse cause minute hemorrhagic points and intense itching and scratching particularly at night in areas such as trunk, neck and groin.
- Pediculosis infestations are treated by application of gamma benzene hexachloride or pyrethrines on different parts of the body.
- Nurses' responsibilities with regard to pediculosis treatment are to teach the person to apply the medicine over the affected part of the body; to treat all family members and contacts at a time; maintain hygiene; and to wash linen, clothings, beddings and combs with hot water.

Scabies

- Scabies is an infestation of skin by the itch mite *Sarcoptes scabiei*.
- Common with people living in unhygienic conditions. Parasites are transmitted by direct physical contact with an infected individual or by sharing of clothing bedding, etc.
- The female mite penetrates the superficial layer of the skin and deposits eggs. Larvae hatch from the eggs in 3 to 4 days and progress to adult mites by 10 days.
- Presence of mite parts, eggs and feces causes allergic reaction and gives rise to severe itching. After contact with the parasites about 4 weeks time is required for the symptoms to appear.
- Scabies manifests as small raised burrows commonly between the fingers, on the flexor surface of wrists, genitals, anterior axillary folds, under breasts, extensor surface of elbows, the knees, edges of the feet, near the groin or gluteal fold; red pruritic eruptions between the adjacent skin areas; secondary lesions such as vesicles, papules, excoriations and crusts; bacterial super infection from constant excoriation of the burrows and papules; severe itching specially at night (Fig. 13.9).
- Diagnosis is confirmed by recovering the mites or the mites' byproducts from the skin and identifying those under microscope.
- Scabies is treated by application of scabicides (5% permethrine) over whole body except face and scalp; antibiotics if bacterial infection and antihistamine to control possible residual itching.
- Nurses' responsibilities are to teach the patient about application of scabicides (apply scabicides after a thorough bath with soap and scrubbing over whole body except face and scalp and leaving it for 12 to 24 hours and repeat application after 1 week); treatment of all family members simultaneously, washing of bed linens, clothing with hot water and maintaining personal hygiene.

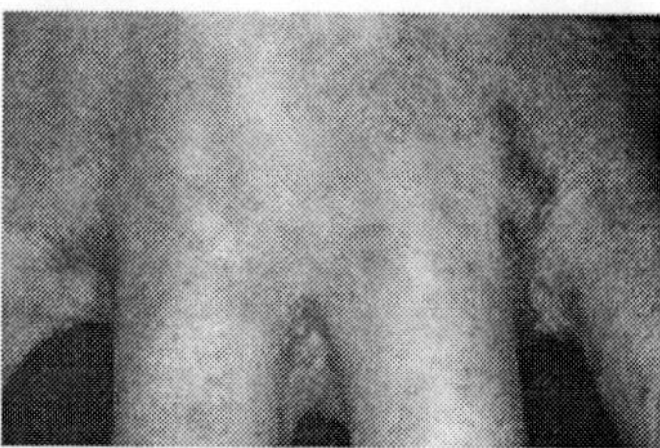

Fig. 13.9: Scabies

ALLERGIC SKIN PROBLEMS

Contact Dermatitis

- Contact dermatitis is an inflammatory reaction of the skin to physical, chemical or biologic agents.
- Irritant contact dermatitis is one of the types of contact dermatitis where non-allergic reaction results from exposure to an irritating substance. Common irritating substances are soaps, detergents, scouring compounds, industrial chemicals. It is the most common type of contact dermatitis.
- The other type of contact dermatitis is allergic contact dermatitis. It is a delayed hypersensitivity reaction occurring to sensitized people on contact with an allergen. Common allergens are poison ivy, nickel, bacitracin, formaldehyde.
- Irritant contact dermatitis manifests as eruptions following contact with irritating substance. Itching and burning, erythema, edema, papules, vesicles and woozing or weeping follow (Fig. 13.10). Alternate drying, crusting, fissuring and peeling occur. Pigmentation or lichenification results due to repeated reactins or due to constant scratching (Fig. 13.10).
- Manifestations of allergic contact dermatitis begin at the site of exposure with itching, stinging, erythema and edema. Eruptions spread to more distant sites. Symptoms may begin within an hour of contact or even after 7 days of contact. Severity of symptoms may vary from mild erythema to vesicles to ulceration.
- Identifying the irritating or allergic substance may be done by patch test.
- Management of contact dermatitis includes—identifying and avoiding the irritating substance or the allergen; applying topical medication or wet dressings; administering antihistaminic agents such as topical or systemic steroids if required.

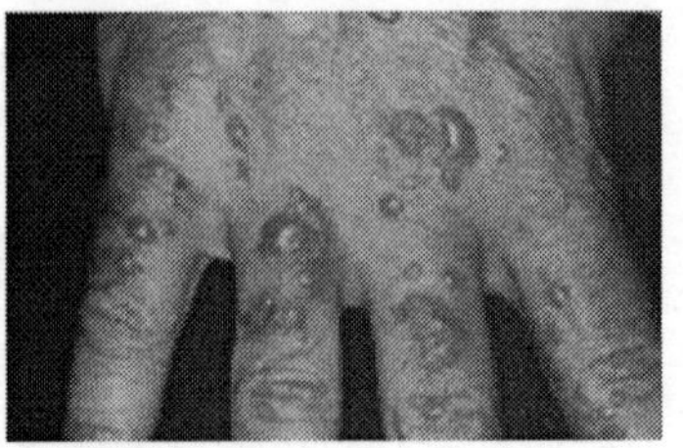

Fig. 13.10: Contact dermatitis

NONINFECTIOUS INFLAMMATORY DISEASE OF SKIN

Psoriasis

Definition

Psoriasis is a chronic recurrent noninfectious inflammatory disorder of the skin that involves excessively rapid turn over of epidermal cells.

Incidence

- It affects approximately 2% of the population.
- Disease may occur at any age but more common in 15 to 50 years.

Causes

- Primary cause is unknown.
- A combination of genetic make up and environmental stimuli may trigger the onset of the disease.
- Periods of emotional stress and anxiety may aggravate the symptoms of the disease.
- Trauma, infections, seasonal and hormonal changes are some of the trigger factors.

Pathophysiology

- The cells in the basal layer of the epidermis divide too quickly, 6 to 9 times faster than normal rate.

- The newly formed psoriatic cells travel from the basal cell layer of the epidermis to the stratum corneum within 3 to 4 days only, where normal cells take 28 to 30 days to complete the same phenomena.
- Due to increased number of basal cell and their very rapid passage to the skin surface, the normal cell growth and maturation cannot take place resulting in impaired formation of the normal protective layer of skin.
- Instead of falling off (shedding) the immature cells in the superficial layer pile up and form lesions.
- Blood vessels dilate with increased blood supply to nourish these cells.

Clinical manifestations

Manifestations vary from mild with cosmetic concern to severe disease with physical disability and disfigurement.

- Lesions appear as red, raised patches of skin covered with silvery scales.
- On scraping of the scales dark red base of the lesion is exposed producing multiple bleeding points.
- Patches are dry and pruritic.
- Appearance of lesions is in bilateral symmetrical fashion and occurs usually on the scalp, extensor surfaces of the elbows and knees, sacral and genital regions (Fig. 13.11).
- A generalized eruption may occur in severe psoriasis vulgaris (Fig. 13.12).
- Generalized sterile cutaneous pustules may appear in a small percentage of patients and is known as pustular psoriasis.
- In Koebner's phenomenon lesion may develop at the site of an injury.
- In palmer plantar psoriasis pustular or plaque type lesion appears only in palms and soles.
- In 50% of patients nails are involved with discoloration, pitting, crumbling beneath the free edges and separation from the nail plate.

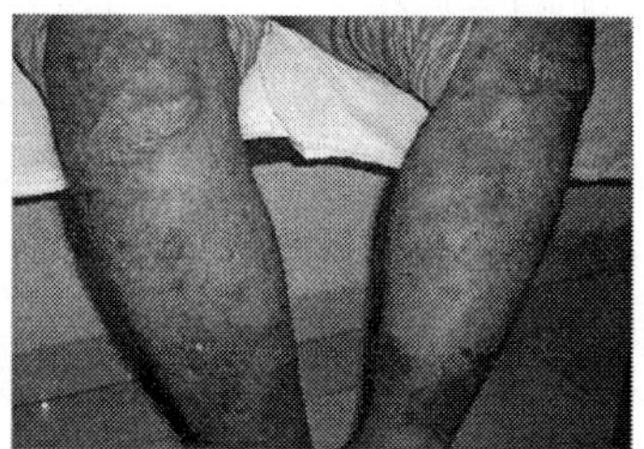

Fig. 13.11: Bilateral lesion in psoriasis

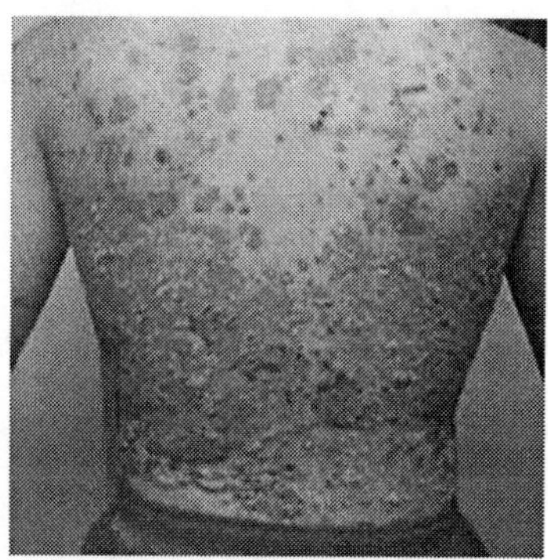

Fig. 13.12: Psoriasis vulgaris

Complications

1. Psoriatic arthritis of distal joints.
2. Exfoliative psoriatic state—Involves whole body surface. Patient is acutely ill with fever, chills and electrolyte imbalance. Complication develops when a patient with chronic psoriasis is affected with infections or exposed to certain medications or is withdrawn from systemic corticosteroids suddenly.

Diagnosis

- Diagnosis is established by signs and symptoms, specially by involvement of scalp and nails.
- Presence of positive family history.

Medical management

There is no known cure. Goals of management are:
1. To slow the rapid turnover of epidermis.
2. To promote resolution of the psoriatic lesions.

Topical treatments
1. Application of topical medications slows the overgrowth of epidermis without affecting other tissues. Medications include corticosteroids, tar preparations, anthralin, salicylic acid, vitamin D preparation, calcipotriene, and a retinoid compound, tazarotene.
2. Intralesional injections of corticosteroids for chronic plaques.
3. Ultraviolet light alone or with topical tripsoralen or oral psoralen (a photosensitizing medication).

Systemic treatments
1. Cytotoxic drugs such as methotrexate, hydroxyurea for extensive lesions that does not respond to other forms of therapy.
2. Immunosuppressant cyclosporin A in severe form of psoriasis that is resistant to other treatments.
3. Oral retinoids (etretinate) in severe pustular psoriasis is helpful.
4. Corticosteroids (only limited use).

Nursing management

- Assist the patient to cope with altered self concept.
- Teach patient—
  - To keep the involved area clean and dry to prevent secondary infections.
  - To use creams or ointments always over the involved area as prescribed.
  - To adopt good nourishing diet, rest and regular exercise to promote health.
  - Treat infections or other illnesses if appear promptly.
  - To keep stress under control.

Acne Vulgaris

Definition

Acne vulgaris is an inflammatory skin disease affecting the tiny pores that cover the face, arms, back and chest and the sebaceous glands attached to them.

Incidence

- Commonly occurs in adolescents and young adults between ages 12 to 35.
- Boys and girls are equally affected but onset is earlier in girls.

Causes

- Genetic, hormonal and bacterial factors seem to be the cause of the condition.
- Presence of family history play a role in the occurrence.

Pathophysiology and clinical manifestations

- Normally sebaceous glands are small and nonfunctioning in childhood. During puberty androgens stimulate sebaceous glands to enlarge and secrete sebum.
- Acne develops when there is an excessive response in the sebaceous glands by androgens resulting in excessive production of sebum that plugs the pilosebaceous ducts.
- Accumulated materials such as impacted lipids and keratin plug the follicles and form characteristic lesion of acne known as comedones (Fig. 13.13).
- Primary lesions of acne, comedones or white heads appear most commonly on face, neck and back. Contents of some closed comedones or white heads are in open communication with the external environment and are known as black heads. Some closed comedones rupture and comes in contact with certain skin bacteria resulting in inflammatory reaction.

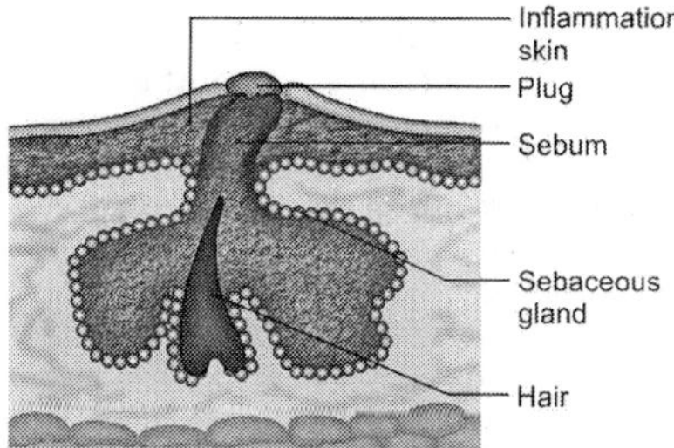

Fig. 13.13: Acne comedones

- These inflammatory reactions seen as erythematous papules, inflammatory pustules and inflammatory cysts. Mild papules and cysts drain and heal on their own. Deeper papules and cysts give rise to scarring of the skin (Fig. 13.14).

Management

Local treatment

- Maintain hygiene. Wash face with cleansing soap twice a day.
- Take balanced diet. Avoid foods that seem to cause flare up of acne such as cola, chocolate, milk products and fried foods.
- Apply topical acne medications—
  - Salicylic acid and benzoyl peroxide gel once a day to remove sebaceous plugs.
  - Benzoyl peroxide, benzoyl erythromycin and benzoyl sulfur combinations may also be used.
  - Preparations containing vitamin A acid (tretinoin) to clear the keratin from the pilosebaceous ducts.
  - Antibiotics preparations, e.g. tetracycline, clindamycin and erythromycin suppress growth of skin bacteria, decrease comedones, papules and pustules.

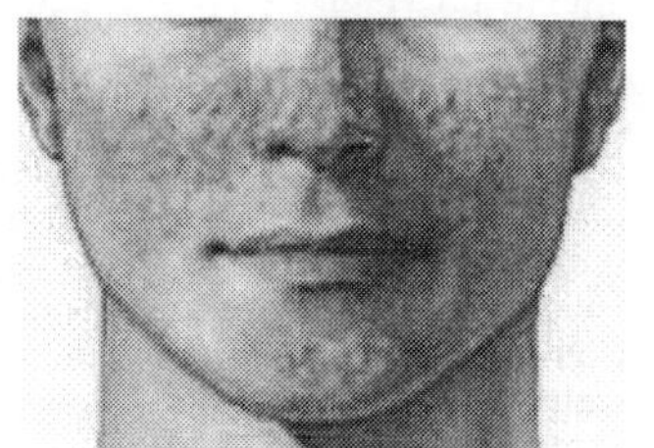

Fig. 13.14: Acne

Systemic treatments

- Oral antibiotics such as tetracycline, doxycycline, and minocycline in small doses over a long period of time may be given in moderate to severe acne.
- Oral retinoids synthetic vitamin A compounds isotretinoin (accutane) reduces sebaceous gland size and inhibits sebum production and epidermal desquamation. It is effective in the treatment of nodular cystic acne unresponsive to other treatments.
- Hormone therapy in the form of estrogen dominant oral contraceptives is given to young women whose acne flares up during menstrual cycle.

Surgical treatments—That may be carried out in severe cases are:

- Extraction of comedo contents.
- Drainage of pustules and cysts.
- Interlesional corticosteroids for anti-inflammatory action.
- Cryotherapy.
- Dermabrasion for scars.
- Laser resurfacing of scars.

NURSING MANAGEMENT OF PATIENTS WITH BURNS

- Burns are injuries or damages to the body's tissues caused by heat, chemicals, electricity or radiation. A burn injury occurs as a result of destruction of the skin from direct or indirect thermal force. Scald burn results from exposure to moist heat (steam or hot fluids) and involves superficial layers.

- Burns are caused by a transfer of energy from heat source to the body. The depth of the injury depends on the temperature of the burning agent and the duration of contact with it. Burns disrupt the skin, which leads to increased fluid loss, infection, hypothermia, scarring, compromised immunity and changes in further appearance and body image.

Incidence

- In India, about 2.4 million people suffer burns annually. It accounts for an estimated 700,000 emergency room visits every year and 45,000 require hospitalization. Between 8,000–12,000 burn patients die and approximately one million sustain substantial or permanent disabilities.

Causes

- Burns are caused by a wide variety of substances and external sources such as exposure to chemicals, friction, electricity, radiation and heat.

Chemicals

- Most chemicals that cause chemical burns are strong acids or bases. Chemical burns can be caused by caustic chemical compounds such as sodium hydroxide or silver nitrate and acids such as sulfuric acid.
- Hydrofluoric acid can cause damage down to the bone and its burns are sometimes not immediately evident.
- Chemical burns can be either first, second, or third degree burns, depending on duration of contact, strength of the substance and other factors.

Electrical

- Electrical burns are caused by either an electric shock or an uncontrolled short circuit (a burn from a hot, electrified heating element is not considered an electrical burn).
- Common occurrences of electrical burns include workplace injuries, or being defibrillated or cardioverted without a conductive gel.
- Lightning is also a rare cause of electrical burns.

Radiation

- Radiation burns are caused by protracted exposure to UV light (as from the sun), tanning booths, radiation therapy (in people undergoing cancer therapy), sun lamps, radioactive fallout, and X-rays.
- The most common burn associated with radiation is sun exposure.
- Tanning booths also emit these wavelengths and may cause similar damage to the skin such as irritation, redness, swelling and inflammation.
- Severe cases of sun burn result in what is known as sun poisoning or "heatstroke".
- Microwave burns are caused by the thermal effects of microwave radiation.

Thermal burns

- Thermal burns which can be caused by flame, flash, or contact with hot objects are the most common types of burn.

Scalds

- Scalding (from the Latin word **calidus**, meaning hot) is caused by hot liquids (water or oil) (Fig.13.15) or gases (steam), most commonly occurring from exposure to high temperature tap water in baths or showers or spilled hot drinks.

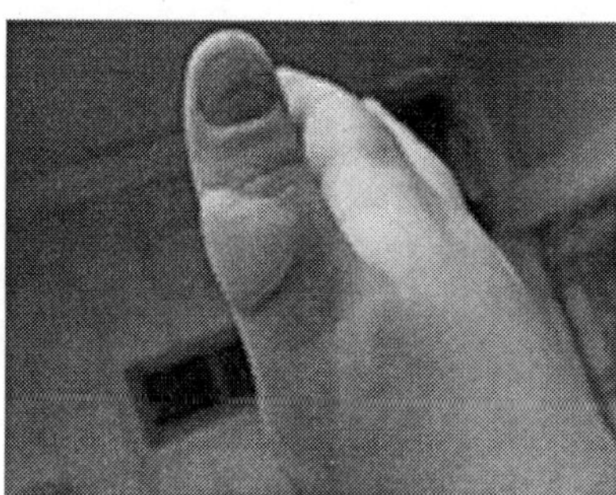

Fig. 13.15: Two-day-old scald caused by boiling radiator fluid

- An immersion scald is created when an extremity is held under the surface of hot water, and is a common form of burn seen in child abuse.
- A blister is a "bubble" in the skin filled with serous fluid as part of the body's reaction to the heat and the subsequent inflammatory reaction. The blister "roof" is dead and the blister fluid contains toxic inflammatory mediators.
- Scald burns are more common in children, specially "spill scalds" from hot drinks and bath water scalds. Generally scald burns are first or second degree burns, but third degree burns can result, specially with prolonged contact.

Smoke and Inhalation injury—Results from the inhalation of hot air and noxious chemicals, cause damage to the tissue of respiratory tract. Inhalation injury and pulmonary complications are common (50–60% of fire deaths occur due to inhalation injury)

Classification of Burn injury

- Burns can be classified by depth, severity, and extent of injury to body surface area.

By depth

- Burns are described according to the depth of injury to the dermis and are classified into first, second, third degree.
  1. *Superficial partial thickness burn (1st degree burn)*: It usually produces a pink to reddish color on the burned skin and very sensitive to touch and the skin will appear blanched when light pressure is applied. It is least serious type of burn and involves minimal tissue damage, only to the epidermis, e.g. sunburn.
     Signs and symptoms are: Pain, redness, swelling and dry without blisters.
  2. *Deep partial thickness burn (2nd degree burn)*: It affects both the epidermis and dermis causing redness, pain, swelling and blisters. Sweat glands and hair follicles are affected. It often produces scarring. If it is not treated properly, swelling and decrease blood flow in the tissues may lead to third degree burn.
  3. *Full thickness burn (3rd degree burn)*: They affect the epidermis, dermis and hypodermis causing charring of skin or a translucent white color with coagulated vessels visible just below the skin surface. Other organs tissues, muscles, or bones may also be affected. They are most serious, healing is very slow and result in extensive scarring.
     Signs and symptoms are: Surface appears dry and can look waxy white leathery, brown or charred. Little or no pain and the area may feel numb at first because of nerve damage.
     The following Table 13.1 describes the degrees of burn injury under this system as well as provides pictorial examples.

Table 13.1: Classification of burn according to the depth of injury

Nomenclature	Layer involved	Appearance	Texture	Sensation	Time to healing	Complications	Example
First degree (superficial partial thickness)	Epidermis	Redness (erythema)	Dry	Painful	1 week or less	None	
Second degree	Extends into superficial (papillary) dermis	Red with clear blister. Blanches with pressure	Moist	Painful	2–3 weeks	Local infection/ cellulitis	
Second degree (deep partial thickness)	Extends into deep (reticular) dermis	Red-and-white with bloody blisters. Less blanching	Moist	Painful	Several weeks—may progress to third degree	Scarring, contractures (may require excision and skin grafting)	
Third degree (full thickness)	Extends through entire dermis	Stiff and white/ brown	Dry, leathery	Painless	Requires excision	Scarring, contractures (may require amputation)	

By Severity of Injury

- Burns can be classified as major, moderate and minor.
- This classification is based on a number of factors, including total body surface area (TBSA) burnt, the involvement of specific anatomical zones, age of the person and associated injuries.

Major

Major burns consist of any one of the followings:

- Partial thickness burns >25% of total body surface area in patient, aged 10–50 years.
- Partial thickness burns >20% of total body surface area in patient, aged <10 or >50 years.
- Full thickness burns >10%.
- Burns involving the hands, face, feet or perineum.
- Burns that cross major joints.
- Circumferential burns to any extremity.
- Any burn associated with inhalational injury.
- Electrical burns.
- Burns associated with fractures or other trauma.
- Burns in infants and the elderly.
- Burns in persons at high-risk of developing complications.

These burns typically require referral to a specialized burn treatment center.

Moderate

- Moderate burns are considered as any one of the followings:
- Partial thickness burns involving 15–25% of total body surface area in patient, aged 10 to 50 years.
- Partial thickness burns involving 10–20% of total body surface area in patient, aged <10 or >50 years.
- Full thickness burns involving 2–10% of total body surface area.

Persons suffering these burns often need to be hospitalized for burn care.

Minor

Minor burns are:

- Partial thickness burns <15% of total body surface area in patient, aged 10 to 50 years
- Partial thickness burns involving <10% of total body surface area in patient aged <10 or >50 years.
- Full thickness burns <2% of total body surface area, without associated injuries.

These burns usually do not require hospitalization.

By Surface Area of Injury

- Burns are also described in terms of total body surface area (TBSA), which is the percentage affected by partial thickness or full thickness burns.
- First degree (erythema only, no blisters) burns are not included in this estimation.
- The rule of nine (Fig. 13.16) and palmar method (Fig. 13.17) is used as a quick and useful way to estimate the affected TBSA.
- More accurate estimation can be made using Lund and Browder chart (Fig. 13.18), which takes into account the different proportions of body parts in adults and children.
- The size of a person's hand print (palm and fingers) is approximately 0.8% of their TBSA, but for quick estimates, medical personnel round this to 1%, slightly overestimating the size of the affected area.

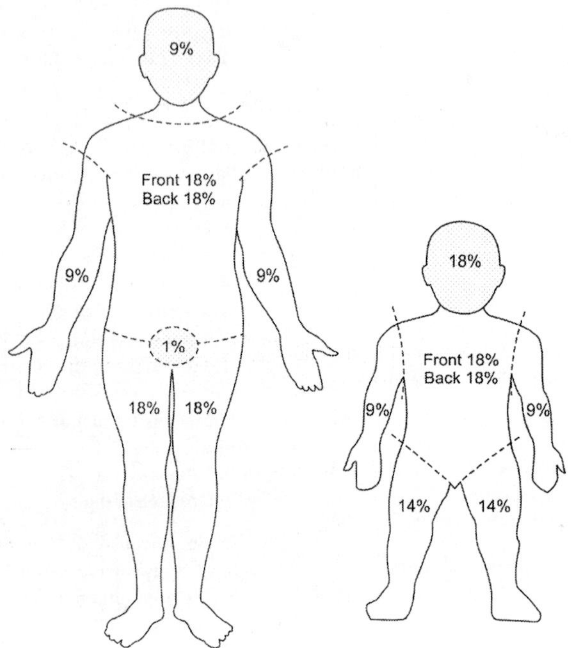

Fig. 13.16: Rule of Nine (Adult)

Child For every year of life after 12 months take 1% from the head and add ½% to each leg, Until the age of 10 years when adult proportions

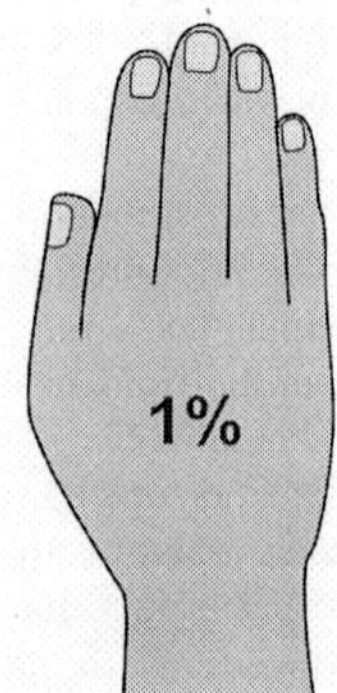

Fig. 13.17: Palmar method

- Burns of 10% in children or 15% in adults (or greater) are potentially life-threatening injuries (because of the risk of hypovolemic shock) and should have formal fluid resuscitation and monitoring in a burns unit.
- Palm and fingers of the patient = 1% TBSA.
- Useful for small and scattered burns.
- Can be used for subtraction, e.g. full arm burnt except for hand–sized area = 8% TBSA.

A BURN CHART

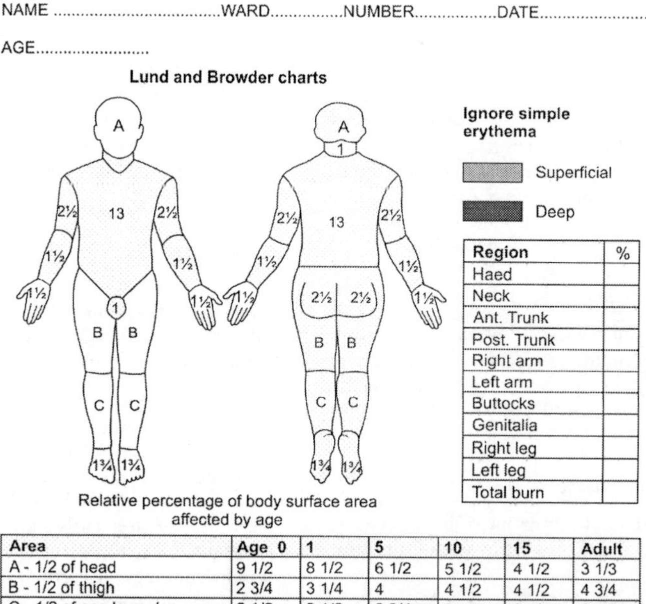

NAME ....................................WARD................NUMBER.................DATE..........................

AGE.........................

Lund and Browder charts

Region	%
Haed	
Neck	
Ant. Trunk	
Post. Trunk	
Right arm	
Left arm	
Buttocks	
Genitalia	
Right leg	
Left leg	
Total burn	

Relative percentage of body surface area affected by age

Area	Age 0	1	5	10	15	Adult
A - 1/2 of head	9 1/2	8 1/2	6 1/2	5 1/2	4 1/2	3 1/3
B - 1/2 of thigh	2 3/4	3 1/4	4	4 1/2	4 1/2	4 3/4
C - 1/2 of one lower leg	2 1/2	2 1/2	2 3/4	3	3 1/4	3 1/2

Fig. 13.18: Lund and Browder chart

Pathophysiology

- Understanding the pathophysiology of a burn injury is important for effective management.
- Burn injuries result in both local and systemic responses.

Local response

- The three zones of a burn (Fig. 13.19) were described by Jackson in 1947.

Zone of coagulation

- Occurs at the point of maximum damage.
- There is irreversible tissue loss due to coagulation of the constituent proteins.

Zone of stasis

- The surrounding zone of stasis is characterized by decreased tissue perfusion. The tissue in this zone is potentially salvageable.
- The main aim of burns resuscitation is to increase tissue perfusion here and prevent any damage becoming irreversible.
- Additional insults—Such as prolonged hypotension, infection, or edema can

convert this zone into an area of complete tissue loss.

Zone of hyperemia

- In this outermost zone tissue perfusion is increased.
- The tissue here will invariably recover unless there is severe sepsis or prolonged hypoperfusion.
- These three zones of a burn are three-dimensional and loss of tissue in the zone of stasis will lead to the wound deepening as well as widening.

Systemic Response

- The release of cytokines and other inflammatory mediators at the site of injury has a systemic effect once the burn reaches 30% of total body surface area.

Cardiovascular changes

- Capillary permeability is increased, leading to loss of intravascular proteins and fluids into the interstitial compartment.
- Peripheral and splanchnic vasoconstriction occurs.
- Myocardial contractility is decreased, possibly due to release of tumor necrosis factor α.
- These changes, coupled with fluid loss from the burn wound, result in systemic hypotension and end organ hypoperfusion.

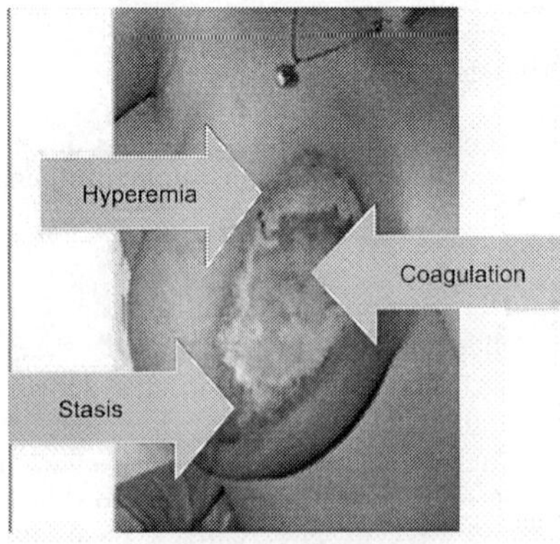

Fig. 13.19: Clinical image of burn zones. There is central necrosis, surrounded by the zones of stasis and of hyperemia

Respiratory changes

- Inflammatory mediators cause bronchoconstriction and in severe burns adult respiratory distress syndrome can occur.

Metabolic changes

- The basal metabolic rate increases up to three times its original rate. This, coupled with splanchnic hypoperfusion, necessitates early and aggressive enteral feeding to decrease catabolism and maintain gut integrity.

Immunological changes

- Nonspecific down regulation of the immune response occurs, affecting both cell-mediated and humoral pathways.

Diagnostic Tests

Blood tests

- CBC (increased / decreased hematocrit, decreased RBCs and leukocytosis).
- ABG: Decreased PaO_2 and $PaCO_2$ may be seen with carbon-dioxide poisoning
- COHb (>15% : CO poisoning).
- Serum electrolytes (potassium and sodium increased/decreased and magnesium decreased).

- Alkaline phosphatase elevated due to fluid shift.
- Serum glucose and serum albumin increases that suggest stress response.
- BUN and creatinine increase that reflects decrease renal perfusion. Creatinine level increases because of tissue injury.
- Urine (albumin, Hb and myoglobin). Presence of albumin, Hb and myoglobin indicates deep tissue damage and protein loss.
- Random urine sodium (>20 mEq/L indicates excessive fluid resuscitation; <10 mEq/L indicates inadequate fluid resuscitation).

Radiologic Studies

- **Chest X-ray**: It may appear normal in early postburn period. However, a true inhalation injury presents as infiltrates, often progressing to white out X-ray.
- **Fiberoptic bronchoscopy**: It is useful in diagnosing extent of inhalation injury.
- **ECG**: Signs of myocardial infarction/ dysrhythmias may occur with electrical burns.

Management

Four major goals relating to burn management are prevention, institution of life saving measures for the severely burned person, prevention of disability and disfigurement and rehabilitation.

Burn management has been organized chronologically into three phases

- Emergent (resuscitative) phase
- Acute (wound healing) phase
- Rehabilitative (restorative) phase.

Emergent (resuscitative) phase

The emergent phase is the period of time required to resolve the immediate life-threatening problems resulting from the burn injury. It begins at the time of injury and ends with the restoration of capillary permeability; phase may last from the time of burn to 3 or more days, usually 24–48 hours and ends with fluid mobilization and beginning of diuresis. The prime goal is to prevent hypovolemic shock and to preserve vital organ functioning. It includes prehospital care and emergency room care.

- The resuscitative and stabilization phase begins with the assessment of the injured person's airway, breathing and circulatory state.
- Aggressive fluid resuscitation is done. If inhalation injury is suspected, intubation is required.
- Once the injured person is stabilized, attention is turned to the care of the burn wound. Until then, it is advisable to cover the burn wound with a clean and dry sheet or dressing.
- Early cooling reduces burn depth and pain, but care must be taken as uncontrolled cooling can result in hypothermia.

Airway management

- Early orotracheal intubation for airway maintenance and oxygenation.
- Ventilatory assistance with PEEP (positive end expiratory pressure)
- ABG (arterial blood gas analysis) suggests the level of hypoxia in tissues. It also reveals metabolic acidosis and alkalosis.
- Extubation, after edema is relieved usually after 3–6 days of burn injury.
- Any smoke inhalation can be diagnosed through fibrooptic bronchoscopy.
- If no intubation administer humidified air, supplemental oxygen (HBOT).
- Place patient in Fowler's position.

- If patient having any history of spinal injury—provide Trendelenburg position.
- Encourage coughing and deep breathing every hour.
- Administer bronchodilators if prescribed.

Fluid therapy (Table 13.2)

- Assess fluid needs of the patient.
- Begin IV fluid replacement.
- Insert urinary catheter to monitor the urinary output every hour.
- If >15% TBSA burn insert 2 large bore IV cannula.
- In >30% TBSA burn maintain central line and arterial line for fluid medication and blood access.

These formulas are guides only and infusions must be tailored to the urine output and central venous pressure. Inadequate fluid resuscitation may cause renal failure and death, but over-resuscitation also causes morbidity.

Nutritional therapy is also one of the major aspects in this phase.

Feeding protocol

- Start 20–40 mL/hr and increase to the goal rate within 24–48 hours.
- Formulas containing arginine supplementation.
- High calorie, high protein, iron, multivitamin is required.

Table 13.2: Fluid calculation formula and types of fluid for burn management

Formula	First 24 hours	Second 24 hours	
	Crystalloids	**colloids**	**Glucose in water**
Brooke army	Lactated Ringer solution	0.5 mL/kg/ %TBSA burn	Amount to replace estimated evaporative losses
Parkland / Baxter (modified	1.5 mL/kg/%TBSA burn; ½ given during 1st 8 hours, ½ given next 16 hours Lactated Ringer solution : 4 mL/kg/%TBSA burn; ½ given during 1st 8 hours, ½ given next 16 hours	20–0% of calculated plasma volume	Amount to replace estimated evaporative losses
Consensus	Lactated Ringer solution	—	Amount to replace estimated evaporative losses
Evans	2–4 mL/kg/%TBSA burn; ½ given during 1st 8 hours, ½ given next 16 hours	1 mL/kg/ %TBSA burn	Amount to replace estimated evaporative losses
Hypertonic saline solutions	Lactated Ringer solution : 1 mL/kg/%TBSA burn; ½ given during 1st 8 hours, ½ given next 16 hours NaCl and lactate (250–300 mEq Na/L)		Amount to replace estimated evaporative losses

- Dietary protein started at 1.2 gm/kg/day and increased with subsequent increase in protein markers.
- Caloric needs to be met according to Harris-Benedict formula (adult), Galveston formula (children) and Currie formula (adult and children).
- Fat – 30% of calories to be provided as fat.
- Supplemental vitamin A, C, E promotes wound healing.
- Minerals iron, zinc promotes cell integrity and hemoglobin formation.
- Increased thirst of burn patients to be relieved by providing protein containing solutions, soy/milk-based supplements, protein-containing fruit drinks.
- Oxandrolone promotes weight gain and preservation of lean body mass.

Acute Phase (wound care)

This phase begins with the mobilization of extracellular fluid, the patient is hemodynamically stable, capillary permeability is restored and diuresis has begun. It usually begins 48–72 hours after the time of injury. Emphasis is placed on restorative therapy and the phase continues until wound closure is achieved (Fig. 13.20). This may take weeks or many months. The main focus is on infection control, wound care, wound closure, nutritional support, pain management and physical therapy.

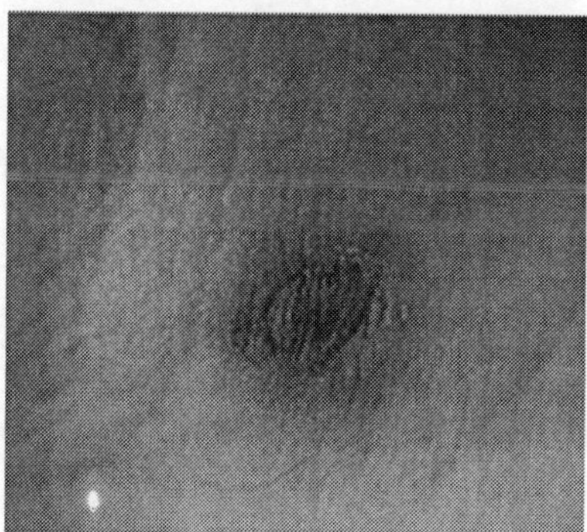

Fig. 13.20: Second degree heat burn, approx 1 cm across center, 6 days after burn

Wound care

- Start hydrotherapy.
- Initiate wound debridement as necessary.
- Assess the extent and depth of burns.
- Initiate appropriate wound care.
- Administer tetanus toxoid or tetanus antitoxin.

Debridement cleaning and then dressings are important aspects of wound care. The wound should then be regularly reevaluated until it is healed. In the management of first and second degree burns little quality evidence exists to determine which type of dressing should be used. Silver sulfadiazine (Flamazine) is not recommended as it potentially prolongs healing time while biosynthetic dressings may speed healing.

Antibiotics

- Intravenous antibiotics may improve survival in those with large and severe burns.

Analgesics

- Analgesics (such as ibuprofen and acetaminophen) and narcotics are administered for pain.
- A local anesthetic may help in managing pain of minor first degree and second degree burns.

Surgery

- Wounds requiring surgical closure with skin grafts or flaps should be dealt with as early as possible.
- Circumferential burns of digits, limbs

or the chest may need urgent surgical release of the burnt skin (escharotomy) to prevent problems with distal circulation or ventilation.

Escharotomy

- A lengthwise incision is made through the burn eschar to relieve constriction and pressure and to improve circulation.
- It is performed for circulation compromise resulting from circumferential burns.
- After eschartomoy, it is important to assess pulses, color, movement, and sensation of affected extremity and control any bleeding with pressure.
- Apply topical antimicrobial agents as prescribed.

Fasciotomy

- An incision is made, extending through subcutaneous tissue and fascia. Performed if adequate tissue perfusion does not return after an escharotomy.
- Performed in operating room under general anesthesia.

Alternative treatments

- Hyperbaric oxygenation may be useful in adjunct to traditional treatments to speed up the healing time.
- Honey has been used since ancient times to aid wound healing and may be beneficial in first and second degree burns, but may cause infection.

Rehabilitation Phase

It is the final phase of burns care. It begins with the initiation of fluids and ends when capillary integrity returns to near normal and large fluid shifts have decreased. The person's burn has healed and he can resume selfcare activities. Goals are to assist the patient in resuming functional role in the society and to accomplish functional and cosmetic reconstructive surgery.

COMPLICATIONS OF BURNS

1. **Infection** is a major complication of burns.
   - Infection is linked to impaired resistance from disruption of the skin's mechanical integrity and generalized immune suppression.
   - The skin barrier is replaced by eschar. This moist, protein-rich avascular environment encourages microbial growth. Migration of immune cells is hampered and there is a release of intermediaries that impede the immune response.
   - Eschar also restricts distribution of systemically administered antibiotics because of its avascularity.

   Risk factors of burn wound infection include—
   - Burn > 30% TBSA.
   - Full-thickness burn.
   - Extremes in age (very young and very old).
   - Preexisting disease, e.g. diabetes.
   - Virulence and antibiotic resistance of colonizing organism.
   - Failed skin graft.
   - Improper initial burn wound care.
   - Prolonged open burn wound.

   Management—
   - Burn wounds are prone to tetanus. A tetanus booster dose is required if individual has not been immunized within the last 5 years.
   - Circumferential burns of extremities may compromise circulation. Elevation of limb may help to prevent dependent edema.
   - An escharotomy may be required.

2. **Acute tubular necrosis** of the kidneys can be caused by myoglobin and hemoglobin released from damaged muscles and red blood cells. This is common in electrical burns or crush injuries where adequate fluid resuscitation has not been achieved.
3. **Burn contracture**: Burn scar contractures refer to the tightening of the skin after a second and third degree burn. When skin is burned, the surrounding skin begins to pull together; resulting in a contracture. Burn scar contracture may improve with the passage of time and physiotherapy and splinting. Release of contracture to be done with techniques such as use of local skin flaps (Z-plasty) or skin grafting.
4. **Scars**: One of the most devastating sequelae of burn injury is the formation of hypertrophic scars. Scar management occurs mainly in the rehabilitative phase after the wounds are closed.
5. **Keloids**: Keloid is an overgrowth of scar tissue that develops around a wound; usually after the wound has healed. Treatment includes application of pressure/and or airtight (occlusive) dressings, surgery, radiotherapy (brachytherapy), cryotherapy and laser therapy.
6. **Failure to Heal**: Failure of the wound to heal may result from many factors, including infection and underlying disease process, shearing, pressure or inadequate nutrition. A serum albumin level of less than 2 gm/dL is usually a factor in impaired healing in the burn patient.

NURSING MANAGEMENT

Nursing Assessment

A detailed history and physical examination is the first step. Evaluate the type, duration and timing of the burn; the burn location, and severity and associated dehydration, disfigurement and infection.

Primary survey

A. **Airway maintenance with cervical spine control**
   - Stabilise the neck for suspected cervical spine injury.
   - Inspect the airway for foreign material/edema. If the patient is unable to respond to verbal commands open the airway with a chin lift and jaw thrust.
   - Keep movement of the cervical spine to a minimum and never hyperflex or hyperextend the head or neck.
   - Insert artificial airway if airway patency is compromised. Think about early intubation.

B. **Breathing and ventilation**
   - Administer 100% oxygen.
   - Expose the chest and ensure that chest expansion is adequate and bilaterally equal.
   - Palpate for crepitus and for rib fractures.
   - Auscultate for breath sound bilaterally.
   - Ventilate via a bag and mask or intubate the patient if necessary.
   - Monitor respiratory rate. Beware if rate <10 or > 20/min.
   - Apply pulse oximeter monitor.
   - Consider carbon monoxide poisoning. Nonburnt skin may by cherry pink in color in a nonbreathing patient (send blood for carboxyhemaglobin.

C. **Circulation with hemorrhage control**
   - Inspect for any obvious bleeding. If bleeding stop with direct pressure.
   - Monitor and record the peripheral pulse for rate, strength (strong and weak) and rhythm.

- Apply capillary blanching test (centrally and peripherally to burnt and nonburnt areas). Normal return is two seconds. Longer return time indicates poor perfusion due to hypotension, hypovolemia or need for escharotomy on that limb; check another limb.
- Monitor circulation of peripheries if there is a circumferential burn present. Firstly elevate the limb to reduce edema and aid blood flow. If this does not prove effective then it may be necessary to perform an escharotomy.

D. Disability: Neurological status

- Establish level of consciousness:
  A - Alert
  V - Response to vocal stimuli
  P - Responds to painful stimuli
  U - Unresponsive.
- Examine pupils' response to light for reaction and size.
- Be alert for restlessness and decreased level of consciousness–hypoxemia, CO intoxication, shock, alcohol, drugs and analgesia influence level of consciousness.

E. Exposure with environmental control

- Remove all clothing and jewellery.
- Keep patient warm.
- Hypothermia can have detrimental effects on the patient. It is important to ensure that the patient is kept warm, specially during first aid cooling periods.
- Log roll patient, remove wet sheets and examine posterior surfaces for burns and other injuries.

F. Fluids resuscitation

- Fluid Resuscitation will be required for a patient who has sustained a burn >10% for children and >15% for adults.
- Estimate burn area using Rule of Nines. For smaller burns the palmar surface (including fingers) of the patient's hand (represents 1% TBSA) can be used to calculate the %TBSA burnt.

Secondary survey

Perform a comprehensive secondary survey.

Collect history on
A - Allergies
M - **M**edications
P - **P**ast Illnesses
L - **L**ast meal
E-**E**vents/environment related to injury.

Mechanism of injury—Gather information from the patient or others about the followings

- Date and time of burn injury, date and time of first presentation.
- Source of injury and length of contact time.
- Clothing worn.
- Activities at time of burn injury.
- Adequacy of first aid.

Head to toe assessment
Reassess **A, B, C, D, E,** and **F** of primary survey.

Other actions

- Record and document.
- Swab all burn wounds and send to microbiology.

Nursing Assessment in Emergent/Resuscitative Phase

- Focus on the major priorities of any trauma patient; the burn wound is a secondary consideration, although aseptic management of the burn wounds and invasive lines continues.
- Assess circumstances surrounding the injury: time of injury, mechanism of burn, whether the burn occurred in a

closed space, the possibility of inhalation of noxious chemicals and any related trauma.

- Monitor vital signs frequently; monitor respiratory status closely; and evaluate apical, carotid and femoral pulses particularly in areas of circumferential burn injury to an extremity.
- Start cardiac monitoring if indicated (e.g. history of cardiac or respiratory problems and electrical injury).
- Check peripheral pulses on burned extremities hourly; use Doppler as needed.
- Monitor fluid intake (IV fluids) and output (urinary catheter) and measure hourly. Note amount of urine obtained when catheter is inserted (indicates preburn renal function and fluid status).
- Assess body temperature, body weight, history of preburn weight, allergies, tetanus immunization, past medical surgical problems, current illnesses and use of medications.
- Arrange for patients with facial burns to be assessed for corneal injury.
- Continue to assess the extent of the burn; assess depth of wound and identify areas of full and partial thickness injury.
- Assess neurologic status, consciousness, psychological status, pain and anxiety levels, and behavior.
- Assess patient's and family's understanding of injury and treatment. Assess patient's support system and coping skills.

Nursing Diagnosis

- Ineffective airway clearance/impaired gaseous exchange related to burn injury.
- Deficient fluid volume related to fluid loss, electrolyte imbalances and fluid shifts.
- Pain and anxiety related to exposed nerves, wound healing and treatments.
- Risk of complications related to emergent phase of burn.

Nursing Interventions

Promoting gas exchange and airway clearance

- Provide humidified oxygen, and monitor arterial blood gases (ABGs), pulse oximetry and carboxyhemoglobin levels.
- Assess breath sounds and respiratory rate, rhythm, depth and symmetry; monitor for hypoxia.
- Observe for signs of inhalation injury, e.g. blistering of lips or buccal mucosa; singed nostrils; burns of face, neck, or chest; increasing hoarseness; or soot in sputum or respiratory secretions.
- Report labored respirations, decreased depth of respirations, or signs of hypoxia to physician immediately; prepare to assist with intubation and escharotomies.
- Monitor mechanically ventilated patient closely.
- Institute aggressive pulmonary care measures: turning, coughing, deep breathing, periodic forceful inspiration using spirometry and tracheal suctioning.
- Maintain proper positioning to promote removal of secretions and patent airway and to promote optimal chest expansion; use artificial airway as needed.

Restoring fluid and electrolyte balance

- Monitor vital signs and urinary output (hourly), central venous pressure (CVP), pulmonary artery pressure and cardiac output.
- Note and report signs of hypovolemia or fluid overload.

- Maintain IV lines and regular fluids at appropriate rates, as prescribed. Document intake, output and daily weight.
- Elevate the head of bed and burned extremities.
- Monitor serum electrolyte levels (e.g. sodium, potassium, calcium, phosphorus, bicarbonate); recognize developing electrolyte imbalances.
- Notify physician immediately of decreased urine output; blood pressure; central venous pressure, pulmonary artery pressure, or pulmonary artery wedge pressures; or increased pulse rate.

Maintaining normal body temperature

- Provide warm environment: use heat shield, heat lights, or blankets.
- Assess core body temperature frequently.
- Work quickly when wounds must be exposed to minimize heat loss from the wound.

Minimizing pain and anxiety

- Use a pain scale to assess pain level (i.e. 1–10); differentiate between restlessness due to pain and restlessness due to hypoxia.
- Administer IV opioid analgesics as prescribed and assess response to medication; observe for respiratory depression in patient who is not mechanically ventilated.
- Provide emotional support, reassurance and simple explanations about procedures.
- Assess patient and family understanding of burn injury, coping strategies, family dynamics and anxiety levels. Provide individualized responses to support patient and family coping; explain all procedures in clear, simple terms.
- Provide pain relief, and give antianxiety medications if patient remains highly anxious and agitated after psychological interventions.

Monitoring and managing potential complications

- **Acute respiratory failure**: Assess for increasing dyspnea, stridor and changes in respiratory patterns; monitor pulse oximetry and ABG values to detect problematic oxygen saturation and increasing CO_2; monitor chest x-rays; assess for cerebral hypoxia (e.g. restlessness and confusion); report deteriorating respiratory status, immediately to physician; and assist as needed with intubation or escharotomy.
- **Distributive shock**: Monitor for early signs of shock (decreased urine output, cardiac output, pulmonary artery pressure, pulmonary capillary wedge pressure, blood pressure, or increasing pulse) or progressive edema. Administer fluid resuscitation as ordered in response to physical findings; continue monitoring fluid status.
- **Acute renal failure**: Monitor and report abnormal urine output and quality, blood urea nitrogen (BUN) and creatinine levels; assess for urine hemoglobin or myoglobin; administer increased fluids as prescribed.
- **Compartment syndrome**: Assess peripheral pulses hourly with Doppler; assess neurovascular status of extremities hourly (warmth, capillary refill, sensation and movement); remove blood pressure cuff after each reading; elevate burned extremities; report any extremity pain, loss of peripheral pulses or sensation; prepare to assist with escharotomies.
- **Paralytic ileus**: Maintain nasogastric tube on low intermittent suction until

bowel sounds resume; auscultate abdomen regularly for distention and bowel sounds.

- **Curling's ulcer**: Assess gastric aspirate for blood and pH; assess stools for occult blood; administer antacids and histamine blockers (e.g. ranitidine [zantac]) as prescribed.

ACUTE/INTERMEDIATE PHASE

The acute or intermediate phase begins 48–72 hours after the burn injury. Burn wound care and pain control are priorities at this stage.

Nursing Assessment

- Focus on hemodynamic alterations, wound healing, pain and psychosocial responses and early detection of complications.
- Measure vital signs frequently; respiratory and fluid status remains highest priority.
- Assess peripheral pulses frequently for first few days after the burn for restricted blood flow.
- Closely observe hourly fluid intake and urinary output, as well as blood pressure and cardiac rhythm; changes should be reported to the burn surgeon promptly.
- For patient with inhalation injury, regularly monitor level of consciousness, pulmonary function and ability to ventilate; if patient is intubated and placed on a ventilator, frequent suctioning and assessment of the airway are priorities.

Nursing Diagnosis

- Impaired skin integrity related to open burn wounds.
- Alteration in comfort related to burn injury and treatment
- Impaired physical mobility related to burn wound edema, pain and joint contractures.
- Risk for infection related to loss of skin barrier and impaired immune response.
- Imbalanced nutrition less than body requirements due to increased metabolic needs following burn injury and wound healing.
- Ineffective individual coping related to fear and anxiety, grieving and forced dependence on health care providers.
- Altered family process related to burn injury.
- Body image disturbance and role strain related to burn injury and appearance.

Nursing Interventions

Promoting skin integrity

- Assess wound status.
- Support patient during distressing and painful wound care.
- Coordinate complex aspects of wound care and dressing changes.
- Assess burn for size, color, odor, eschar, exudate, epithelial buds (small pearl-like clusters of cells on the wound surface), bleeding, granulation tissue, the status of graft take, healing of the donor site and the condition of the surrounding skin; report any significant changes to the physician.
- Inform all members of the health care team of latest wound care procedures in use for the patient.
- Assist, instruct, support and encourage patient and family to take part in dressing changes and wound care.

Relieving pain and discomfort

- Frequently assess pain and discomfort; administer analgesic agents and anxiolytic medications, as prescribed, before the pain becomes severe. Assess and document the patient's response to medication and any other interventions.

- Teach patient relaxation techniques. Provide frequent reassurance.
- Use guided imagery and distraction to alter patient's perceptions and responses to pain; hypnosis, music therapy and virtual reality are also useful.
- Assess the patient's sleep patterns daily; administer sedatives, if prescribed.
- Work quickly to complete treatments and dressing changes.
- Encourage patient to use analgesic medications before painful procedures.
- Promote comfort during healing phase with oral antipruritic agents, a cool environment, frequent lubrication of the skin with water or a silica-based lotion, exercise and splinting to prevent skin contracture and diversional activities.

Promoting physical mobility

- Prevent complications of immobility (atelectasis, pneumonia, edema, pressure ulcers and contractures) by deep breathing, turning and proper repositioning.
- Modify interventions to meet patient's needs. Encourage early sitting and ambulation. When legs are involved, apply elastic pressure bandages before assisting patient to upright position.
- Make aggressive efforts to prevent contractures and hypertrophic scarring of the wound area after wound closure for a year or more.
- Initiate passive and active range-of-motion exercises from admission until after grafting, within prescribed limitations.
- Apply splints or functional devices to extremities for contracture control; monitor for signs of vascular insufficiency, nerve compression and skin breakdown

Preventing infection

- Provide a clean and safe environment; protect patient from sources of cross contamination (e.g. visitors, other patients, staff and equipment).
- Closely scrutinize wound to detect early signs of infection.
- Monitor culture results and white blood cell counts.
- Practice clean technique for wound care procedures and aseptic technique for any invasive procedures. Use meticulous hand hygiene before and after contact with patient.
- Caution patient to avoid touching wounds or dressings; wash unburned areas and change linens regularly.

Maintaining adequate nutrition

- Initiate oral fluids slowly when bowel sounds resume; record tolerance. If vomiting and distention do not occur, fluids may be increased gradually and the patient may be advanced to a normal diet or to tube feedings.
- Collaborate with dietitian to plan a protein and calorie-rich diet acceptable to patient. Encourage family to bring nutritious and patient's favorite foods. Provide nutritional and vitamin and mineral supplements if prescribed.
- Document caloric intake. Insert feeding tube if caloric goals cannot be met by oral feeding (for continuous or bolus feedings); note residual volumes.
- Weigh patient daily and graph weights.

Restoring normal fluid balance

- Monitor IV and oral fluid intake; use IV infusion pumps.

- Measure intake and output and daily weight.
- Report changes (e.g. Blood pressure and pulse rate) to physician.

Strengthening coping strategies

- Assist patient to develop effective coping strategies. Set specific expectations for behavior, promote truthful communication to build trust, help patient practice coping strategies and give positive reinforcement when appropriate.
- Demonstrate acceptance of patient. Enlist a noninvolved person for patient to vent feelings without fear of retaliation.
- Include patient in decisions regarding care. Encourage patient to assert individuality and preferences. Set realistic expectations for selfcare.

Supporting patient and family processes

- Support and address the verbal and nonverbal concerns of the patient and family.
- Instruct family in ways to support patient.
- Make psychological or social work referrals as needed.
- Provide information about burn care and expected course of treatment.
- Initiate patient and family education during burn management. Assess and consider preferred learning styles; assess ability to grasp and cope with the information; determine barriers to learning when planning and executing teaching.
- Remain sensitive to the possibility of changing family dynamics.

Monitoring and managing potential complications

- Heart failure: Assess for fluid overload, decreased cardiac output, oliguria, jugular vein distention, edema, or onset of S_3 or S_4 heart sounds.
- Pulmonary edema: Assess for increasing CVP, pulmonary artery and wedge pressures and crackles; report promptly. Position comfortably with head elevated unless contraindicated. Administer medications and oxygen as prescribed and assess response.
- **Sepsis**: Assess for increased temperature, increased pulse, widened pulse pressure and flushed, dry skin in unburned areas (early signs), and note trends in the data. Perform wound and blood cultures as prescribed. Give scheduled antibiotics on time.
- **Acute respiratory failure and acute respiratory distress syndrome (ARDS)**: Monitor respiratory status for dyspnea, change in respiratory pattern and onset of adventitious sounds. Assess for decrease in tidal volume and lung compliance in patients on mechanical ventilation. The hallmark of onset of ARDS is hypoxemia on 100% oxygen, decreased lung compliance and significant shunting; notify physician of deteriorating respiratory status.
- **Visceral damage (from electrical burns)**: Monitor electrocardiogram (ECG) and report dysrhythmias; pay attention to pain related to deep muscle ischemia and report. Early detection may minimize severity of this complication. Fasciotomies may be necessary to relieve swelling and ischemia in the muscles and fascia; monitor patient for excessive blood loss and hypovolemia after fasciotomy.

REHABILITATION PHASE

- Rehabilitation should begin immediately after the burn has occurred. Wound healing, psychosocial support, and restoring maximum functional activity remain priorities. Maintaining fluid and electrolyte balance and improving nutrition status continue to be important.

Nursing Assessment

- In early assessment, obtain information about patient's educational level, occupation, leisure activities, cultural background, religion and family interactions.
- Assess self concept, mental status, emotional response to the injury and hospitalization, level of intellectual functioning, previous hospitalizations, response to pain and pain relief measures and sleep pattern.
- Perform ongoing assessments relative to rehabilitation goals, including range of motion of affected joints, functional abilities in ADLs, early signs of skin breakdown from splints or positioning devices, evidence of neuropathies (neurologic damage), activity tolerance and quality or condition of healing skin.
- Document participation and selfcare abilities in ambulation, eating, wound cleaning and applying pressure wraps.
- Maintain comprehensive and continuous assessment for early detection of complications, with specific assessments as needed for specific treatments, such as postoperative assessment of patient undergoing primary excision.

Nursing Diagnosis

- Activity intolerance related to pain on exercise, limited joint mobility, muscle wasting and limited endurance.
- Disturbed body image related to altered appearance and self-concept.
- Deficient knowledge of postdischarge home care and recovery needs.

Collaborative Problems/Potential Complications

- Contractures.
- Inadequate psychological adaptation to burn injury.

Planning and Goals

- Goals include increased participation in ADLs; increased understanding of the injury, treatment and planned follow-up care; adaptation and adjustment to alterations in body image, self-concept, and lifestyle; and absence of complications.

Nursing Interventions

Promoting activity tolerance

- Schedule care to allow periods of uninterrupted sleep. Administer hypnotic agents, as prescribed, to promote sleep.
- Communicate plan of care to family and other caregivers.
- Reduce metabolic stress by relieving pain, preventing chilling or fever and promoting integrity of all body systems to help conserve energy. Monitor fatigue, pain and fever to determine amount of activity to be encouraged daily.
- Incorporate physical therapy exercises to prevent muscular atrophy and maintain mobility required for daily activities.
- Support positive outlook, and increase tolerance for activity by scheduling diversion activities in periods of increasing duration.

Improving body image and self-concept

- Take time to listen to patient's concerns and provide realistic support; refer patient to a support group to develop coping strategies to deal with losses.

- Assess patient's psychosocial reactions; provide support and develop a plan to help the patient handle feelings.
- Promote a healthy body image and self-concept by helping patient practice responses to people who stare or ask about the injury.
- Support patient through small gestures such as providing a birthday cake, combing patient's hair before visitors, and sharing information on cosmetic resources to enhance appearance.
- Teach patient ways to direct attention away from a disfigured body to the self within.
- Coordinate communications of consultants, such as psychologists, social workers, vocational counselors and teachers during rehabilitation.

Monitoring and managing potential complications

- **Contractures**: Provide early and aggressive physical and occupational therapy; support patient if surgery is needed to achieve full range of motion.
- **Impaired psychological adaptation to the burn injury**: Obtain psychological or psychiatric referral as soon as evidence of major coping problems appears.

Teaching self-care

- Throughout the phases of burn care, make efforts to prepare patient and family for the care they will perform at home. Instruct them about measures and procedures.
- Provide verbal and written instructions about wound care, prevention of complications, pain management and nutrition.
- Inform and review with patient specific exercises and use of elastic pressure garments and splints; provide written instructions.
- Teach patient and family to recognize abnormal signs and report them to the physician.
- Assist the patient and family in planning for the patient's continued care by identifying and acquiring supplies and equipment that are needed at home.
- Encourage and support follow-up wound care.
- Refer patient with inadequate support system to home care resources for assistance with wound care and exercises.
- Evaluate patient status periodically for modification of home care instructions and/or planning for reconstructive surgery.

Expected Patient Outcomes

- Demonstrates activity tolerance required for desired daily activities.
- Adapts to altered body image.
- Demonstrates knowledge of required selfcare and follow-up care.
- Exhibits no complications.

14

Nursing Management of Patients with Disorders of Musculoskeletal System

NURSING ASSESSMENT OF PATIENT WITH MUSCULOSKELETAL DISORDERS

Subjective Data

Symptoms of musculoskeletal impairment include pain, weakness, deformity, limitation of movement, stiffness, joint crepitation.

- **Past health history**: Collect history regarding occurrence of tuberculosis, poliomyelitis, diabetes mellitus, parathyroid problems, hemophilia, rickets, scurvy, soft tissue, infection, neuromuscular disabilities.Any history of trauma, gout, arthritis, SLE, osteomalacia, osteomyelitis, and fungal infection of the bones, or joints. Any secondary bacterial infection such as the ears, tonsils, teeth, sinuses, lungs or genitourinary.
- **Medications**: Patients should be asked in details about the use of certain drugs such as skeletal muscle relaxants, opioids, NSAID's systemic and topical corticosteroids.
- **Surgery**: Detailsofemergencytreatment any surgical procedure, postoperative course and complications.
- **Nutrition**: Collect history regarding dietary habits. Adequate amounts of vitamins C and D, calcium and protein are essential for healthy, intact musculoskeletal system. Abnormal nutritional patterns can predispose individuals to problems such as osteomalacia and osteoporosis. Obesity places extrastress on weight bearing joints such as the knees, hips and spine.
- **Activity-exercise patterns**: Obtain history type, duration and frequency of exercise and recreational activities. Ask patient about limitations in movement, pain, weakness, clumsiness, crepitus or any change in the bones or joints that interferes with daily activities.
- **Elimination**: Use of any assistive devices such as elevated toilet seat, or a grab bar for accomplishing toileting.

Objective Data

Physical examination involves observation, palpation, motion and muscular assessment.

Inspection

1. Inspect head, neck, upper extremities and trunk.
2. Inspect the skin for color, scar and signs of previous injury or surgery.

3. General body build, muscle configuration, and symmetry of joints are noted.
4. Observe for any swelling, deformity, nodules or masses, and discrepancies in limb length or muscle size.
   - **Palpation of muscles and joints**—Evaluation of skin temperature, local tenderness, swelling and crepitation.
   - **Motion**—Evaluate both passive and active range of motion, common movements that occur at the synovial joints, including abduction, adduction, flexion and extension.
   - **Muscle strength testing**—Assess the strength of individual muscles or groups of muscles during contraction. Normal muscle strength should be 5 bilaterally, with full resistance to the force exerted.
   - **Measurement**—Obtain limb length and circumferential muscle mass measurements when length discrepancies or subjective problems are noted.
   - **Others**—Note any assistive devices used by the patient such as walker or cane. Observe the posture and gait of the individual by watching the patient walk, stand, and sit. Musculoskeletal and neurologic problems can result in abnormal gait patterns.

Diagnostic Studies

- **X-ray**—It is used to assess musculoskeletal problems and to monitor the effectiveness of treatment. It provides information about bone deformity, joint congruity, bone density and calcification in soft tissue.
- **CT scan or MRI**—It is used to identify soft tissue abnormalities, bony abnormalities and various musculoskeletal trauma. Useful in diagnosing of avascular necrosis, disk disease, tumors, osteomyelitis, ligament tears, etc.
- **Bone scan**—It involves injection of radioisotope that is taken up by bone, a uniform uptake of the isotope is normal. Increase uptake is seen in osteomyelitis, osteoporosis, primary metastatic malignant lesions of bone and certain fractures.
- **Arthroscopy**—It is used directly to examine the interior of a joint cavity and a biopsy of the synovium or cartilage can be obtained.
- **Arthrocentesis or joint aspiration**—It is usually performed for a synovial fluid analysis.
- **Bone mineral density (BMD)**—Measurements use to diagnose metabolic bone disease and to monitor changes in bone density with treatment.
- **Electromyogram**—It evaluates electrical potential associated with skeletal muscle contraction related to lower motor neuron dysfunction and primary muscle disease.
- **Laboratory tests**—
  - Blood tests for alkaline phosphatase, calcium, phosphorous. Elevated levels of alkaline phosphatase are found in healing fractures, bone cancers, osteoporosis, etc.
  - Blood for serologic studies such as rheumatoid factor, erythrocyte sedimentation rate (ESR), antinuclear antibody, uric acid, C- reactive protein.
  - Blood for markers of muscle injury such as creatinine kinase, potassium and aldolase.

FRACTURES

Musculoskeletal trauma can result in fractures, joint dislocations, soft tissue edema, hemorrhage into muscle and joints, nerve tendon and vascular damage and injuries to body organs.

Definition

A fracture is any disruption, complete or incomplete in the continuity of a bone.

Incidence

- Fractures constitute a high proportion of musculoskeletal injuries.
- Fractures occur in all age groups, at any point of the skeletal system, and they may result in a significant change in an individual's quality of life.
- They can cause activity restriction, disability, impairment, handicap and economic loss.

Pathophysiology

Predisposing factors

- Stress is the amount of force (load) applied to a bone.
- Strain is the reaction within the bone to the stress. The amount and frequency of stress applied and the no. of repetitions play on determining when a fracture will occur. The amount of force required a bone varies with the biologic, extrinsic and intrinsic factors present.
- Biologic factors are conditions that alter the composition and strength of the bone.
- Age affecting the amount of force required to produce a fracture. As age increases the bone becomes more brittle, the amount of force required to produce a fracture decreases. The amount of force required also varies with the size of the bone involved.
- Extrinsic factors include the magnitude, duration and direction of the force as well as the rate of loading.
- Intrinsic factors are properties of bone, such as its size, energy, absorbing capacity, elasticity, fatigue, strength, size and density.
- Behavioral factors that may predispose the individual to fracture include a high-risk activities (e.g. parachuting, skateboarding) in which the individual engages for either recreation or employment.

Mechanism of injury

A fracture occurs when bone is subjected to more stress than it can absorb.

- It is caused by direct or indirect force or by stress or fatigue of the bone.
- Pathologic in origin.

Direct force: Causing tapping, crush or penetrating fractures.

- A tapping fracture is caused by a small force applied to a small area, such as kick or blow with a blunt instrument.
- Crush fractures are caused by a large amount of force being applied to a small area and are generally accompanying by extensive soft tissue damage.
- Penetrating fractures are caused by a large amount of force acting on a small area, as in projectile injuries, e.g. gun shot wound.

Indirect trauma: It is a force applied distant from the fracture site.

- Causes include traction or tension forces, angulation forces, rotational forces, vertical compression forces or any combination of these.
- Traction or tension fracture (e.g. ankle sprain with avulsed fragment) result when a muscle contracts and force is exerted simultaneously tissues loss.
- Closed fractures are those in which there is loss of bone continuity internally but no break in the skin.

Classification of Fractures

Fractures are classified as the following:

- Open or closed.
- By the type of fracture line.
- By the anatomical location of the fracture bone.

- By the appearance.
- Position.
- Alignment of the feature fragments and by classic name (Colles' fracture).
  a. An open fracture is one in which there is loss of continuity of the bone is internally and external wound communicating directly to the fracture site, that is a fragment protruding through the skin. Referred to as compound or complex fracture and can be further subdivided by the degree or severity of soft tissue injury. These fractures are commonly associated with severe soft tissue damage.
  b. Impacted fracture occurs when a direct force causes a fracture and telescopes the fragment with the smaller diameter. Fragments of the fracture move in unison and rapid union occurs.
  c. Avulsed fractures are those which bone fragments and tissues are pulled away from bone at the insertion site.
  d. A transverse fracture line crosses the shaft of the bone involved at a 90° angle and is usually caused by angulation force. Transverse are generally stable after reduction.
  e. Oblique fractures lines occur diagonally across the bone and are usually produced by a twisting force. Oblique fracture may slip following reduction unless traction is maintained or the fracture surfaces allow the fragments to interlock.
  f. Spiral fracture lines are caused by a twisting force with an upward thrust and are continuation of an oblique fractures line coiling around the bone.
  g. Green stick fractures are incomplete fractures that occur when the cortex of the bone bends one side and buckles on the other. Green stick fracture may be caused by a compression force on the long axis of the bone or angulated force.
  h. Compressions fractures are produced by a force applied parallel to the long axis of cancellous bone and usually result in a tubular bone changing rapidly in size and shape.
  i. Communited fractures are produced by high energy forces, such as crush or penetrating injuries, producing more in the opposite direction.
     - Angulation fractures: When the lever (bone) is forced into angulation, e.g. night stick fractures.
     - Rotational fractures produce spiral fracture line either with or without splintering and commonly occurs in the distal third of the tibia.
     - Compression fractures of long bones produce T-or Y-shaped fractures and occasionally may cause a longitudinal displaced fracture.
     - Stress fractures occur after normal everyday activities when there is no evidence of trauma to explain occurrence of the fracture.
     - Pathologic fractures: occur when a bone weakened by preexisting fractures in response to an amount of stress that would leave a normal bone intact.

Diagnostic evaluation: It is based on client's symptoms, history of trauma, physical examination and radiologic findings.

Physical examination reveal deformity, mobility of bone fragments, crepitus, muscle spasm, edema or eccymosis.

Management

Assessment of fractures

- The mechanism of injury and accident history assist in determining the nature and extent of known injuries and may help in the identification of injuries that might otherwise be overlooked.

- Individuals at the accident scene, assess level of consciousness, response to stimuli, orientation, position of the body, and head and movement of the limbs.
- Previous illness or injuries, allergies, the last date of tetanus inoculation and current medication should be determined and recorded.
- The physical examination is the most important aspect of assessing the trauma client.

  Include the presence of deformity, shortening of a limb and discoloration and soft tissue damage. Clinical findings include pain, loss of function, and degree of deformity, restriction of posture and movement, abnormal mobility, crepitus and neurovascular change.
- Radiologic examination of a suspected limb fracture includes the joint above and the joint below the suspected fracture site.
- Neurologic examination of the trauma client is related to the type of injury known or suspected. Multiple trauma clients should always have X-ray films or CT scan taken of the chest and pelvis. A femoral fracture may cause or loss of 1 to 2.5 L of blood volume, and a tibial fracture result in a loss of 0.5 to 1.5 L of blood.
- Soft tissue damage and associated open fracture wounds is covered with a sterile normal saline dressing. Irrigation of open wounds is performed in OT to avoid contamination of the wound.
- All open wound tissue should be sent for culture and sensitivity tests. Injection tetanus toxoid is administered if needed.
- Neurovascular assessment of the involved extremities should be performed and documented at frequent intervals. A comprehensive assessment includes the peripheral pulses, color, temperature, capillary refill and edema. Peripheral neurologic assessment includes sensation and motor function. Peripheral tissue perfusion is an integral component of nursing care.

Emergency management: It is governed by basic principles of trauma care.

Assessment and treatment are carried out simultaneously. Initial primary assessment includes:

- General condition of the client, including respiratory status.
- Bleeding or shock.
- Stabilization of any potential life-threatening injuries.
- Assessment of neurovascular status and followed by splinting.
- When a closed fracture is suspected, a splint should be applied, if possible, before the extremity or the client is moved.
- Splinting minimizes bleeding, swelling and pain and also helps prevent further damage to nerves, vessels, muscles and tendons.
- In addition, it is more difficult to transport the client and to perform X-ray, examination.
- Fractures sites are left unsplinted. Before splints are applied open fracture should be covered with sterile compression dressings to help control bleeding and to prevent further contamination.
- Methods available for controlling pelvic bleeding included pneumatic antishock, anterior external fixation, angiography with operative control of hemorrhage, retroperitoneal packing.

Management of Fracture

Method of treatment

- Require closed or open reduction, traction, splinting, casts, internal fixation, external fixation bracing, amputation, etc.

- The basis of the treatment of fractures is reduction and immobility.
- For bony union to occur, the fragments should be in approximation and alignment and must be held relatively immobile during the period of healing.

Objectives

Closed reduction includes reduction of the fracture and immobilization. It is the alignment of the fracture fragments through manual manipulation or traction.

Indications

- To ensure recover of limb function.
- To prevent or delay degenerative changes in joints.
- To reduce a fracture is to minimize the deforming effects of the injury.

Immobilization

Closed reduction of fracture is followed by immobilization.

Purposes

- Relieve pain.
- Prevent rotation.
- Shearing at the fracture site.
- Maintain the position of the fracture by preventing displacement or angulation until bony union occurs, permits active muscle contraction, and commonly allow free movement of uninvolved joints. It may be accomplished by application of casts, traction, splints, braces, or internal fixators.
- Casts may be of plaster of paris or fiber glass
- Traction types are skin, skeletal, plaster or combination of pin and plaster.

Open Treatment

Indicated in delayed union, multiple fracture, pathologic fracture and fracture in which closed treatment is known to be ineffective.

Internal fixation

- Open reduction of a fracture is usually followed by internal fixation to stabilize the fracture and allow fracture healing to occur.
- Wires and pins may be implanted to provide internal fixation either percutaneously or through open methods.
- One advantage of wires and pins is that they can be left protruding through the skin and may then be removed easily with local anesthesia. Examples (Figs 14.1A to C):
  - Bone screws
  - Cortical screws
  - Malleolar screws
  - Plates
  - Nail and sliding screw plate
  - Intramedullary nailing.

Open reduction and internal fixation (ORIF)

- Open reduction should be performed when closed methods have failed or would be ineffective, when articular surfaces are fractured and displaced, or when the fracture is secondary to tumor metastasis, and when there are associated arterial injuries or multiple injuries.

  Advantages—Early mobilization
—Restoration of the anatomic shape of the bone
—Decreased costs
—Shorter hospital stays.
- Open fractures present special problems in their care and treatment.
- They may occur as a result of the piercing of skin by a sharp bone fragment or through disruption of the tissue by the force that causes the fracture.

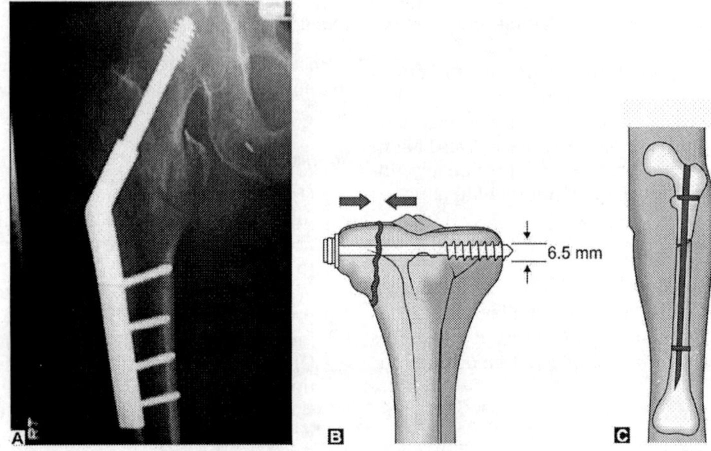

Figs 14.1A to C: (A) Sliding screw and plate; (B) Bone screw and (C) Intramedullary nailing

- Open fracture should be covered with sterile dressing in the emergency department following preliminary examination and should remain covered until the client is transferred to the OT.
- Antibiotic therapy should begin as soon as possible after the injury (2–3 days).

Fracture healing

Bone healing is a unique process in the human body. Healing occurs through regeneration of tissue rather than the scar tissue formation. (Table 14.1)

The most important factors in bone healing are:

- Adequate circulation and immobilization of the fracture site.
- Fracture in an infant may heal in as little as 4 to 6 weeks, whereas the same fracture in adolescents taken 6 to 10 weeks to heal.

Table 14.1: Stages of fracture healing

Stage	Description	Length
I	Hematoma formation—Fracture occurs and hematoma forms at site	1–3 days
II	Fibrocartilage formation—Granulation tissue invades the hematoma	3 days–2 weeks
III	Callus formation—Granulation tissue matures	2–6 weeks
IV	Ossification—Callus bridges the gap between fracture fragments; callus gradually replaced by bone	3–6 months
V	Consolidation and remodeling—Bone is reshaped to meet its mechanical requirements	6 weeks–1 year

Goal: To achieve union of the fracture fragments and to restore the normal anatomy and function of the bone.

Types of healing

Clinical healing: It refers to the point in the healing process when the fracture has achieved enough stability and strength to resume its function, the fracture site is free of pain and there is no gross movement across the site and X-ray films show bone crossing the fracture site.

Biologic healing: It is said to have occurred when the maximum strength of the bone is reached.

Complications

Immediate complications
- Shock
- Fat embolism
- Compartment syndrome
- DVT, pulmonary embolism
- Infection.

Delayed complications
- Joint stiffness.
- Posttraumatic arthritis.
- Dystrophy, complex regional pain syndrome (CRPS).
- Myositis ossificans.
- Malunion.
- Delayed union.
- Nonunion.
- Loss of reduction of fracture fragments.
- Refraction and osteomyelitis.
- **Gas gangrene** is a rare but extremely serious complication that may occur following open fracture. Gas gangrene can develop from the clostridium spore in 72 hours.
  - **Symptoms**: Severe pain, swelling at the fracture site, tachycardia, hypertension, fever, disorientation and agitation. Muscle necrosis and crepitus are usually present.

Treatment
- Hyperbaric oxygenation or immediate surgical exploration.
- Excision of all areas of necrosis.
- IV administration of penicillin.
- Limb salvage may be possible, but amputation is often required
- If salvage is chosen, debridement of the wound should be performed in the operating room under sterile conditions and the fracture should be stabilized
- Debridement of the wound includes detection and removal of all non-vital tissues and foreign material. This reduces bacteria contamination to create a wound capable of dealing with any residual bacterial contamination
- Debridement may be repeated in 24 to 72 hours.

NURSING MANAGEMENT

Nursing Assessment

Subjective data

- History of any traumatic injury, bone or systemic disease, prolonged immobility, use of corticosteroid, analgesics, surgery or first aid treatment of fracture, previous musculoskeletal surgeries. Loss of motion or weakness of affected areas, muscle spasm, sudden and severe pain in the affected area increases with activity, numbness, tingling and loss of sensation distal to injury.

Objective data

- On assessment patient is apprehensive, guarding the injured site. Skin laceration, pallor or cool skin, bluish and warm skin distal to injury, eccymosis, hematoma, edema at the

site of fracture. Reduced or absent pulse distal to injury, decrease skin temperature, delayed capillary refill. Parasthesias absent or decrease sensation, hypersensation, restricted or lost function of the affected part, local bony deformities, shortening, rotation, crepitation of the affected part.
- Localization and extent of fracture on X-ray, bone scans and CT scan or MRI.

Nursing Diagnosis

- Acute pain related to edema, movement of bone fragments, muscle spasm, as evidenced by pain description, guarding and crying.
- Impaired physical mobility related to pain, spasms or fear of movement, as evidenced by limited ROM, inability of move and inability to bear weight.
- Self-care deficit related to mobility impairment following hip fracture as evidenced by difficulty in bathing/ hygiene, dressing/grooming.
- Ineffective therapeutic regimen related to lack of knowledge regarding muscle atrophy, exercise program, care of plaster cast or external immobilizers as evidenced by questioning regarding long term use of cast, devices and prognosis of treatment.
- Risk of impaired skin integrity related to mobility limitations as evidenced by presence of skeletal traction, plaster casts.
- Risk for infection related to loss of primary defenses and malnutrition (if present).
- Risk for peripheral neurovascular dysfunction related to lower extremity edema or positioning.
- Risk of constipation related to impaired physical mobility and side effects of opioids analgesics.

PLANNING OUTCOMES/GOALS

- Demonstrate comfort after surgery.
- Demonstrate improved physical mobility.
- Resume preinjury level of independence in meeting self-care needs.
- Understands the disease process and participates in treatment and rehabilitation program.

Nursing Interventions

Demonstrate comfort after surgery

- Use of patient controlled analgesia (PCA), or epidural analgesia.
- Provide ice application over the dressed surgical wound.
- Administer analgesic (nonopioid, NSAIDS) for pain and also before physical therapy or activities such as transferring to the chair.
- Be aware of any weight bearing imitations ordered for the client before transfer.
- Pay careful attention to the operated extremity during transfer to ensure client is following weight bearing requirements.

Demonstrate improved physical mobility

- Assist the client during bathing and other hygienic needs.
- Ask the physiotherapist to help the client with ambulation and muscle strengthening exercise.
- Use a pressure ulcer risk assessment tool to determine risk level.
- Change the position of the client at least every 2 hours, the client can be turned to either side but is usually comfortable on the nonoperative side with a pillow to support the operative leg.
- Assess the skin over bony prominences such as the sacrum, coccyx, scapulae, elbows and heels.

- Place a pressure reducing mattress on the client's bed.

Resume preinjury level of independence in meeting self-care needs

- Assess the client and the wound for any local and systemic signs of infection.
- Provide high carbohydrate and high protein diet for adequate healing.
- Administer antibiotics before, during and after the surgical intervention.
- Use aseptic technique during dressing.
- Assess the neurovascular function of the operative extremity at least every 4 hours.
- Assessment includes the presence and quality of bilateral pedal pulse, skin color, and the temperature of the extremity, capillary refill in the toes, sensation and movement in the toes and the client's ability to perform dorsi-plantar flexion of the foot.
- Advise the client to report any pallor or coolness, numbness or tingling or inability to move the extremity.
- Regular assessment and implementation of proactive bowel program are important for minimizing client's concerns about bowel elimination.
- Encourage the client for plenty of fluids and fiber if not contraindicated.
- Administer laxative to stimulate the return to normal bowel elimination.
- Assist the client to transfer to a bedside commode or ambulate to the bathroom when ever possible.

OSTEOMYELITIS

Definition

Osteomyelitis is a severe infection of the bone, bone marrow and surrounding soft tissue.

Causes

- *Staphylococcus aureus*
- *Staphylococcus epidermidis.*
- *Staphylococcus viridans.*
- *Mycobacterium tuberculosis.*
- Pseudomonas.
- Salmonella.
- Fungi.

Pathophysiology

Route of entry indirect and direct

Indirect entry: (Hematogenous) of microorganism in osteomyelitis most frequently affects growing bone in boys less than 2 years and is associated with higher incidence of blunt trauma.

Site of trauma and infection

- Distal femur.
- Proximal tibia.
- Humerus.
- Radius.
- In case of adults with vascular insufficiency disorders (e.g. diabetes mellitus) and genitorinary and respiratory infections the chance is increase for primary infection to spread via the blood to the bone.
- The pelvis, tibia and vertebra, which are vascular rich sites of bone; are the most common sites of infection.

Direct entry

- It occurs at any age when there is open wound (e.g. penetrating wounds, fractures) and microorganism enters through that wound to the body.
- It also can occur in presence of a foreign body such as implant or an orthopedic prosthetic device (e.g. total joint prosthesis) (e.g. plate, total joint prosthesis).
  - Indirect or Direct Invasion (from blood to the bone).
  - Microorganism multiplies in the bone and there is decrease blood circulation.
  - Increase in presence because of non-expanding nature of most bone.

- Ischemia and vascular compromise of the periosteum.
- Infection passes through the bone cortex and marrow cavity ultimately resulting in cortical devascularization and necrosis and subsequently bone dies.
- Area of devitalized bone eventually separates from the surrounding living resulting in bone forming sequestra.
- Sequestra which is a part of the periosteum that continues to have blood supply forms a new bone called involucrum.
- Once formed, a sequestrum continues to be an infected island of bone surrounded by pus.
- Difficult for blood borne antibiotic or WBC to reach the sequestra.
- A sequestrum may enlarge and serve as a site for microorganism that spread to other sites including lungs and brain.
- Chronic osteomyelitis is either a continuous, persistent problem (a result of inadequate acute treatment) or a process of exacerbations and remmisions.

Clinical manifestations (Table 14.2)

Table 14.2: Clinical manifestations

Acute osteomyelitis	Chronic osteomyelitis
Initial infection Duration: Less than 1 month Systemic and local clinical manifestations Systemic manifestations: Fever, night sweats, chills, restlessness, nausea, malaise Local manifestations: Constant bone pain that is unrelieved by rest, worsens with activity swelling, tenderness and warmth at the infection site and restricted movement of the affected part. Later signs: Drainage from sinus tracts to the skin and or the fracture site	Bone infection persists for increase one month or an infection that has failed to respond the initial course of antibiotic therapy Systemic signs may be dimished with local signs of infection more common, including constant bone pain, swelling, tenderness and warmth at the infection site

Diagnostic Tests

- A bone or soft tissue biopsy to determine causative organism.
- Blood/wound culture and sensitivity to identify the causative organism.
- Blood routine examination: Increase WBC and increase ESR.
- X-ray: Radiologic signs of osteomyelitis usually do not appear until 10 day to weeks after the appearance of clinical features.
- Radionuclide bone scan: Positive in the area of infection.
- MRI or CT scan: It may be used to help identify the extent of the infection, including soft tissue involvement.

Management

Acute osteomyelitis medical management

- Vigorous and prolonged antibiotic therapy is the treatment of choice.
- Antibiotics used are: Penicillin, nafcillin, neomycin, vancomycin, cephalexin, cefazolin,gentamycin, tobramycin.
- If antibiotic therapy is delayed, surgical debridement and decompression is done.

- Home care: Central venous catheter is kept for 3 to 6 months and antibiotic therapy is continued for 4 to 6 weeks.

Chronic osteomyelitis

Oral therapy with a fluoroquinolone (Ciprofloxacin) for 6 to 8 weeks is given instead of IV antibiotics.

Surgical Management

- Removal of the poorly vascularized tissue and dead bone and the extended use of antibiotics.
- Antibiotics impregnated polymethacrylate bead chains are also implanted to fight against infection.
- After debridement of the devitalized and infected tissue, the wound is closed and a suction irrigation system is inserted.
- Intermittent or constant irrigation of the affected bone with antibiotics is required.
- Protection of the limb or surgical part with casts or braces is frequently done.

Wound VAC/negative pressure wound therapy (NPWT)

Used in cases of acute or chronic traumatic wounds, surgical wounds that have contaminated, pressure ulcers and chronic ulcers.

- It is type of therapy use over the site of infection to draw the wound together.
- It uses suction to remove the drainage and speed wound healing.
- The wound is cleaned and special dressings consisting of sponges packed with tubing are placed into the wound to absorb drainage.
- Tubing from the wound is then attached to a pump which creates negative pressure in the wound bed.

Hyperbaric oxygen therapy

- It the delivery of oxygen at an increased atmospheric pressures.
- It is given systematically with the patient placed in an enclosed chamber where 100% oxygen is administered at 1.5 to 3 times the normal atmospheric pressures.
- An alternative approach is to topically administer hyperbaric oxygen by creating a chamber around the injured limb.
- The topical treatments can last 20 minutes twice a day or 4 to 6 hours daily.
- Hyperbaric oxygen accelerates granulation tissue formation and wound healing.

Complications

- Septicemia
- Septic arthritis
- Pathologic fracture
- Amyloidosis.

NURSING MANAGEMENT

Nursing Assessment

Objective data

General: Restlessness, high spiking temperature, night sweats.

Integumentary: Diaphoresis, erythema, warmth and edema at infected bone.

Musculoskeletal: Restricted movement, wound drainage and spontaneous fracture.

Nursing Diagnosis

- Acute pain related to inflammatory process, secondary to infection as evidenced by guarding, moaning, crying, restlessness.
- Ineffective therapeutic regimen management related to knowledge re-

garding long-term management of osteomyelitis.
- Impaired physical mobility related to pain, immobilization devices, or unwillingness to change positions, and ambulate with assistive devices.

PLANNING OUTCOMES/GOAL

- Have satisfactory pain and fever control.
- Not experience any complication associated with osteomyelitis and cooperate with the treatment plan.

Nursing Interventions

Have satisfactory pain, and fever control

- Do a comprehensive pain assessment including location, characteristics, onset, duration, frequency, quality, intensity or severity of pain and precipitating factors of pain.
- Administer analgesic to relieve pain.
- Teach nonpharmacologic techniques (e.g. relaxation, guided imagery, distraction)
- Immobilize or support affected body part.
- Position the client in proper body alignment.
- Elevate affected body part to reduce swelling and provide comfort.

Not experience any complication associated with osteomyelitis and cooperate with the treatment plan

- Demonstrate skills (e.g. wound care, aseptic technique, antibiotic administration)
- Instruct patient to perform activities one step at a time.
- Assist patient to stand and ambulate specified distance.
- Apply or provide assistive devices, e.g. cane, walker, wheel chair for ambulation.

OSTEOMALACIA

- Osteomalacia is a rare condition of adult bone associated with vitamin D deficiency, resulting in decalcification and softening of bone.
- This disease is the same as rickets in children except that the epiphyseal growth plates are closed in the adult.
- Vitamin D, with its complex actions and method of synthesis, is required for the absorption of calcium from the intestine.
- Insufficient vitamin D intake can interfere with the normal mineralization of bone, causing failure or insufficient calcification of bone, which results in bone softening.

Causes

- Lack of exposure to UV rays (needed for vitamin D synthesis).
- GI malabsorption
- Extensive burns
- Chronic diarrhea
- Pregnancy
- Kidney disease
- Drugs – Phenytoin (dilantin).

Clinical Manifestations

- Localized pain.
- Difficulty rising from a chair and walking.

Others

- Low back and bone pain
- Progressive muscular weakness specially in the pelvic girdle, weight loss, and progressive deformities of the spine (kyphosis) or extremities.
- Fracture is very common. Mineralization may take 2 to 3 months.

Diagnostic Tests

- Serum calcium and phosphorous level to increase.

- Serum 25 hydroxy vitamin D.
- Increase alkaline phosphatase.
- Radiologic (X-ray)findings.
- Demonstrate the effects of generalized bone mineralization especially loss of calcium in the bone of the pelvis and the presence of associated bone deformity.
- Losser's transformation zones (ribbons of decalcification) in bone found on X-ray are diagnosis of osteomalacia.

Management

- Correction of vitamin D deficiency.
- Administer vitamin D3(cholecalciferol) and vitamin D2 (ergocalciferol).
- Calcium salts or phophorous supplments may be given.
- Diet: Eggs, low fat milk, fish, vegetable
- Weight bearing exercise.

Nursing Interventions

- Focus on careful positioning, ambulation, and prescribed exercises.
- Monitor pain scale.
- Give vitamin D supplementation as per order.
- Give analgesics as per doctor order.
- Include the patient and his family in all phases of care.
- Check the patient's skin daily for redness, warmth, and new painsites.
- Monitor the patient's pain level, and assess her response to analgesic's.
- Explain all treatments, tests, and procedure to the patient.
- To teach clients and her family clearly understand the prescribed drug regimen.
- To provide emotional support clients and her family.

NURSING MANAGEMENT OF PATIENT WITH AMPUTATION

Definition

Amputation is the removal of a body extremity by trauma, prolonged constriction, or surgery.

- As a surgical measure, it is used to control pain or a disease process in the affected limb, such as malignancy or gangrene.
- It is carried out on individuals as a preventive surgery for such problems. A special case is that of congenital amputation, a congenital disorder, where fetal limbs have been cut off by constrictive bands.
- A transplant or a prosthesis are the only options for recovering the loss.

Types

Leg amputations

- Amputation of digits.
- Partial foot amputation.
- Ankle disarticulation.
- Below-knee amputation, abbreviated as BKA.
- Knee disarticulation.
- Above-knee amputation (Fig. 14.2).
- Van-ness rotation/rotationplasty (foot being turned around and reattached to allow the ankle joint to be used as a knee).
- Hip disarticulation.
- Hemipelvectomy/hindquarter amputation.

Arm amputations

- Amputation of digits.
- Metacarpal amputation.
- Wrist disarticulation.
- Forearm amputation (transradial).

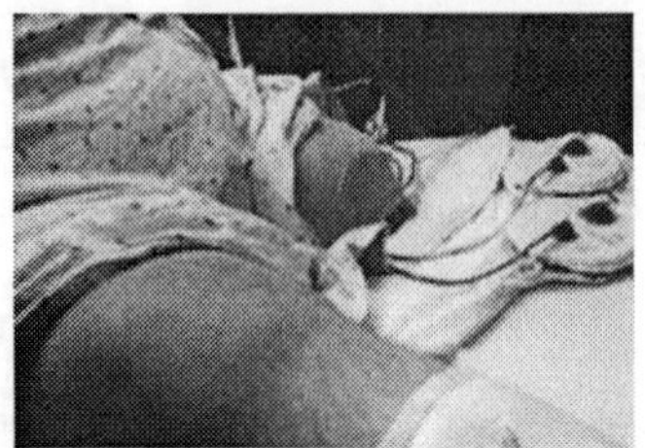

Fig. 14.2: Transfemoral amputation due to liposarcoma

- Elbow disarticulation.
- Above-elbow amputation (transhumeral).
- Shoulder disarticulation and forequarter amputation.
- Krukenberg procedure.

Other amputations

- Face
  - Amputation of the ears.
  - Amputation of the nose (rhinotomy).
  - Amputation of the tongue (glossectomy).
  - Amputation of the eyes (blinding).
- Breasts
  - Amputation of the breasts (mastectomy).
  - Genitals amputation.
  - Amputation of the scrotum.
  - Amputation of the testicles (castration).
  - Amputation of the penis (penectomy).
  - Amputation of the foreskin (circumcision).

Causes

Circulatory disorders

- Diabetic foot infection or gangrene (the most frequent reason for infection-related amputations).
- Sepsis with peripheral necrosis.

Neoplasm

- Cancerous bone or soft tissue tumors (e.g. osteosarcoma, osteochondroma, fibrosarcoma, epithelioid sarcoma, Ewing's sarcoma, synovial sarcoma, sacrococcygeal teratoma, liposarcoma).
- Melanoma.

Trauma

- Severe limb injuries in which the limb cannot be saved or efforts to save the limb fail.
- Traumatic amputation (an unexpected amputation that occurs at the scene of an accident, where the limb is partially or entirely severed as a direct result of the accident, for example a finger that is severed from the blade of a table saw).
- Amputation in utero (amniotic band).

Deformities

- Deformities of digits and/or limbs, e.g. proximal femoral focal deficiency.
- Extra digits and/or limbs, e.g. polydactyly.

Infection

- Bone infection (osteomyelitis).
- Diabetes.
- Frostbite.

Surgical Amputation

Method

- The first step is ligating the supplying artery and vein, to prevent hemorrhage (bleeding).
- The muscles are transected, and finally the bone is sawed through with an oscillating saw.
- Sharp and rough edges of the bone(s) are filed down, skin and muscle flaps are then transposed over the stump,

occasionally with the insertion of elements to attach a prosthesis.

Traumatic Amputation

It is the partial or total avulsion of a part of a body during a serious accident, like traffic, labor, or combat.

Traumatic amputation of a human limb, either partial or total, creates the immediate danger of death from blood loss.

Causes

Traumatic amputation is rare in humans (1 per 20, 804 population per year). Loss of limb usually happens immediately during the accident, but sometimes a few days later after medical complications.

- Amputations in traffic accidents (cars, motorcycles, bicycles, trains, etc.).
- Amputations in labor accidents (equipments, instruments, cylinders, chain saws, press machines, meat machines, wood machines, etc.).
- Amputations in agricultural accidents, with machines and power equipments.
- Amputations from electric shock hazard.
- Amputations from guns, weapons, and explosives, dynamite, bombs, fireworks, terrorism attacks, etc.
- Amputations from violent rupture of ship rope or industry wire rope.
- Amputations from ring traction (ring amputation, de-gloving injuries).

Treatment

A traumatic amputation can be taken care with these choices, depending from patient's trauma and clinical situation:

- 1st choice: Surgical amputation-break-prosthesis.
- 2nd choice: Surgical amputation—Transplantation of other tissue - Plastic reconstruction.
- 3rd choice: Replantation-Reconnection - Revascularization of amputated limb, by Microscope (after year 1969).
- 4th choice: Transplantation of cadaveric hand (after year 2000).

NURSING MANAGEMENT

Nursing Assessment

Subjective data

Health problems (such as dehydration, anemia, heart failure, chronic respiratory problems, diabetes mellitus) need to be identified and treated so that the patient is in the best possible condition to withstand the trauma of surgery.

Objective data

- Evaluate the extremity's neurovascular and functional status through history and physical assessment.
- If the patient has experienced a traumatic amputation, assess the residual limb's condition and function.
- Assess the unaffected extremity's circulatory status and function.
- If infection or gangrene develops, the patient may have associated enlarged lymph nodes, fever, and purulent drainage.
- A culture is taken to determine the appropriate antibiotic therapy.
- Assess the patient's psychological status.
- Need to determine emotional reaction to amputation and resulting disability to plan his care effectively.

Nursing Diagnosis

- Impaired physical mobility related to loss of a limb (particularly a lower extremity); pain/discomfort; perceptual impairment (altered sense of balance)

as evidenced by Reluctance to attempt movement, impaired co-ordination; decreased muscle strength, control, and mass.
- Risk for Infection related to inadequate primary defenses (broken skin, traumatized tissue) invasive procedures; environmental exposure chronic disease, altered nutritional status.
- Risk for ineffective peripheral tissue perfusion, related to reduced arterial/ venous blood flow; tissue edema, hematoma formation hypovolemia.
- Self-esteem, situational low related to loss of body part/change in functional abilities as evidenced by anticipated changes in lifestyle; fear of rejection/ reaction by others, negative feelings about body, focus on past strength, function or appearance, feelings of helplessness, powerlessness.

PLANNING OUTCOMES/GOALS

- Verbalize understanding of individual situation, treatment regimen and safety measures.
- Maintain position of function as evidenced by absence of contractures.
- Demonstrate techniques/behaviors that enable resumption of activities.
- Achieve timely wound healing, be free of purulent drainage or erythema and be afebrile.
- Maintain adequate tissue perfusion as evidenced by palpable peripheral pulses, warm/dry skin and timely wound healing.
- Begin to show adaptation and verbalize acceptance of self in situation (amputee). Recognize and incorporate changes into self-concept in accurate manner without negating self-esteem.
- Develop realistic plans for adapting to new role/role modifications.

Nursing Interventions

Demonstrate techniques/behaviors that enable resumption of activities

- Provide stump care on a routine basis, e.g. inspect area, cleanse and dry thoroughly, and rewrap stump with elastic bandage or air splint, or apply a stump shrinker (heavy stockinette sock), for delayed prosthesis.
- Measure circumference periodically.
- Rewrap stump immediately with an elastic bandage, elevate if immediate/ early cast is accidentally dislodged. Prepare for reapplication of cast.
- Assist with specified ROM exercises for both the affected and unaffected limbs beginning early in postoperative stage.
- Encourage active/isometric exercises for upper torso and unaffected limbs.
- Provide trochanter rolls as indicated.
- Instruct patient to lie in prone position as tolerated at least twice a day with pillow under abdomen and lower-extremity stump.
- Caution against keeping pillow under lower-extremity stump or allowing BKA limb to hang dependently over side of bed or chair.
- Demonstrate/assist with transfer techniques and use of mobility aids, e.g. trapeze, crutches or walker.
- Assist with ambulation.
- Refer to rehabilitation team.

Achieve timely wound healing; be free of purulent drainage or erythema; and be afebrile

- Maintain aseptic technique when changing dressings/caring for wound
- Inspect dressings and wound: Note characteristics of drainage.
- Maintain patency and routinely empty drainage device.
- Cover dressing with plastic when using the bedpan or if incontinent.

- Expose stump to air; wash with mild soap and water after dressings are discontinued.
- Monitor vital signs.
- Obtain wound/drainage cultures and sensitivities as appropriate.
- Administer antibiotics as indicated.

Maintain adequate tissue perfusion as evidenced by palpable peripheral pulses, warm/dry skin, and timely wound healing

- Monitor vital signs. Palpate peripheral pulses, noting strength and equality.
- Perform periodic neurovascular assessments (sensation, movement, pulse, skin color and temperature).
- Inspect dressings/drainage device, noting amount and characteristics of drainage.
- Apply direct pressure to bleeding site if hemorrhage occurs. Contact physician immediately.
- Investigate reports of persistent/ unusual pain in operative site.
- Evaluate nonoperated lower limb for inflammation, positive Homans sign.
- Encourage/assist with early ambulation.
- Administer IV fluids/blood products as indicated.
- Apply antiembolic/sequential compression hose to nonoperated leg, as indicated.
- Administer low-dose anticoagulant as indicated
- Monitor laboratory studies, e.g. Hb/Hct; PT/activated partial thromboplastin time (aPTT).

Begin to show adaptation and verbalize acceptance of self in situation (amputee). Recognize and incorporate changes into self-concept in accurate manner without negating self-esteem

- Assess/consider patient's preparation for and view of amputation.
- Encourage expression of fears, negative feelings, and grief over loss of body part.
- Reinforce preoperative information including type/location of amputation, type of prosthetic fitting if appropriate (i.e. immediate, delayed), expected postoperative course, including pain control and rehabilitation.
- Assess degree of support available to patient.
- Ascertain individual strengths and identify previous positive coping behaviors.
- Encourage participation in ADLs. Provide opportunities to view/care for stump, using the moment to point out positive signs of healing.
- Encourage/provide for visit by another amputee, specially one who is successfully rehabilitating.
- Note withdrawn behavior, negative self-talk, use of denial, or over concern with actual/perceived changes. Discuss availability of various resources, e.g. counseling, occupational therapist.

Index

Page numbers followed by *f* refer to figure and *t* refer to table

A

B

D

H

I

M

N

R

S

U

V

W

X

Y

Z